29.99
WA152 STA

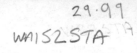

HOT TOPICS

in

General Practice

Fifth Edition

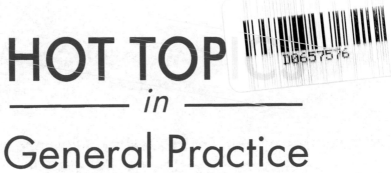

MRCGP WORKBOOK
and courses

By the author of *Hot Topics in General Practice* and *Critical Reading Questions for the MRCGP...*

- An absolute must for those sitting the MRCGP exam.

- The MRCGP workbook will guide you in a step-by-step fashion through your written paper revision.

- The workbook contains: critical reading questions and statistics, multiple essay questions, hot topics questions, as well as MCQs and other essential tips.

- All answers and comprehensive explanations are included.

- Your complete self-contained companion for the MRCGP. An ideal complement to the other texts in the BIOS series.

To order contact
www.mrcgpexam.co.uk

HOT TOPICS

in

General Practice

Fifth Edition

Ese Stacey
MBBS, MRCGP, DCH, DRCOG, MSc Sports Medicine, LF Hom (Med)
General Practitioner and Sports Physician, London

Scion

Fifth Edition © Scion Publishing Ltd, 2004
Fourth Edition © BIOS Scientific Publishers Ltd, 2002

First Published 1996 (ISBN 1 85996 210 6)
Reprinted 1997
Second Edition 1998 (ISBN 1 85996 251 3)
Reprinted 1999
Third Edition 2000 (ISBN 1 85996 129 0)
Reprinted 2001
Fourth Edition 2002 (ISBN 1 85996 073 1)
Reprinted 2003
Fifth Edition first published by Scion Publishing Ltd, 2004 (1 904842 00 3)

A CIP catalogue record for this book is available from the British Library.

Scion Publishing Limited
Bloxham Mill, Barford Road, Bloxham, Oxfordshire OX15 4FF
www.scionpublishing.com

This book is dedicated to my Lord Jesus Christ

Important Note from the Publisher

The information contained within this book was obtained by Scion Publishing Ltd from sources believed by us to be reliable. However, while every effort has been made to ensure its accuracy, no responsibility for loss or injury whatsoever occasioned by the authors or publishers.

The reader should remember that medicine is a constantly evolving science and while the authors and publishers have ensured that all dosages, applications and practices are based on current indications, there may be specific practices which differ between communities. You should always follow the guidelines laid down by the manufacturers of specific products and the relevant authorities in the country in which you are practising.

Production Editor: Andrea Bosher
Typeset by The Charlesworth Group, Huddersfield, UK
Printed by Biddles Ltd, King's Lynn, UK

CONTENTS

Abbreviations	**vii**
Preface	**xi**
Acknowledgements	**xii**
ACE inhibitors	1
Alcohol	4
Antimicrobials	10
Antiplatelet therapy	16
Asthma	21
Back pain	37
Bereavement	43
Breast cancer	45
Burnout	51
Cannabis	54
Cervical cancer	58
Children	62
Chlamydia	71
Chronic disease	74
Chronic fatigue syndrome	82
Chronic obstructive pulmonary disease	86
Complementary medicine	88
Continuing professional development (CPD)	94
Contraception	100
Deprivation	105
Diabetes mellitus	111
Diet	128
Doctor–patient relationship	130
Drug misusers	145
Elderly	148
Ethnic minorities	162
Evidence–based medicine	166
Heart disease	171
Helicobactor pylori	190
Hormone replacement therapy	197
Hypertension	200
Immunization	210
Lipids	218
Medicalisation	225
Mental illness	230
Musculoskeletal	250
Myocardial infarction	259
NHS	265
Obesity	285
Osteoporosis	290

Out-of-hours care   293
Postnatal depression   297
Practice nurse   299
Prescribing   301
Primary care   306
Prostate disease   319
Respiratory infections   322
Smoking   332
Stroke   338
Teenagers   341
Women's health   346

ABBREVIATIONS

ACE	angiotensin-converting enzyme
ADA	American Diabetes Association
ADHD	attention deficit hyperactivity disorder
AF	atrial fibrillation
AIDS	acquired immunodeficiency syndrome
BHS	British Hypertension Society
BMI	body mass index
BMJ	British Medical Journal
BPH	benign prostatic hypertrophy
BTS	British Thoracic Society
C:B	corticosteroid: bronchiodilator
CAD	coronary artery disease
CAM	complementary and alternative medicine
CASH	Consensus Action on Salt and Hypertension
CBT	cognitive behavioural therapy
CCU	coronary care unit
CFS	chronic fatigue syndrome
CG	clinical governance
CHD	coronary heart disease
CHI	Commission for Health Improvement
CI	confidence interval
CIN	cervical intraepithelial neoplasia
CME	Continuing Medical Education
COAD	chronic obstructive airways disease
CPD	Continuing Professional Development
CRP	C-reactive protein
CSAG	Clinical Standards Advisory Group
CSM	Committee on Safety of Medicines
CT	cognitive therapy
CT	computed tomography
CV	cardiovascular
CVD	cardiovascular disease
CXR	chest X-ray
D & C	dilatation and curettage
DCCT	Diabetes Control and Complications Trial
DDC	Defeat Depression Campaign
DEXA	dual-energy X-ray absorptiometry
DOH	Department of Health
DSH	deliberate self-harm
DTB	Drug and Therapeutics Bulletin
EAG	expert advisory group
EBM	Evidence-Based Medicine
ECHO	echocardiography
ECR	extra contractual referral

EIB	exercise induced bronchoconstriction
ELISA	enzyme linked immunosorbent assay
EPDS	Edinburgh postnatal depression scale
FHSA	Family Health Services Authority
FOB	faecal occult blood
GABHS	group A β-haemolytic streptococci
GMC	General Medical Council
GRASSIC	Grampian asthma studies on integrated care
HD	heart disease
HDL	high-density lipoprotein
HERS	Heart and Estrogen/Progestin Replacement Study
HMO	Health Maintenance Organization
HP	*Helicobacter pylori*
HPV	human papillomavirus
HS	heartsink
IDDM	insulin-dependent diabetes mellitus
IHD	ischaemic heart disease
IMS	intercontinental medical statistics
INR	International Normalized Ratio
ISAAC	International Study of Asthma and Allergies in Childhood
ISIS	International Study of Infarct Survival
LDL	low-density lipoprotein
LIMIT-2	Leicester intravenous magnesium intervention trial-2
LRTi	lower respiratory tract illness
LRTI	lower respiratory tract infection
LTA	leukotriene antagonists
MA	meta-analysis
MAAG	Medical Audit Advisory Group
MAPP	Maudsley Alcohol Pilot Project
MDI	metered dose inhaler
MI	myocardial infarction
MMR	mumps, measles and rubella (vaccine)
MPP	major polypharmacy
MRC	Medical Research Council
MRCGP	Member of the Royal College of General Practitioners
MRSA	methicillin-resistant *staphylococcus aureus*
NICE	National Institute of Clinical Excellence
NIDDM	non-insulin-dependent diabetes mellitus
NNH	number needed to harm
NNS	number needed to screen
NNT	number needed to treat
NSAIDS	non-steroidal anti-inflammatory drugs
OCP	oral contraceptive pill
OPCS	Office of Population Censuses and Surveys
OR	odds ratio
OTC	over-the-counter
PACT	prescribing analysis and cost (data)
PCG	primary care group

PCT	primary care trust
PEFR	peak expiratory flow rate
PGEA	postgraduate education allowance
PHCT	primary health care team
PID	pelvic inflammatory disease
PND	postnatal depression
PPA	Prescription Pricing Authority
PSA	prostate-specific antigen
PUFA	n-3 polyunsaturated fatty acid
RCGP	Royal College of General Practitioners
RCP	Royal College of Physicians
RCT	randomized controlled trial
RR	relative risk
RSV	respiratory syncytial virus
SERM	selective oestrogen receptor modulator
SI	sexual intercourse
SIDS	sudden infant death syndrome
SMAC	Standing Medical Advisory Committee
SSRI	selective serotonin re-uptake inhibitor
STAR-PU	specific therapeutic group age-sex related prescribing units
STOP	Swedish trial of old patients with hypertension
TCA	tricyclic anti-depressant
TENS	transcutaneous nerve stimulation
TIA	transient ischaemic attack
UKPDS	UK Prospective Diabetes Study
URTI	upper respiratory tract infection
UTI	urinary tract infection
VLCD	very low calorie diet
VT	venous thromboembolism
WNCCC	Women's National Cancer Centre Campaign

Preface

As a general practice registrar sitting the MRCGP exam, I was surprised to find only a handful of books to guide me. I was part of a small study group and it was a very daunting and time-consuming task to find and read through 2 years worth of *BMJ*s and *BJGP*s. Needless to say, I spent an inordinate amount of time on the 'hot topics' section of the exam and not so much on the rest. I hope that this book takes some of the drudgery out of working for the exam and replaces it with a real insight into the developments in medicine, health, politics and social welfare.

The book is a good read for anyone wishing to keep up with current developments, including general practice registrars, trainers, principals as well as medical students and those working for the MRCP exam.

The book consists of the popular ('hot') topics from four major journals: *British Medical Journal, British Journal of General Practice, Drug and Therapeutics Bulletin* and *Evidence-based Medicine*.

Where appropriate, each topic begins with a summary box containing the key points that stand out after reading the papers. Rather than lose the valuable background information from older papers, where appropriate, I have presented these papers as background information, at the beginning of the topic.

Summaries are presented of relevant articles from around 1999 onwards. I must stress that the summaries are not a critical appraisal of the paper. They are purely my summaries, with no additional analysis. Each summary has a full reference so that the reader can find and examine the original article in more detail if necessary.

Under the heading 'Further Reading', at the end of the topic, I have included references, but no summary for related papers.

Acknowledgements

I would like to thank the medical students who are invaluable in writing summaries for the book; without them the project would have long ceased.

I would also like to thank Simon, my constant support and Luke and Harry for keeping my feet on the ground.

ACE INHIBITORS

- HOPE study found that ramipril reduced risk of fatal strokes by 61%
- ACE inhibitors may reduce renal disease progression in non-diabetic patients
- Angiotensin II Receptor Blockers do not confer significant reductions in mortality and hospital admission rates in patients with heart failure

Review: angiotensin receptor blockers do not reduce mortality or hospital admission rates in heart failure. Kitzman, Dalane W. MD. Wake Forest School of Medicine, Winston-Salem, NC, USA.
Evidence-based Medicine, 7(5): 141, 1 September 2002.

Question: In patients with heart failure, do angiotensin receptor blockers reduce mortality and hospital admission rates?

The following article is briefly presented:
Angiotensin receptor blockers in heart failure: meta-analysis of randomized controlled trials. Demers, J.P., McKelvie, R.S., *et al.*
***J. Am. Coll. Cardiol.* 39:** 463–470, 6 Feb. 2002.

Seventeen papers were included in this review.
- They found that angiotensin receptor blockers were no better than ACE is or placebo for reducing mortality or hospital admission.

Commentary
It was found that mortality was reduced if the patient was not already receiving an ACE Inhibitor or a Beta Blocker, it was slightly reduced if the patient was already receiving either an ACE Inhibitor or a Beta Blocker, and if the patient was already receiving an ACE Inhibitor and a Beta Blocker, the addition of an Angiotensin II receptor blocker actually increased rates of hospital admission and death.

Further to studies such as these, guidelines now suggest ACE Inhibitors as first-line and angiotensin II receptor blockade only in the event of contraindication or intolerance of an ACE Inhibitor. Many patients intolerance of ACE Inhibitors can be overcome with counselling regarding the importance of the drug for their condition.

Use of ramipril in preventing stroke: double blind randomised trial. Bosch, J., Yusuf, S. and Pogue, J. *et al.* on behalf of the HOPE investigators.
BMJ, **324**(7339): 699-688, 23 March 2002.

and

EDITORIAL – Preventing stroke. Schrader, J. and Luder, S. Medizinische Klinik, St Josefs Hospital, Cloppenburg, Germany.
BMJ, **324**(7339): 687-688, 23 March 2002.

The aim of this part of the HOPE study was to evaluate the effect of ramipril on the secondary prevention of stroke. The HOPE study is a double blind RCT with a 2 by 2 design, whereby patients receive either 10 mg of ramipril, 400 IU of vitamin E or both or placebo. Just under 9300 patients (average age 66) from 19 countries take part in the study. All patients have vascular disease or diabetes plus one extra risk factor. Follow up was for 4.5 years.

- They found that fatal stroke was reduced by 61% and any non-fatal stroke by 24% in the ramipril group compared with placebo.
- Those who did suffer with a stroke were better off if they were taking ramipril. Cognitive and functional status, sleep and swallowing were better in the ramipril group.
- The effect on blood pressure was minimal (3.8 mmHg/2.8 mmHg).
- The reduced risk of stroke was seen across all blood pressure ranges, even in those with a normal blood pressure.

The Editorial highlights several points.

- The HOPE study is not a hypertension study. They excluded anyone with uncontrolled blood pressure. They point out that hypertension is still the primary risk factor for stroke. The PROGRESS study (Lancet 2001) using perindopril and indapamide, found that a 9/4 mmHg reduction in blood pressure resulted in a 28% reduction in risk of stroke.
- This and other studies suggest that ACE inhibitors have an effect on blood vessels which prevents the development of atherosclerotic plaques.
- The higher dose of 10 mg of ramipril worked better than the 2.5 mg dose.
- Patients taking aspirin or with a previous history of a cerebral event do less well on ramipril.
- It is unclear whether one would get the same effect from other ACE inhibitors.

The HOPE authors suggest that ACE inhibitors be used for the primary and secondary prevention of stroke.

REVIEW: Angiotensin-converting enzyme inhibitors reduce the progression of non-diabetic renal disease. Berns, J. Presbyterian Medical Centre, Philadelphia, PA, USA. *Evidence-based Medicine, 7*(1): 13, Jan./Feb. 2002.

Question: In patients with non-diabetic renal disease, are antihypertensive regimens with angiotensin-converting enzyme (ACE) inhibitors effective for slowing the progression of disease?

The following article is briefly presented
Angiotensin-converting enzyme inhibitors and progression of nondiabetic renal disease. A meta-analysis of patient-level data. Jafar, T.H., Schmid, C.H., Landa, M. *et al.* for the ACE Inhibition in Progressive Renal Disease Study Group.
Ann. Intern. Med. **135:** 73-87, 17 July 2001.

This meta-analysis involved 11 studies (around 1800 patients).
  • The incidence of renal disease was lower in the ACE inhibitor group than in the control group.

Commentary
ACE inhibitors slow the progression of renal disease in type 1 and probably type 2 diabetics. In half of the trials studied above, ACE inhibitors had no effect on renal disease progression. In addition ACE inhibitor use was associated with lower blood pressures than the control group. Hence, the ACE inhibitor effect may be due to its blood pressure lowering action. This study and others also found that ACE inhibitors reduce urinary protein excretion even after controlling for blood pressure effects. One important point to take from analyzing these studies is that most of them were conducted on patients who were white.

ALCOHOL

- According to a study performed in Belgium, the Five-Shot alcohol questionnaire is an ideal tool for screening for problem drinkers in primary care
- GPs and practice nurses have a poor knowledge of the alcohol content of drinks and the recommended safe drinking levels
- Increasing use of alcohol increases the all-cause death risk for men and women. Deaths at younger ages could be prevented by focusing on lowering risky patterns of alcohol use
- Naltrexone does not reduce drinking in alcohol-dependent patients
- One study found that only half of those identified as being risk drinkers, were offered brief alcohol intervention by their GP.
- Screening for excessive alcohol use in general practice creates more problems than it solves
- Brief interventions reduce drinking in patients not seeking treatment

BACKGROUND

Ischaemic heart disease

The relative risk of ischaemic heart disease (IHD) in moderate drinkers is 0.5-0.7. In men IHD is lowest in those drinking seven units per week. There is a U-shaped curve which describes the relationship between IHD and alcohol consumption. However, the U-shaped curve has a flat bottom and IHD is not raised until >40 units per week are consumed. However, deaths from accidents, strokes and liver disease are raised when more than seven units per week are consumed.

The French Paradox describes the situation in France, whereby there exists a low incidence of IHD in spite of high intakes of saturated fats. The modifying effects of alcohol may be responsible for this paradox.

Cancer

Alcohol is second in importance to smoking as a proved cause of cancer. Most morbidity and mortality occurs in moderate and heavy drinkers. There is an increased risk of cancer of the mouth, oropharnyx, larynx and liver. The effects of alcohol are synergistic with smoking and low intake of fruit and vegetables.

Reducing consumption

Population based strategies for decreasing alcohol consumption include:
- increasing tax on alcohol;
- advertising control;
- drink-driving campaign;
- licensing law;
- occupational health strategies in the workplace.

A general practitioner approach which targets those at high risk could also be employed. A Department of Health (DOH) systematic review estimated that £20 was all that was needed to detect a problem drinker and deliver a brief intervention! A 5–10 minute brief intervention plus a leaflet will result in a 25–35% reduction in alcohol consumption which is still evident 1 year later. An MRC study estimates that 250 000 men and 67 500 women could be encouraged to reduce their alcohol consumption from excessive to moderate levels. It seems however that GPs are reluctant to get involved in treating alcohol problems. Diagnosis and treatment of disease is preferred to health promotional work.

A GP approach that targets those at high risk could also be employed. A 5–10 min intervention plus a leaflet will result in a 25–35% reduced alcohol consumption, which is still evident 1 year later.

Patient and practitioner characteristics predict brief alcohol intervention in primary care. Kaner, E.F.S., Heather, N. and Brodie, J. *et al.* Department of Primary Health Care, School of Health Sciences, The Medical School, Newcastle upon Tyne, UK.
Br. J. Gen. Pract., 51(471): 822-827, 1 October 2001.

The aim of this study was to assess which characteristics of both patients and GPs help to predict the likelihood of the patient receiving a brief alcohol intervention. The 48 GPs who took part in this study had taken part in a previous trial concerning brief alcohol interventions. The GPs screened all adults attending the surgery over a 3 month period. The AUDIT questionnaire was used and around 4000 'risk' drinkers were identified.

- Of those identified only half received brief alcohol intervention.
- Brief intervention was more likely in females, the unemployed, technically trained people (as compared with university trained people).
- GP characteristics which increased the likelihood of a brief intervention were: solo GP; non-RCGP member; GPs who had received training in alcohol interventions; GPs with longer consultation times.

Screening properties of questionnaires and laboratory tests for the detection of alcohol abuse or dependence in a general practice population. Aertgeerts, B., Buntix, F., Ansoms, S. and Fevery, J. Department of General Practice, Clinical Epidemiology Unit, University Hospital Gasthuisberg, Catholic University of Leuven, Belgium.
Br. J. Gen. Pract., 51(464): 206-217, March 2001.

The authors claim that this is one of the largest studies of its kind to look at the screening of problem drinkers in primary care. The study was performed in Belgium and involved nearly 100 GPs and nearly 2000 patients. The aim of the study was to compare the diagnostic accuracy of several questionnaires (including CAGE, AUDIT and several derivatives) and laboratory blood tests (e.g. GGT, MCV, CDT). Patients were seen by their GP who administered the CAGE questionnaire. They then completed the other self-administered questionnaires.

- Nearly 9% of the population tested had had an alcohol problem in the previous year (3:1 male to female). This is consistent with findings from other studies.
- The CAGE questionnaire, was the least able to identify problem drinkers. The best questionnaire was the Five-Shot test which uses three CAGE questions and two AUDIT questions. AUDIT was powerful in men but poor in women.
- All laboratory tests were poor at identifying problem drinkers.

The authors recommend that the Five-Shot be used routinely in primary care.

General practitioners' and practice nurses' knowledge of how much patients should and do drink. Webster-Harrison, P.J., Barton, A.G., Barton, S.M. and Anderson, S.D. Postgraduate Medical School, University of Plymouth, Plymouth, UK.
Br. J. Gen. Pract., **51**(464): 200-218, March 2001.

This study was a postal questionnaire designed to assess general practitioners' and practice nurses' knowledge of the alcohol content of six different drinks, and also to assess their knowledge of the recommended safe drinking levels. Questionnaires were sent to nearly 500 GPs and just over 300 practice nurses. The response rate was 63%.

- Most were unable to accurately determine the alcohol content of all six drinks. Less than 50% were able to determine the alcohol content of five out of six of the drinks.
- Only 50% were recommending safe limits of 21 units for men and 14 units for women (as per guidelines for the Royal Colleges and the BMA). Over 40% were recommending limits higher than these.

The authors argue that the government should legislate for the bold labelling of 'units' on alcoholic drinks.

HEART DISEASE AND MORTALITY

Alcohol consumption and mortality: modelling risks for men and women at different ages. White, I.R., Altmann, D.R. and Nanchahal, K. Medical Statistics Unit, London School of Hygiene and Tropical Medicine, London, UK.
BMJ, **325**(7357): 191-197, 27 July 2002.

This study used statistical models relating alcohol consumption and death risk to estimate the all-cause risk for men and women from varying age groups, in England and Wales. Data was gathered from previously published reviews, relating to cause specific relative risks, distribution of alcohol consumption, and distribution of cause of death.

- Women have a positive relation between alcohol use and all-cause mortality until age 35–44, with a "U" shaped curve at age 45–54.

- Men have a steeper positve relationship below age 35, and the "U" shape appears at age 35–44.
- Using alcohol at Royal Colleges recommended limits increases risk by 9% and 23%, respectively for men and women; government limits increase risk by 15% and 32%, respectively.

The authors acknowledge several sources of error, most significantly that the results are averages so may not apply to individuals. The authors conclude the following,

Women should limit drinking each day to:
- 1 unit in those aged less than 44.
- 2 units in those aged between 45 and 74.
- 3 units in those aged over 75.

Men should limit drinking to:
- 1 unit in those aged less than 34.
- 2 units in those aged between 35 and 44.
- 3 units in those aged between 45 and 54.
- 4 units in those aged between 55 and 84.
- 5 units in those age over 85.

While those aged 54–84, not using alcohol, are at greater risk, they should not be encouraged to drink to prevent imposing a greater burden on public health services. Most alcohol related deaths at young ages are from injuries, so efforts should focus on minimising risky patterns of alcohol use.

OTHERS

Primary Care: Screening and brief intervention for excessive alcohol use: qualitative interview study of the experiences of general practitioners. Beich, A., Gannik, D. and Malterud, K. Department of General Practice, University of Copenhagen, Copenhagen, Denmark.
BMJ, 325(7369): 870-875, 19 October 2002.

A study was conducted in Denmark to see whether screening for excessive alcohol use and any subsequent intervention should be conducted in General Practice. Thirty-nine Danish GPs were chosen to implement a screening and intervention programme over 8 weeks. Around 8000 patients were screened using an alcohol questionnaire and this showed over 1000 drank excessively with 200 of these patients suspected of alcohol dependency. Nine hundred of the patients who drank excessively were randomised to and intervention or control group. The main purpose overall was to look at the GPs experiences of implementing the screening programme. This was done by asking a series of structured questions and interviewing the GPs as groups and also individually. Feedback from the doctor raised a number of issues.
- Doctors felt the problems of young drinkers should be dealt with more by the family and community rather than doctors.

- Many doctors felt that heavy drinkers often lied when answering the screening questionnaire.
- Some felt asking questions regarding personal habits created uneasiness and embarrassment in the doctor-patient relationship.
- Doctors felt that screening made it more difficult to develop a rapport with patients to ensure compliance with interventions.
- Doctors considered there to be a lack of time and training for the programme to be effective.

Doctors felt unable to recommend the screening programme in the future labelling it as awkward and creating too much extra workload.

Brief interventions reduce drinking in patients not seeking treatment. Graham, A.
Kaiser Permante Health Plan of Colorado, Denver, Colorado, USA.
Evidence-based Medicine, 7(5): 150-151, Sept./Oct. 2002.

Question: In people with alcohol problems, are brief interventions effective for reducing drinking?

The following article is briefly presented:
Brief interventions for alcohol problems: a meta-analytic review of controlled investigations in treatment seeking and non-treatment seeking populations.
Moyer, A., Finney, J.W., Swearingen, C.E., *et al.*
Addiction **97**: 279-292 March 2002

Previously completed studies were isolated using database searches. Data was extracted and analysed, including participants and intervention. Outcomes were measured in terms of quantity and time of consumption of alcohol, abstinence and drinking without problems. They found the following:
- Brief interventions in people not actively seeking treatment were shown in 34 out of the 56 studies to produce benefits lasting from 3 to 12 months.
- Effect after 12 months was not statistically significant.
- No difference in benefit was seen between brief interventions or extended treatment in people actively seeking treatment for problem drinking.

Commentary
The above findings are well acknowledged but implementation is prevented by lack of data exploring the cost efficacy of such schemes. Although the benefits are statistically significant they are nevertheless modest. Brief interventions may appear easily affordable and requiring less staff input than other healthcare programmes. The reality however, is quite the opposite.

Naltrexone for 3 or 12 months did not reduce drinking in alcohol dependence.
Chick, J. Royal Edinburgh Hospital, Edinburgh, Scotland, UK.
Evidence-based Medicine, 7(4): 125, July/Aug. 2002.

Question: In patients with alcohol dependence and a recent history of drinking to intoxication, is treatment with naltrexone for 3 or 12 months in addition to standard psychosocial treatment more effective than placebo for reducing alcohol consumption?

The following article is briefly presented
Naltrexone in the treatment of alcohol dependence. Krystal, J.H., Cramer, J.A., Krol, W.F. *et al.* Veterans Affairs Conecticut Healthcare System, West Haven, Connecticut, USA.
N. Engl. J. Med. **345:** 1734-1739, 13 Dec. 2001.

This study was an RCT conducted in 15 Veterans Affairs medical centres in the US. Six hundred and twenty-seven outpatients with alcohol dependence and a recent history of drinking to intoxication were randomised to receive either naltrexone for 3 months, naltrexone for 12 months, or placebo. All patients received standardised psychosocial support. Main outcome measures were time to relapse, percentage of drinking days, and number of drinks per drinking day.
• There were no differences between the three groups for any of the three outcome measures.
The authors concluded that treatment of alcohol-dependent patients with naltrexone for 3 or 12 months was not more effective than placebo for reducing alcohol consumption.

Commentary
Chick comments that evidence exists both for and against the efficacy of naltrexone in the treatment of alcohol dependence. He suggests that the negative findings reported in this study support the need for further trials of opiate antagonist treatment with alternative types of adjuvant psychotherapy.

ANTIMICROBIALS

- Antibiotics improve the rate of remission for acute bacterial conjunctivitis
- A study by P. Little found that high penicillin prescribing was associated with reduced admissions for quinsy and mastoiditis
- Bacteriotherapy may be an alternative to antibiotics in certain conditions
- A study found that probiotics given pre- and post-natally to women with a history of atopy, reduced the prevalence of atopy in their offspring
- Probiotics may be effective in preventing antibiotic associated diarrhoea
- The short and long term risks of antibiotic treatment for cystitis need to be explored in more detail

BACKGROUND

Antimicrobials are generally not indicated. However, when GPs perceive that a patient wants a prescription they are 10 times more likely to write one (*BMJ*, 97, Australian and south east London studies).

Acute bronchitis is usually caused by a virus (meta-analysis 800 patients). Acute exacerbations of COPD are associated with viruses in 20% of cases. Antibiotics do not work for URTIs (Cochrane review 1900 patients 1998) and cough (review *BMJ*, 1998). Antiviral agents are effective for the treatment of influenza. However, a Cochrane review found that amantadine and rimantadine reduced the illness by just 1 day.

Prescribing for URTIs may encourage re-attendance (Little *et al.*, *BMJ*, 97). The standing medical advisory group (SMAC) have issued the following guidelines.

- Do not prescribe antibiotics for simple coughs and colds and viral sore throats.
- Limit prescribing for uncomplicated cystitis to 3 days.
- Limit over-the-telephone prescribing to exceptional cases.

Antimicrobial resistance is becoming an increasing problem. *S. pneumonia* which can cause otitis media, pneumonias and meningitis has resistance rates of 5-10% in this country and higher in others.

The House of Lords Select Committee for Science and Technology have highlighted the problem of increasing antibiotic resistance. Tackling resistance will involve:

- education;
- regulate use of antibiotics e.g. no OTC use;
- improve surveillance;
- research;
- public health measures e.g. sanitation and use in cattle.

A Drug and Therapeutics Bulletin article (February 1999) looked at tackling antimicrobial resistance. Exposure to cephalosporins is associated with rapid acquisition of MRSA by hospital patients. Poor adherence to antibiotic prescribing guidelines aggravates the problem of antibiotic resistance, as does the widespread availability of over-the-counter antibiotics. Resistant bacteria in one patient can spread to other patients.

EDITORIAL – Antibiotic treatment for cystitis. Leibovici, L., Department of Medicine E, Beilinson Campus, Rabin Medical Center, Petah-Tiqva, Israel.
Br. J. Gen. Pract., 52(482): 708-710, 1 Sept. 2002.

Antibiotics have been used for many years in the treatment of cystitis. Much controversy surrounded the use of placebos in a recent trial, carried out by Christiaens *et al.*, to treat women suffering with symptomatic cystitis. Not least the fact that in addition to being given placebos, participants were not provided with written information, or asked for written consent.

It has been argued however, that giving antibiotics in the treatment of cystitis is not without its own problems. For example, the cost of treatment and the increase in antibiotic resistance to which it contributes. In addition to this we have no certain evidence that short-term antibiotic treatment in any way affects long term morbidity. These antibiotics also carry a significant risk of adverse side effects, some of which may necessitate hospital admission yet how many patients are warned about these when they are prescribed?

Successful treatment of cystitis was based on symptom control and not bacterial cure. Whilst not advocating further placebo controlled studies on treatment of cystitis it is vital to recognize the valuable data gathered by the Christiaen *et al.* study and the important questions it has raised for the basis of further work.

Probiotics in prevention of antibiotic associated diarrhoea: meta-analysis.
D'Souza, A.L., Rajkumar, C. and Cooke, J. Care of the Elderly Section, Imperial College School of Medicine, Hammersmith Hospital, London, UK.
BMJ, 324(7350): 1361, 8 June 2002.

The aim of this meta-analysis was to find the efficacy of probiotics in the prevention of antibiotic associated diarrhoea. Nine RCTs met the inclusion criteria. The treatment groups were given antibiotic and probiotic and controls were given antibiotic and placebo. Study sizes varied between 388 and 20 patients. Four studies used yeast, four used lactobacilli, and one used a strain of enterococcus.

Results showed an odds ratio in favour of probiotics over placebo of:
  • for the yeast 0.39
  • for lactobacilli and enterococcus 0.34
  • for all nine trials together 0.37 (CI: 0.26 to 0.53; $P< 0.001$)

The authors suggest that the potential of probiotics in treating colitis associated with *Clostridium difficile* infection secondary to the use of antibiotics should be re-examined. They conclude by pointing out the desirability of probiotics given their "increasing availability, lower costs, and relative lack of side effects" when compared to antibiotics.

Antibiotic prescribing and admissions with major suppurative complications of respiratory tract infections: a data linkage study. Little, P., Watson, L., Morgan, S. and Williamson, I. Community Clinical Sciences, Primary Medical Care Group, University of Southampton, Aldermoor Health Centre, Southampton, UK.
Br. J. Gen. Pract., **52**(476): 187-193, 1 March 2002.

The aim of this study was to assess the effect of penicillin prescribing on hospital admissions for complications of respiratory infections. They use hospital admissions and PACT data from 96 health authorities in England. Admissions for rheumatic fever were rare.
- High penicillin prescribing was associated with reduced admissions for quinsy and mastoiditis.
- High penicillin prescribing was also associated with increased admissions for tonsillectomy.
- For a practice of 10 000 patients, 2000 extra items of penicillin per year would need to be prescribed to prevent one admission for quinsy or mastoiditis.

Other more specific methods need to be identified to reduce the complications of respiratory infections. Increased prescribing of penicillin is not feasible.

Reducing antibiotic use for acute bronchitis in primary care: blinded, randomised controlled trial of patient information leaflet. Macfarlane, J., Holmes, W. and Gard, P. Respiratory Medicine, Nottingham City Hospital, Nottingham, UK.
BMJ, **324**(7329): 91-94, 12 January 2002.

This study assesses the usefulness of delayed prescribing (issuing a prescription but telling the patient to use it only if they get worse) and leaflet information to reduce the use of antibiotics in the management of acute bronchitis. Patients were nearly 260 patients from general practices in Nottingham. Just over 200 previously well patients presenting with acute bronchitis were given a prescription and told to use it only if symptoms got worse. Half of these patients were also given an information leaflet. Patients deemed to need antibiotics were told to use them.
- For those given a leaflet, there was a nearly 25% reduction in antibiotic use.

They comment that a reduction of 25% can make quite an impact at a community level.

Antibacterial prescribing and antibacterial resistance in English general practice: cross sectional survey. Priest, P., Yudkin, P., McNulty, C. and Mant, D. Department of Primary Health Care, University of Oxford, Oxford, UK.
BMJ, **323**(7320): 1037-1041, 3 November 2001.

This study involving specimens from around 400 practices in the north and south of England, examines the relationship between antibiotic prescribing and resistance rates.
- For urinary coliforms they found a low correlation between prescribing and resistance rates.
- Prescribing explained less than 20% of the variation in resistance rates.
- A 20% reduction in antibiotic prescribing would be expected to reduce resistance by 1%.

They offer a number of explanations for these findings.
- Avoidance of those drugs known to have high resistance rates.
- Other antibacterial uses e.g. agriculture.
- Time lag between prescribing and development of resistance.

They conclude that reducing antibiotic prescribing may not reduce community resistance rates

Prenatal and postnatal administration of Lactobacillus GG reduced the occurrence of atopic disease in offspring. Williams, H. Centre of Evidence-Based Dermatology, Queen's Medical Centre, Nottingham, UK.
Evidence-based Medicine, **6**(6): 178, Nov./Dec. 2001.

Question: In offspring at risk for atopic disease, does oral administration of Lactobacillus GG (LGG), given prenatally to mothers and postnatally to their infants, prevent atopic eczema?

The following article is briefly presented
Probiotics in primary prevention of atopic disease: a randomised placebo-controlled trial. Kalliamäki, M., Salminen, S., Arvilommi, H. *et al.*
Lancet **357**: 1076-1079, April 2001.

The study is an RCT with 2 years follow up. It involves around 160 pregnant women with atopy or a family history of atopy. Just over 130 women and the same number of children completed follow up. The intervention group received probiotic capsules 2–4 weeks before delivery and after delivery if breast feeding. Babies who were not breast fed received capsule contents mixed with water for 6 months.
- Atopy was less common in the probiotics group than the placebo group.

Commentary
The commentator highlights some flaws in the study e.g. no intention to treat analysis, atopy is poorly defined. It is also not clear whether

probiotics prevent atopy or simply delay its onset. He suggests further studies should be completed before recommending probiotics in this situation.

EDITORIAL – Bacteriotherapy: the time has come. Huovinen, P. Antimicrobial Research Laboratory, National Public Health Institute, Turku, Finland.
BMJ, 323(7309): 353-354, 18 August 2001.

It is already known that antibiotics themselves may encourage bacterial infection by disturbing the balance of normal flora. Several recent studies have highlighted the benefits of using bacteriotherapy rather than antibiotics in the treatment of certain conditions. This involves giving harmless bacteria which will displace pathogenic bacteria. It has been successfully used in the following situations:
- to reduce recurrent otitis media in children as well as streptococcal tonsillitis;
- prophylaxis against antibiotic induced diarrhoea in children;
- in the management of acute diarrhoea in children;
- in the treatment of ulcerative colitis (with non-pathogenic *E. coli*).

More research needs to be done to look at long term and population effects of bacteriotherapy.

Topical antibiotics for acute bacterial conjunctivitis: a systematic review. Sheikh, A. and Hurwitz, Department of Primary Health Care and General Practice, Imperial College School of Medicine, London, UK.
Br. J. Gen. Pract., 51(467): 473-477, June 2001.

This was a meta-analysis designed to assess the efficacy of topical antibiotics for the treatment of acute bacterial conjunctivitis. Three trials involving around 500 patients met the inclusion criteria. There was a degree of heterogeneity between the studies. A range of antimicrobials were used.
- They found that acute bacterial conjunctivitis is a self-limiting condition.
- Antibiotics improve the rate of remission and improve the rate of eradication of pathogen.

When issues of cost and antibiotic resistance are considered, a delayed prescribing strategy may be appropriate for this condition. However, the possibility of adverse sequelae occurring if the condition is left untreated cannot be ruled out.

FURTHER READING

Decision making, evidence, audit and education: case study of antibiotic prescribing in general practice. Lipman, T. and Price, D. Westerhope Medical Group, Newcastle upon Tyne.
BMJ, 320(7242): 1114–1118, 22 April 2000.

Tackling antimicrobial resistance.
Drug and Therapeutics Bulletin, **2**(37): 9-16, Feb. 1999.

See 'Respiratory infections' for

Symptoms, signs and prescribing for acute lower respiratory tract illness. Department of Respiratory Medicine, Nottingham City Hospital, Nottingham.
Br. J. Gen. Pract., **51**(464): 177-181, March 2001.

and

Pragmatic randomised controlled trial of two prescribing strategies for childhood acute otitis media. Community Clinical Sciences (Primary Medical Care Group), University of Southampton, Aldermoor Health Centre, Southampton.
BMJ, **322**(7282): 336-342, 10 Feb. 2001.

and

A randomised controlled trial of delayed antibiotic prescribing as a strategy for managing uncomplicated respiratory tract infection in primary care. Tayside Centre for General Practice, University of Dundee, Dundee.
Br. J. Gen. Pract., **51**(464): 200-205, March 2001.

ANTIPLATELET THERAPY

- In high risk patients, antiplatelet therapy results in a reduction in the risk of
  - non-fatal myocardial infarcts by one-third
  - non-fatal strokes by one-third
  - vascular deaths by one-sixth
- Antithrombotic Trialist' Collaborators conclude that aspirin should be given to anyone with medium or high risk of a occlusive vascular event (> 2% per year), whether it be primary or secondary prevention
- Cleland concludes that "The reader should not accept the conclusions of the Antithrombotic Trialists Collaboratioin uncritically..."
- Patients who are over the age of 65 and those with cardiovascular risk factors should receive low dose aspirin
- Aspirin may be useful in the primary prevention of coronary artery disease in high risk patients
- Combination therapy of Warfarin and aspirin post MI conferred no extra benefit to a single therapy of aspirin alone

Warfarin combined with low dose aspirin in myocardial infarction did not provide clinical benefit beyond that of aspirin alone. Oh, Vernon M. National University Hospital, Singapore, Republic of Singapore.
Evidence-based Medicine, 7(5): 140, Sept./Oct. 2002.

Question: In patients who have survived an acute myocardial infarction (MI), is warfarin combined with aspirin more effective than aspirin alone?

The following article is briefly presented:
Department of Veterans Affairs Cooperative Studies Program Clinical Trial comparing combined warfarin and aspirin with aspirin alone in survivors of acute myocardial infarction. Primary results of the CHAMP study. Fiore, L.D., Ezekowitz, M.D., Brophy, M.T. *et al.*
Circulation **105:** 557-563, 5 Feb. 2002.

This was a randomised controlled, unblinded trial carried out across 78 Department of Veterans Affairs medical centres in the United States. Approximately 5000 patients within 14 days of an acute MI were targeted. Half were assigned warfarin and aspirin, half were assigned aspirin alone. Follow up was carried out at a median of 2.7 years.
  - Warfarin combined with aspirin was no better than aspirin alone.
  - Major bleeding was more common in the combined group.

Commentary
More work needs to be done to assess the potential benefit of a combination therapy of aspirin and clopidogrel in the post MI setting.

Review: aspirin reduces CAD events in people with no history of cardiovascular disease, but it increases gastrointestinal bleeding. Jain, M. and Rosenberg, M. Providence Portland Medical Center, Portland, OR, USA.
Evidence-based Medicine, 7(4): 111, July/Aug. 2002.

Question: What are the benefits and harm of aspirin use to prevent coronary artery disease (CAD) events in people with no history of cardiovascular disease?

The following article is briefly presented
Aspirin for the primary prevention of cardiovascular events: a summary of the evidence for the U.S. Preventive Services Task Force. Hayden M, Pignone M, Phillips C, *et al.* University of North Carolina Hospital, Chapel Hill, NC, USA.
Ann. Intern. Med. **136:** 161-172, 15 Jan. 2002

This meta-analysis used the results of five RCTs (n=53035), all comparing the use of aspirin versus placebo/no-aspirin in participants with no history of cardiovascular disease. Rates of myocardial infarction, stroke and mortality in the treatment and non-treatment groups were compared. In addition, case control studies, RCTs and systematic reviews of aspirin related harm were systematically reviewed.

- Aspirin treatment reduced the combined outcome of non-fatal myocardial infarction or death from coronary artery disease.
- Aspirin treatment did not affect the following outcomes: Coronary artery disease mortality; all-cause mortality; stroke.
- Previous meta-analyses (that included the five RCTs) showed that aspirin increased the risk of major gastrointestinal bleeding

The authors concluded that in patients with no history of cardiovascular disease, aspirin reduces the risk for coronary artery disease events, but does not affect risk for mortality or stroke. Aspirin increases the risk for gastrointestinal bleeding.

Commentary
This meta-analysis was used by the US Preventive Services Task Force as evidence to support the recent recommendation that aspirin should be used for the primary prevention of cardiovascular events in high-risk patients. Jain and Rosenberg comment that other primary preventive measures, such as smoking cessation, dietary modification, and treatment of hypertension, may be more important in prevention as they are based on a wealth of strong evidence, do not increase the risk of bleeding, and have lower numbers needed to treat.

Collaborative meta-analysis of randomised trials of antiplatelet therapy for prevention of death, myocardial infarction, and stroke in high risk patients.
Antithrombotic Trialist' Collaboration.
BMJ, 324(7329): 71-86, 12 January 2002.

This meta-analysis (MA) by the Antithrombotic Trialist Collaborators, is an update on previous meta-analyses and contains randomized trials available before September 1997. The aim of the MA is to assess the usefulness of antiplatelet therapy in the prevention of primary or secondary cardiovascular events in those at high risk (over 3% per year). Just over 280 studies were identified (135 000 patients in antiplatelet vs. control studies, 77 000 in comparisons between different antiplatelets).

- Combined outcomes for any serious vascular event were reduced by 25%.
- Non-fatal MIs were reduced by a third.
- Non-fatal strokes were reduced by 25%.
- Vascular mortality was reduced by one sixth.
- The benefits of treatment outweighed the risk of adverse events.
- Low doses (aspirin 75-150 mg per day) were as effective as higher doses.
- Clopidrogel reduced risk of vascular event by 10% compared with aspirin.

Aspirin should be given to anyone with medium or high risk of an occlusive vascular event (> 2% per year), whether it be primary or secondary prevention.

EDUCATION AND DEBATE SECTION: Preventing atherosclerotic events with aspirin.
Cleland, J. Department of Cardiology, Castle Hill Hospital, Kingston upon Hull, UK.
BMJ, 324(7329): 103-105, 12 January 2002.

Cleland states that the above MA contains serious flaws.

- He notes that individual trials of antiplatelet agents rarely reduce fatal events.
- Antiplatelets reduce non-fatal events but in doing so, their mechanism of action may actually conceal or even cause fatal events. For example, aspirin is an analgesic and also causes dyspepsia. Hence, symptoms of an MI may be masked by these two features. Trials show that aspirin can increase the risk of sudden death by up to 6%, which may represent these 'silent' events. Additionally non-fatal events may be converted to fatal events by inducing haemorrhage as a complication of MI or cerebral infarction.
- Up to 25% of patients were lost to follow up in some trials. If these people were counted as 'died', it would neutralise the beneficial effect found in ISIS-2 (Lancet, 1998).
- Several sources of bias in the analysis of studies are highlighted by Cleland. There is evidence of publication bias. In addition, when they

reanalyzed trials, some numbers seemed to have changed since the original analysis.

- Cleland comments that "Most interventions probably help some people some of the time and harm others some of the time". With this statement in mind, it is difficult to tell how aspirin's benefits occur. For example, aspirin may provide a small benefit to lots of people or a large benefit to a few people and harm to the rest. Alternatively aspirin could provide short term benefit followed by long term harm.
- Cleland notes that the adverse interactions between aspirin and ACE inhibitors in the SOLVD and HOPE studies is also worrying.
- The trial population is not characteristic of the usual treatment population. People at risk of adverse events from aspirin were excluded. The patients tended to be younger and have less co-morbidity.
- Cost implications need to be assessed, taking the cost of managing adverse events into account. A Scottish study put the cost of primary prevention of an event with aspirin at £80 000 (£3000 for secondary prevention).

Cleland concludes that "The reader should not accept the conclusions of the Antithrombotic Trialists Collaboratioin uncritically..."

Aspirin but not vitamin E prevented cardiovascular events in patients at risk.
Gluckman, R. Providence-St Vincent Medical Center, Portland, OR, USA.
Evidence-based Medicine, 6(4): 112, July/Aug. 2001.

Question: In patients with = 1 cardiovascular risk factor but no history of cardiovascular disease, how effective is treatment with aspirin and vitamin E in preventing cardiovascular events?

The following article is briefly presented
Low-dose aspirin and vitamin E in people at cardiovascular risk: a randomised trial in general practice. Collaborative Group of the Primary Prevention Project (PPP).
Lancet 357: 89-95, 13 Jan. 2001.

The PPP study is a RCT with 3.6 years follow up, involving nearly 4500 patients from 315 general practices and 15 hospitals in Italy. Patients had at least one cardiovascular risk factor.

- The trial was stopped prematurely because aspirin was found to have obvious benefits.
- Vitamin E did not effect outcome.

Commentary
Gluckmann suggests that patients who are over the age of 65 and those with cardiovascular risk factors should have aspirin. The effects of vitamin E are either very small or require longer follow up to detect changes in outcome.

Clopidogrel reduced recurrent ischaemic events in patients with previous cardiac surgery more than aspirin. Groeneveld, P.W. and Hlaky, M.A. Stanford University School of Medicine, Palo Alto, CA, USA.
***Evidence-based Medicine, 6**(4): 114, July/Aug. 2001.*

Question: In patients with recent ischaemic stroke, recent myocardial infarction (MI), or peripheral arterial disease and previous cardiac surgery, is clopidogrel more effective than aspirin in reducing recurrent ischaemic events?

The following article is briefly presented
Superiority of clopidogrel versus aspirin in patients with prior cardiac surgery. Bhatt, D.L., Chew, D.P., Hirsch, A.T. *et al.*
***Circulation* 103:** 363-368, 23 Jan. 2001.

This was a subgroup analysis of another larger study (Clopidogrel vs. Aspirin in Patients at Risk of Ischaemic Events: CAPRI). The subgroup analysis involved 1480 patents randomised to receive either clopidogrel or aspirin. Follow up was for 1–3 years.
   • Vascular end points were significantly reduced in the clopidogrel group compared with the aspirin group.

Commentary
The absolute risk reduction (ARR) in cardiovascular events with clopidogrel amounts to 0.51% (3.3% in those who have recently had a stenting procedure). Clopidogrel is more expensive than aspirin and has haematological side effects. They suggest that it be reserved for those people for whom aspirin is contraindicated and in people who have recently had coronary stenting.

ASTHMA

MANAGEMENT
- One practice found that a third of women and one fifth of men had symptoms suggestive of dysfunctional breathing
- On demand use of inhaled short acting β2-agonist is just as good as regular scheduled doses
- High dose inhaled steroid is as effective as oral steroids in patients discharged from emergency departments after an exacerbation of asthma
- Action plans for asthma management are viewed positively by patients
- Addition of long-acting beta agonists is more appropriate than increasing corticosteroid doses in patients with poorly controlled asthma

DRUGS
- High quality evidence from a meta-analysis supports the combination of ipratropium bromide and β-agonist for the management of acute asthma in adults
- In patients discharged from the casualty with acute asthma, the addition of inhaled budesonide to a fixed dose of oral prednisolone reduces relapses
- An Australian study has shown that peer led programmes could be an important way to reduce the burden of asthma in the community
- Two studies have shown that "as needed" formoterol use provides more clinical benefit than using the shorter-acting β2 agonists
- Sensitization and exposure to allergens together with viral infection are associated with an increased risk of admission to hospital with an acute episode of asthma
- Pressurised MDIs do not differ from other hand held devices for most clinical outcome measures
- The dose-response curve for fluticasone in the management of asthma begins to plateau at 100–200 µg per day and reaches a peak at 500 µg per day. These figures are lower than those recommended in national guidelines
- For patients with acute severe asthma (peak flow less than 30% predicted) oxygen should be given before, during and after use of nebulized β2 agonist
- Anti-IgE (omalizumab) reduced inhaled corticosteroid use and asthma exacerbation in children with allergic asthma
- Australian researchers have developed an asthma score which may help to identify which children have asthma
- A Manchester study estimated that, in their particular population, between 3.5 and 8% of children were potentially undiagnosed asthmatics
- Runny noses and viral infections before age 1, are associated with reduced likelihood of asthma at age 7

EPIDEMIOLOGY
- A multicentre cross sectional study has shown that the severity of asthma is associated with sensitisation to moulds such as *A. alternata* and *Cladosporium herbarum*
- Migraine and asthma are associated in the United Kingdom
- A German study found that it was not possible to use medications to reliably identify asthma patients in general practice
- Fluticasone propionate treatment is associated with a greater growth rate in asthmatic children compared with beclomethasone dipropionate treatment.

BACKGROUND

Non-drug management

- Previously, asthma self-monitoring was seen as the way forward in asthma management. In 1994, the GRASSIC studies (*BMJ*, 1994) were published. One of the studies found that self monitoring did not improve asthma outcomes. In fact self-monitoring was associated with increased GP consultations compared with standard care.
- Integrated GP and hospital care produced good results in the GRASSIC studies (*BMJ*, 1994). Integrated care was as effective as hospital only care.

Newer drug treatment for asthma: Leukotriene antagonists (LTAs)

The two drugs are Montelukast (M) and Zafirlukast (Z). M is licensed as an add-on therapy for adults and children (aged 6 and over) with mild and moderate asthma, who are not controlled on inhaled steroids and as required short acting β-agonists. It is also licensed for prophylaxis against exercise-induced asthma. Z is licensed for the 'treatment' of asthma in adults and children over 12 years.

Leukotrienes are important mediators of asthma. Their release is activated by eosinophils, basophils and mast cells, resulting in increased mucus production, airway oedema and bronchoconstriction. They are especially important mediators in people with aspirin-sensitive asthma. LTAs are absorbed orally, with peak plasma concentrations, between 2 and 3 hours after ingestion. A Drug and Therapeutics article (Sept. 1998) concluded that, as yet there is little or no evidence for their use as an add-on therapy in the management of asthma.

ASTHMA IN CHILDREN

It is generally thought that the prevalence of asthma in industrialized countries is on the increase.

Undiagnosed asthma

Several studies evaluate the level of undiagnosed asthma in different populations. The ISAAC study (*BMJ*, Jan. 1998) looking at prevalence in around 27000 12-14 year old children in the UK found that a third of those with nocturnal wheeze had no diagnosis of asthma. The Odense School child study (*BMJ*, Feb. 1998), involving around 1400 children, also found that a third of asthma sufferers were undiagnosed. In this study undiagnosed asthma was associated with:

- low physical activity;
- high body mass index;
- serious family problems;
- passive smoking;
- absence of rhinitis.

Other researchers would question the proposed increase in prevalence of asthma. Magnus (*BMJ*, June 1997) suggests several factors can explain the increase in prevalence figures.

Study methodology:
- selection bias;
- poor use of objective measures of airway responsiveness.

Drug factors:
- it is postulated that asthma drugs may increase the response to histamine challenge.

Risk factors

Some independent risk factors for the development of asthma are:
- atopy:
- female:
- first attack after 2 years of age:
- more than 10 attacks as a child:
- low peak flow:
- parental history of asthma:

Poor growth is thought to be associated with asthma and its treatment. A Scottish study investigated this further. They evaluated over 2000 children over a 4 year period. Social deprivation was more important than drug treatment or diagnosis of asthma. Children receiving high doses of inhaled corticosteroids had lower than normal growth rates (*BMJ*, Feb. 1998).

MANAGEMENT

Low dose budesonide improved asthma control in mild asthma; adding formoterol improved control in corticosteroid treated patients. Grosser, D. and Smith, B. Queen Elizabeth Hospital Woodville, South Australia, Australia.
***Evidence-based Medicine, 7**(4): 120, July/Aug. 2002.*

Question: In patients with mild asthma, do regular low doses of inhaled budesonide, with or without low doses of inhaled formoterol, reduce severe exacerbations and improve asthma control?

The following article is briefly presented
Low dose inhaled budesonide and formoterol in mild persistent asthma: the OPTIMA randomised trial. O'Byrne, P.M., Barnes, P.J., Rodriguez-Roisin, R., *et al.* St. Josephs Healthcare, Hamilton, Ontario, Canada.
Am. J. Respir. Crit. Care Med. **164:** 1392-1397, 15 Oct. 2001.

This study was a RCT conducted in 198 centres in 17 countries. Almost 2000 patients were included. These patients were separated into those previously taking inhaled corticosteroids for >3 months, and those not. Both groups were then separately randomised to receive either budesonide, budesonide plus formoterol, or placebo (all via twice daily inhalation for 1 year). The main outcome measures were time to first severe asthma exacerbation, and number of poor asthma days.

- In patients not previously taking inhaled corticosteroids, budesonide alone reduced the risk of severe exacerbations and poor asthma days.
- Adding formoterol to the budesonide did not significantly improve outcomes in these patients.
- In patients previously taking inhaled corticosteroids, budesonide alone did not reduce the risk of severe exacerbations and poor asthma days.
- Adding formoterol significantly improved both outcomes in these patients.

The authors concluded that inhaled budesonide improved asthma control in patients with mild asthma not previously on corticosteroids, and that addition of formoterol improved control in those already taking inhaled corticosteroids.

Commentary

Grosser and Smith comment that the effects of these medications on underlying disease processes are still unknown. However, they recommend that following initiation of corticosteroid therapy, any further deterioration of asthma should prompt addition of long acting beta-agonists rather than increasing the dose of inhaled corticosteroids, given the potential for long term side effects that high dose monotherapies carry.

A qualitative study of action plans for asthma. Douglass, J., Aroni, R. and Goeman, D. *et al.* Department of Asthma, Allergy and Clinical Immunology, Alfred Hospital and Monash University, Prarhan, Victoria, Australia.
BMJ, **324**(7344): 1003-1014, 27 April 2002.

This hospital based, qualitative study sought to evaluate patient's views on action plans, given to them by doctors, for the management of their asthma. Sixty-two consecutive patients who presented to the emergency department of a city and a rural hospital over a 2 month period were recruited to the study, and interviewed. They found that

- only 29 of the 62 patients had action plans
- patients felt that, when deciding to seek medical help, the decision should be based on their symptoms and not solely their Peak Flow reading
- patient's misconceptions about asthma and its symptoms may compromise the efficacy of asthma action plans
- the more recently the plan had been devised the less confident the patient was is in using the plan
- most patients without action plans had not been offered one by their doctor
- patients generally had a positive view of plans, finding it helped them manage their asthma
- patients without plans developed their own "plans" based on personal experiences of their disease.

Prevalence of dysfunctional breathing in patients treated for asthma in primary care: cross sectional survey. Thomas, M., McKinley, R.K., Freeman, E. and Foy, C. Surgery, Minchinhampton, Stroud, Gloucestershire, UK.
***BMJ,* 322**(7294): 5 May 2001.

This study assesses the prevalence of dysfunctional breathing in a population of asthma patients registered with a semi-rural UK practice. Just over 300 patients were identified and sent the Nijmegen questionnaire (response rate 74%). This questionnaire assesses symptoms associated with abnormal breathing.

- They found that a third of women and one fifth of men had scores suggestive of dysfunctional breathing.
- Asthma in these patients ranged from mild to moderately severe.

They discuss the limitations of the study. The Nijmegen questionnaire has limitations and there is no gold standard diagnostic tool to identify dysfunctional breathing.

DRUGS

Dose-response relation of inhaled fluticasone propionate in adolescents and adults with asthma: meta-analysis. Holt, S., Suder, A. and Weatherall, M. Wellington Asthma Research Group, Wellington School of Medicine, Wellington, New Zealand.
***BMJ,* 323**(7307): 253-256, 4 August 2001.

The aim of this MA was to examine the dose-response relationship for fluticasone in the management of asthma in adolescents and adults. Eight studies met the inclusion criteria.

- The dose-response curve began to plateau at a dose of 100–200 μg per day.
- A peak in response was seen at 500 μg per day.
- Few studies examined the dose-response relationship beyond 500 μg per day.

They conclude that guidelines will need to be altered to cater for lower doses of fluticasone. Given the option to either increase the dose of inhaled corticosteroid or add-in a long acting β agonist, the latter should be chosen.

Formoterol was more effective than terbutaline when taken as needed for moderate to severe asthma. Commentator, O'Byrne, P.M. McMaster University and St Joseph's Hospital, Hamilton, Ontario, Canada.
***Evidence-based Medicine,* 6**(6): 105, July/Aug. 2001.

Question: In patients with moderate to severe asthma who use an inhaled corticosteroid but still require as needed medication, is formoterol (a long acting β2 agonist) more effective than terbutaline (a short acting β2 agonist) when used as needed?

The following article is briefly presented
Comparison of formoterol and terbutaline for as-needed treatment of asthma: a randomised trial. Tattersfield, A.E., Löfdahl, C.G., Postma, D.S. *et al.*
Lancet **357**: 257-261, 27 Jan. 2001.

This study was an RCT involving 362 patients who had had asthma ≥6 months, from 35 centres in Greece, the Netherlands, Norway and Sweden. Patients had been treated with a constant dose of inhaled corticosteriod for ≥4 weeks. They were allocated inhaled formoterol or inhaled terbutaline for 12 weeks, and were instructed to use as needed.
- Time to first severe exacerbation was greater in the formoterol group.
- Morning and evening PEFR decreased in terbutaline group and increased in formoterol group.
- Formoterol group had fewer inhalations of relief medication.

Commentary
A previous study agrees that the time to first exacerbation increases with formoterol use (Pauwels *et al.*, *N. Engl. J. Med.* 1997). Formoterol is unique in that although it is long acting (> 12 hours), it has a short onset of action. This means that it can be used as an "as needed" preparation. O'Byrne therefore concludes that "as needed" formoterol use provides more clinical benefit than using the shorter-acting drug terbutaline.

EDUCATION AND DEBATE SECTION: Oxygen treatment for acute severe asthma.
Inwald, D., Roland, M. and Kuitert, L. Portex Department of Anaesthesia, Intensive Care and Respiratory Medicine, Institute of Child Health, London, UK.
BMJ, **323**(7304): 98-100, 14 July 2001.

This is a review of 24 papers analyzing the dangers of giving nebulized β2 agonist in air to patients suffering with acute severe asthma. Studies have shown that nebulized β2 agonist in air can cause or worsen hypoxaemia. This happens because the β2 agonist causes pulmonary vasodilatation resulting in a ventilation-perfusion mismatch, together with increased cardiac output. They postulate that the continuing trickle of deaths from asthma may be due this β2 action. They state that β2 agonist can be used as usual in mild to moderate in asthma either via nebulizer or by spacer. However, for those with acute severe asthma (peak flow less than 30% predicted) oxygen should be given before, during and after use of nebulized β2 agonist. They suggest that every GP practice should have oxygen available and certain patients should have oxygen available at home.

On demand use of β2–agonists led to better asthma control than regular use in moderate to severe asthma. Commentator, Peter Honig, Food and Drug Administration, Maryland, USA.
Evidence–based Medicine, 6(1): 15, Jan./Feb. 2001.

Question: In patients with moderate to severe asthma, is on demand use of β2-agonists as effective and safe as regular use?

The following article is briefly presented
Effects of on–demand β2 agonist inhalation in moderate–to–severe asthma. A randomized controlled trial. Richter, B., Bender, R. and Berger, M.
J. Intern. Med., **247:** 657–666, June 2000.

This was a German study involving 80 patients with moderate to severe asthma. The aim of the study was to compare asthma morbidity in those taking regular short acting inhaled β2-agonists with those taking on demand short acting inhaled β2-agonists. It was a 24 week RCT crossover study.
 • The groups did not differ in terms of asthma exacerbations.
 • Use of β2-agonist was less in the on demand group.
 • The on demand group had fewer days taking oral prednisolone.
 • Lung function was better in the on demand group.

Commentary
The commentator discusses the flaws in the study including, inadequate blinding, no washout period and inadequate assessment of compliance. He concludes that regular use has no benefit over on demand use.

INHALER DEVICES

Systematic review of clinical effectiveness of pressurised metered dose inhalers versus other hand held inhaler devices for delivering corticosteroids in asthma. Brocklebank, D., Wright, J. and Cates, C. on behalf of the National Health Technology Assessment Inhaler Review Group.
BMJ, **323**(7318): 896-900, 20 October 2001.

This was a systematic review whose aim was to compare pressurised metered dose inhalers (MDIs) with other hand held devices for the delivery of corticosteroids. Twenty-four RCTs met the inclusion criteria.
 • They found no difference between pressurised MDIs and other hand held devices for pulmonary function, symptoms, exacerbation rates, systemic bioavailability and adverse effects.
 • They note, however that some of the confidence intervals do include clinically significant differences.
Further studies will need to examine differences in children, and looking at other dry powder inhalers and also the effect of using and not using a spacer device.

Systematic review of clinical effectiveness of pressurised metered dose inhalers versus other hand held inhaler devices for delivering β2 agonist bronchodilators in asthma. Ram, F.S.F., Wright, J. and Brocklebank, D. *et al.* on behalf of the National Health Technology Assessment Inhaler Review Group.
***BMJ*, 323**(7318): 901-905, 20 October 2001.

This was a systematic review whose aim was to compare pressurised metered dose inhalers (MDIs) with other hand held devices for the delivery of β2 agonists. Eighty four RCTs met the inclusion criteria.

- They found no difference between pressurised MDIs and other hand-held devices for most outcomes e.g. lung function, systemic bioavailability, inhaled steroid requirement, and symptoms. They note that some of the confidence intervals may include clinically important differences.
- In adults, pulse rate was lower for pressurised MDIs compared with turbohalers.
- Hydrofluoralkane pressurised MDIs reduced the need for rescue courses of oral steroids. However, they point out that bias may have affected this result.

ASTHMA IN CHILDREN

Growth rate was greater with fluticasone propionate than with beclomethasone dipropionate in children with asthma. Ducharne, Francine. McGill University, Montreal, Quebec, Canada.
***Evidence-based Medicine*, 7**(4): 114, July/Aug. 2000.

Question: In children with chronic asthma, what are the effects of fluticasone propionate compared with those of beclomethasone dipropionate on growth rates?

The following article is briefly presented.
Effects of 2 inhaled corticosteroids on growth. Results of a randomised controlled trial. De Benedictis, F.M., Teper, A., Green, R.J. *et al.* Clinica Pediatrica, Policlinico Monteluce, Perugia, Italy.
Arch. Pediatr. Adolesc. Med. **155**: 1248-1254, Nov. 2001

This study was a multi-centre RCT conducted in 7 countries: The Netherlands, Hungary, Italy, Poland, Argentina, Chile, and South Africa. Three hundred and forty-three children (4–11 years old), requiring treatment with fluticasone propionate, beclomethasone dipropionate or budesonide prior to the study, and having a peak expiratory flow rate (PEFR) less than 85% their maximum achievable response, were randomised to inhaled fluticasone or inhaled beclomethasone groups. Patients received albuterol sulphate for use on an as-needed basis.

Treatment continued for 52 weeks. The main outcome measure was change in height.
- Mean growth rate was greater in the fluticasone group than in the beclomethasone group.

Commentary

Ducharne comments that there are two possible reasons for the observed difference in growth rates: Improved control of asthma in the fluticasone group; or increased growth as a direct result of the drug. She comments that further research is needed to determine which of the two is responsible for the difference in growth rate.

Budesonide and nedocromil did not improve lung function in children with asthma.
Commentator, Ducharme, F.M., McGill University, Montreal, Quebec, Canada.
Evidence-based Medicine, **6**(3): 84, May/June 2001.

Question: In children with asthma, does continuous, long term treatment with budesonide or nedocromil improve lung function?

The following article is briefly presented
Long-term effects of budesonide or nedocromil in children with asthma. The Childhood Asthma Management Program Research Group.
N. Eng. J. Med. **343**: 1054-1063, 12 Oct. 2000.

This was an RCT conducted in several centres in America and Canada and involving over 1000 children aged 5–12 with mild to moderate asthma. Subjects received either placebo, twice daily inhalations of budesonide, or twice daily inhalations of nedocromil. Follow up was just over 4 years.
- Budesonide and nedocromil were better than placebo in terms of need for urgent care and courses of prednisolone.
- FEV was not improved by the interventions.
- Budesonide improved airway responsiveness.
- The budesonide group were around 1 cm shorter than the placebo group.

Commentary

This study is well designed and has a 98% follow up rate. The predicted final heights for all thre groups were the same. One in five of the placebo group needed inhaled steroids or other medication. Budesonide is still the treatment of choice in mild to moderate asthma.

Omalizumab reduced inhaled corticosteroid use and exacerbation in childhood allergic asthma. Commentator, Mazer B., Meakins Christie Laboratories, Montreal, Quebec, Canada.
Evidence-based Medicine, 7(1): 12, Jan./Feb. 2002.

Question: In children with moderate to severe allergic asthma who require daily inhaled corticosteroid (ICS) treatment, is omalizumab (anti-immuno-globulin E [anti-IgE] antibody) more effective than placebo for reducing steroid use and asthma exacerbations?

The following article is briefly presented
Treatment of childhood asthma with anti-immunoglobulin E antibody (omalizumab). Milgrom, H., Berger, W., Nayak, A. *et al.*
Pediatrics **108:** e36, Aug. 2001.

This was an RCT with 34 weeks follow up, involving around 330 asthmatic patients aged 2–6 years, who were well controlled on ICS prior to the study. Patients either received subcutaneous omalizumab or placebo.
- Reduction in ICS was more marked in the omalizumab group than the placebo group.
- Fewer patients in the omalizumab group experienced asthma exacerbations compared with the placebo group.

Commentary
This study confirms the findings of other similar studies. Further studies are needed to explore the use of anti-IgE in the management of asthma.

Effect of peer led programme for asthma education in adolescents: cluster randomised controlled trial. Shah, S., Peat, J.K., Mazurski, E.J. and Wang, H. *et al.* Primary Health Care Education and Research Unit, Auburn Hospital and Community Health Services, Auburn, Australia.
BMJ, **322**(7286): 583-585, 10 March 2001.

This Australian study was performed to determine whether a peer led asthma education programme could improve asthma morbidity in school children. It was a cluster randomised controlled trial, involving six high schools (around 1500 children). In a three step programme (called triple A), year 11 students were taught how to educate year 10 students about asthma. Year 10 students then made a presentation using drama and song etc. to year 7 students. A quality of life questionnaire was the main outcome measure.
- Quality of life improved more in the intervention group than the control group.
- There was a significant decrease in school absenteeism in year 10 in the intervention. There was no difference in the control group.
- Asthma attacks at school increased in the year 10 control group.
- The asthma intervention had no effect on year 7.

Eight students would need to be educated for one child to report a quality of life improvement. Peer led programmes could be an important way to reduce the burden of asthma in the community.

Childhood asthma: can computers aid detection in general practice? Kable, S., Henry, R., Sanson-Fisher, R. and Ireland, M. *et al.* University of Newcastle, New South Wales, Australia. *Br. J. Gen. Pract.*, **51**(463): 112-116, February 2001.

The aim of this Australian study was to develop a tool to assess whether or not a child is likely to have asthma. A touch-screen, computerized questionnaire with 30 questions was used and was situated in the GP's waiting room. Patients also filled in written questionnaires and were invited to a hospital clinic to have bronchial challenge or skin testing performed.

- Around 320 children completed the computerized questionnaire and just over half of these went on to have bronchial challenge or skin testing.
- Of the 30 questions, 6 items were independently associated with the presence of asthma. These were: parent or self-reported asthma; previous diagnosis of asthma; wheeze in the past year; physical activity affected by symptoms; night cough in the past year; visits to a GP in the past year.
- An asthma score was developed from this which was able to predict the severity and likely frequency of asthma. The higher the score, the more severe the asthma.
- In the pre-school age group, the asthma score had 100% specificity and 83% sensitivity. In the 5–17 year age group the score had 78% specificity and 73% sensitivity.

They conclude that the asthma score is a "valid indicator of asthma".

The use of a screening questionnaire to identify children with likely asthma. Frank, P.I., Frank, T.L., Cropper, J. and Hirsch, S. *et al.* North West Lung Research Institute, Wythenshawe Hospital, Manchester, UK. *Br. J. Gen. Pract.*, **51**(463): 117-120, February 2001.

The aim of this questionnaire survey was to determine the potential workload involved if all undiagnosed cases of childhood asthma were identified. The study took place in two general practice populations in Manchester. Two simple scoring systems were developed to identify those with likely asthma and those with likely severe asthma. Around 3100 questionnaires were sent to parents of the children in the practice populations. The response rate was just over 65%. Case notes were then examined to identify those who were potentially undiagnosed.

- Using the first scoring system, just over 20% were identified as potentially having asthma. Of these, just over one third (123 children) were potentially undiagnosed.

- Using the second scoring system, used to identify more severe asthma, around 15% were identified as potentially having asthma. Of these, one quarter (61 children) had no evidence of an asthma diagnosis in the case notes.
- They estimate that between 3.5 and 8% of children in these practices would need further attention from their GPs to confirm or refute a diagnosis of asthma.

The potential resource implications would need to be weighed against the benefits of treating this proportion of undiagnosed asthmatics.

The protective effect of childhood infections. Johnston, S.L. and Openshaw, P.J.M. Department of Respiratory Medicine, National Heart and Lung Institute, Imperial College School of Medicine at St Mary's, Norfolk Place, London, UK.
BMJ, **322**(7283): 376-377, 17 February 2001.

In 1989 Strachan proposed the "hygiene hypothesis" which stated that our modern and cleaner environments were responsible for the increase in asthma in children. One example of this is the different rates of asthma in East and West Germany before unification. The lower rates in East Germany are now increasing to catch up with their cleaner neighbours. Children are born with a strong type 2 Ig E producing immunological response. The type 1 response develops in the first year of life in response to environmental challenge from viral infections. It is the type 1 response that is thought to be protective. The type 1 response is poor in children of atopic parents. The following conditions promote immunological maturity:
- having older siblings;
- attending daycare;
- contact with pets and animals;
- having measles;
- orofaecal infections, e.g. Hep A.

Early childhood infectious diseases and the development of asthma up to school age: a birth cohort study. Illi, S., von Mutius, E., Lau, S. and Bergmann, R. *et al.* Department of Pulmonology and Allergology, University Children's Hospital, Munich, Germany.
BMJ, **322**(7283): 390-395, 17 February 2001.

This longitudinal Germany study involved following a cohort of around 1300 children from birth to 7 years of age. They were followed at regular intervals. Parents were interviewed. Blood tests and a bronchial challenge were also performed.
- Children with more that two episodes of runny nose, and those with more than one viral infection of the herpes type (exanthema subitum,stomatitis, herpes, varicella), before age 1, were less likely to have asthma at age 5–7 than those with less than one episode of runny nose or less than one viral infection.
- Recurrent lower respiratory tract infections were positively associated with a diagnosis of asthma later on.

• There was a non-significant inverse relationship between measles and asthma at age 7. The numbers in this analysis were small.

Further analysis of these results and other studies suggest that early exposure of the immature immuological system to allergens has a protective effect in later childhood. The relationship between lower respiratory tract infections suggests a "reverse causation", whereby children with asthma are more likely to have or be diagnosed as having a lower respiratory tract infection. The measles association has been found in other studies.

EPIDEMIOLOGY

Sensitisation to airborne moulds and severity of asthma: cross sectional study from European Community respiratory health survey. Zureik, M., Neukirch, C. and Leynaert, B. *et al.* National Institute of Health and Medical Research, Faculte de Medecine Xavier Bichat, Paris, France.
BMJ, 325(7361): 411-417, 24 August 2002.

The aim of this study was to assess whether the severity of asthma is associated with sensitisation to airbourne moulds rather than to other seasonal or perennial allergens. This was a multicentre cross-sectional study involving 1132 adults taken from the European Community respiratory health survey. The subjects, aged 20–44 with current asthma, underwent skin prick tests with the following allergens: *A. alternata, Cladosporium herbarum,* timothy grass, birch, olive, pellitory-of-the-wall, common ragweed, house dust mite and cat. The severity of asthma was given a score based on forced expiratory volume in one second, number of asthma attacks, hospital admissions for breathing problems, and use of corticosteroids.

• The frequency of sensitisation to moulds, *A. alternata* or *Cladosporium herbarum* or both, increased significantly with increasing asthma severity (odds ratio 2.34 (95% confidence interval 1.56 to 3.52) for either for severe vs. mild asthma).

• There was no association between asthma severity and sensitisation to pollens or cats.

• Sensitisation to house dust mite was positively associated with severity.

The authors conclude that sensitisation to moulds is a powerful risk factor for severe asthma in adults. And this information should be used in primary prevention, management and patients education of asthma.

OTHERS

The predictive value of asthma medications to identify individuals with asthma - a study in German general practices. Himmel, W., Hummers-Pradier, E. and Schumann, H. *et al.* Department of General Practice, University of Gottingen, Gottingen, Germany.
Br. J. Gen. Pract., **51:** 879-883, November 2002.

Previously, evaluation of prescribing performance has relied upon the assumption that the drugs a patient receives can be used to identify his or her disease. The aim of this study was to identify the predictive value of certain drugs in the diagnosis of asthma and hence evaluate the validity of this assumption. This cross-sectional study used eight general practices and one community respiratory practice centre in a town in Germany and in total 942 prescriptions for asthma drugs were identified. The main results were:

- In general practices, inhaled betamimetics had a moderate marker function for asthma.
- In the respiratory practice, the diagnosis of asthma was strongly marked by a fixed combinations of cromoglycate plus betamimetics, whereas in contrast inhaled steroids proved to contradict the diagnosis of asthma.

The authors conclude that 'the limited specificity of drugs for a disease (e.g. asthma) should be taken into account when analysing prescribing data that are not diagnosis linked'.

Association between migraine and asthma: matched case-control study. Davey, G., Sedgwick, P. and Maier, W. *et al.* Department of Public Health Sciences, St Georges Hospital Medical School, Cranmer Terrace, London, UK.
Br. J. Gen. Pract., **52**(482): 723-727, September 2002.

Various research has suggested associations between migraine or severe headache and asthma or wheezing. This study examined whether the occurrence of migraine and asthma are associated in the UK.

A matched case-control study design was used, with analysis of data from the General Practice Research Database (over 5 million patients). Subjects with diagnosed migraine were identified from the database, and matched with non-migraine controls of the same general practice, sex and age. Case-control pairs were analysed for occurrence of asthma, other respiratory diseases and symptoms, eczema and hay fever. Almost 65 000 case-control pairs were studied

- The relative risk of asthma among definite cases of migraine was 1.59
- In addition, the relative risks of chronic obstructive pulmonary disease, respiratory symptoms, eczema and hayfever were all raised in migraine cases.
- The association between asthma and migraine was stronger in patients not diagnosed with hayfever.

The authors conclude that migraine and asthma are associated in the UK, although it is suggested that frequent attendance to a GP surgery may confound these results.

> **Synergism between allergens and viruses and risk of hospital admission with asthma: case-control study.** Green, R.M., Custovic, A. and Sanderson, G. *et al.* North West Lung Centre, Wythenshaw Hospital, Manchester, UK.
> ***BMJ, 324**(7340): 763-766, 30 March 2002.*

The aim of this case-control study of adult patients was to evaluate the role of exposure to allergens, sensitisation to allergens and viral infections in precipitating admission to hospital for acute asthma. Controls were those with stable asthma and non-asthmatic hospital in patients. They use skin prick tests to assess sensitization, dust samples from the patients' homes to assess exposure and nasal lavage to identify viral infections.

- Patients admitted to hospital with an acute asthma episode were more likely to have viral infections plus both sensitization and exposure to allergens.
- Detection of virus alone was not significantly associated with an increased risk of hospital admission with an acute episode of asthma.

They conclude that we should aim to reduce exposure to both viruses and allergens in order to reduce acute admissions for asthma.

> **The prevalence of asthma and heart disease in transport workers: a practice-based study.** Fleming, D.M. and Charlton, J.R.H. Birmingham Research Unit, Royal College of General Practitioners, Birmingham, UK.
> ***Br. J. Gen. Pract.,** 51*(469): 638-643, August 2001.

The aim of this study was to analyze the relationship between occupation and cardiac and respiratory diseases. In particular, they wanted to examine the relationship between air pollution and asthma. They use data from the 4th national morbidity survey, which combines occupational data with data concerning consultation rates in general practice, as well as smoking habits. They found that:

- Subjects working in motor vehicle occupations had slightly increased asthma rates compared with all working men. However, this difference was not significant when compared with occupation matched controls.
- Car mechanics had a low levels of asthma.

They conclude that increasing asthma prevalence cannot be due to motor vehicle pollution.

FURTHER READING

Undiagnosed and untreated wheezing in a cohort of adolescents with a family history of allergic disease. Department of Public Health, Bro Taf Health Authority, Cardiff, UK.
Br. J. Gen. Pract., **51**(469): 664-665, August 2001.

Cross-sectional observations on the natural history of asthma. Tayside Centre for General Practice, University of Dundee, Dundee, UK.
Br. J. Gen. Pract., **51**(466): 361-365, May 2001.

Spacer made from sealed cold-drink bottles were as effective as conventional spacers in children with acute asthma. University of Texas Houston Health Science Center, Houston TX, USA.
Evidence-based Medicine, **5**(3): 79, May 2000.

The use of inhaled corticosteroids in childhood asthma.
Drugs and Theraputics Bulletin, **37**(10): 73-77, October 1999.

BACK PAIN

- Most people with chronic low back pain want an X-ray despite the fact that it does not change outcome
- Intensive multidisciplinary biopsychosocial rehabilitation, involving more than 100 hours of therapy, is beneficial for disabling low back pain, of at least 3 months duration
- A Dutch study found positive SLR, duration of symptoms greater than 30 days and positive reverse SLR were predictors of poor outcome in sciatica.
- A Swedish study found that early active treatment with small range rotational movements of the neck, was more effective than standard treatment for the management of acute whiplash injury.
- X-rays for back pain should only be performed if there is a history of cancer or two red flags.

BACKGROUND

Management

In 1992 the Clinical Standards Advisory Group (CSAG) made 3 recommendations concerning back pain management. These were:
1. there needs to be a change in the attitude of both doctors and patients towards back pain;
2. there needs to be more resources for treatment;
3. there needs to be more services for acute and continuing pain.

In 1996 the Royal College of General Practitioners issued guidelines concerning back pain management. They recommended that:
- patients should stay as active as possible and that bed rest is not recommended;
- X-ray and specialist referral is not indicated;
- referral for spinal manipulation should be considered, within 6 weeks of onset;
- refer for exercise programme, if patient has not returned to work within 6 weeks.

Back pain lasting more than 6 weeks is likely to become chronic. At 6 months only 50% go back to work.

One of the aims of the CSAG was to increase access to physical therapy in order to reduce claims for sick benefit. They hence recommended 8 services:
- locally agreed contact for emergency referral;
- suspected serious pathology to be seen by a consultant within 2 weeks;
- unresolved sciatica after 6 weeks should be seen by a consultant within 2 weeks;
- simple back pain to be seen by physical therapist within 72 hours of urgent telephone referral;
- routine referrals to be seen within 2 weeks;

- severe acute back pain to be seen by acute pain relief service within 48 hours of a telephone referral;
- patients with simple acute low back pain should be seen by a physical therapist before they have been off work for 6 weeks;
- patients with chronic low back pain should be seen by a multidisciplinary team before they have been off work for 6 months.

During initial examination doctors need to be aware of signs of serious disease e.g. cauda equina syndrome, fracture, progressive neurological disease. A study performed in 1996 (*BMJ*, Feb. 1996), found that a minority of GPs were not aware of the signs of serious pathology in back pain sufferers.

One of the most striking changes in the management of acute back pain in most recent years is the advice to stay active. A systematic review in 1997 (*BJGP*, Oct. 1997) found that people with back pain who remained active had less disability and health care use and less time off work than those who were advised bed rest.

EDITORIAL – X-rays for back pain? Little, P.D. Community Clinical Sciences, University of Southampton, UK.
Br. J. Gen. Pract., **52**(480): 534-535, 1 July 2002.

The author shows that routine X-ray for first presentation does not improve pain but may provide psychological support. However, routine X-rays for this reason are 'difficult to justify' in view of the increased risk of fatal cancers by higher radiation doses in lumbar X-ray. Guidelines in 1989 suggested that unless there are 'red flags' symptoms X-rays should be delayed for 6 weeks. An algorithm based on 13 patients suggests performing X-rays when:
- there is a history of previous cancer
- two red flags (raised ESR, failure to improve after 6 weeks, unexplained weight loss, systemic signs such as lymphadenopathy).

This would limit X-rays to 22% but maintain 100% sensitivity. More evidence of predictive factors is required, but until then the author suggests that it is reasonable to follow this algorithm. The author also suggests that X-rays should not be arranged for the psychosocial reasons of patient reassurance and satisfaction. Instead providing information to increase patient understanding will improve pain, functioning and satisfaction.

An active exercise and posture protocol reduced pain in acute whiplash injuries.
Commentator, Robert Hawkins. Wright State University, Centreville, OH, USA.
Evidence-based Medicine, 6(3): 76, May/June 2001

Question: In patients with acute whiplash injuries, is an active treatment protocol more effective than standard treatment for reducing pain? Is early initiation better than delayed initiation of treatment?

The following article was briefly presented

Early intervention in whiplash-associated disorders. A comparison of two treatment programmes. Rosenfeld, M., Gunnarson, R. and Borenstein, P. *Spine 25* 1782–1787, 15 July 2000

This was a randomized controlled trial with 6 months follow up involving nearly 30 primary care centres, three emergency departments and just over 100 patients. The study was conducted in Sweden. Patients were allocated to early (within 4 days) or late (after 2 weeks) active treatment or early or late standard treatment. Active treatment involved an individual treatment programme including small range rotational movements of the neck. Standard treatment involved giving a leaflet containing advice about whiplash injuries.

- Early active treatment reduced pain whereas standard treatment increased pain.
- Early active treatment was better than late active treatment

Commentary

This study supports current advice for 'early mobilization as tolerated' for the management of both whiplash and acute low back pain and it may help to reduce the progression to chronic whiplash syndrome.

Predicting the outcome of sciatica at short-term follow-up. Vroomen, P.C.A.J., de Krom, M.C.T.F.M. and Knotterus, J.A. Department of Clinical Neurophysiology, Maastricht University Hospital, Maastricht, Netherlands.
Br. J. Gen. Pract., 52(457): 119-123, February 2002.

This Dutch study assessed predictors of poor outcome (at 3 months) in patients with sciatica. Just over 180 patients took part in the study, which was a prospective study. The study was performed alongside a RCT of bed rest. Predictors of poor outcome were:

- positive straight leg raise (SLR) test;
- duration of symptoms greater than 30 days;
- positive reverse SLR test (femoral stretch).

A previous study (Carragee, Spine 1997) found that duration of pain greater than 6 months, workers compensation claim and older age, were predictors of poor outcome. Patients with a workers compensation claim pending were excluded from this present study and older age was not found to be a predictor of poor outcome in this study.

Randomised trial of acupuncture compared with conventional massage and 'sham' laser acupuncture for treatment of chronic neck pain. Irnich, D., Behrens, N., Molzen, H., König, A. and Gleditsch, J. Department of Anaesthesiology, Ludwig-Maximilians University, Munich, Germany.
***BMJ,* 322**(7302): 1574-1578, 30 June 2001.

This German study involved around 180 patients and its aim was to compare acupuncture with massage and 'sham' acupuncture performed using an inactivated laser pen, for the management of chronic neck pain. Patients received five treatments and follow up occurred immediately, 1 week later and 3 months after treatment.

- One week post treatment, acupuncture was better than massage but not 'sham' acupuncture for pain related to motion. This was particularly so for people with pain lasting more than 5 years, and those with myofacial syndrome.
- For secondary outcomes, acupuncture had better results than the other two groups. At 3 months these differences were not significant.

The lack of a difference between acupuncture and 'sham' acupuncture may be because the therapist still needs to palpate the acupuncture points when using the laser. The palpation may confer some beneficial effects similar to conventional acupuncture. They conclude that acupuncture is effective for the relief of pain and to improve neck mobility.

Multidisciplinary rehabilitation for chronic low back pain: systematic review. Guzmán, J., Esmail, R., Karjalainen, K. and Malmivaara, A. *et al.* Institute for Work and Health, Toronto, Canada.
***BMJ,* 322**(7301): 1511-1516, 23 June 2001.

This study was a systematic review of studies comparing intensive (>100 hours) multidisciplinary biopsychosocial rehabilitation with less intensive multidisciplinary biopsychosocial rehabilitation or non-multidisciplinary biopsychosocial rehabilitation, for the treatment of chronic low back pain. Ten studies involving nearly 2000 patients met the inclusion criteria. All subjects had disabling low back pain for at least 3 months.

- Those in the intensive group did better (in terms of function and pain) than those receiving less intensive therapy or non-multidisciplinary therapy.

They conclude that patients should not be referred for multidisciplinary therapy until the content of therapy is known.

Population based intervention to change back pain beliefs and disability: three part evaluation. Buchbinder, R., Jolley, D. and Wyatt, M. Department of Clinical Epidemiology, Cabrini Hospital and Monash University Department of Epidemiology and Preventative Medicine, Victoria, Australia.
BMJ, **322**(7301): 1561-1520, 23 June 2001.

This study was a population-based intervention whose aim was to alter beliefs, management and costs related to back pain. Two neighbouring Australian states acted as intervention and control populations. The intervention population were subject to a television advertising campaign involving well known personalities and sporting stars. Doctors in the intervention group also received evidence-based guidelines concerning the management of back pain.

- After 2.5 years follow up, the intervention population had significantly more positive beliefs about back pain.
- Doctors in the intervention group also had more positive beliefs about back pain.
- Workers' claims for back pain compensation declined in the intervention group by 15%.

They conclude that population based strategies are effective in causing a positive attitude towards back pain.

Radiography of the lumbar spine in primary care patients with low back pain: randomised controlled trial. Kendrick, D., Fielding, K., Bently, E. and Kerslake, R. *et al.* Division of General Practice, School of Community Health Sciences, University Park, Nottingham, UK.
BMJ, **322**(7283): 400-405, 17 February 2001.

There are four different sets of guidelines concerning the use of diagnostic X-rays in the management of low back pain. These are:

- Agency for Health Care Policy and Research: suggests X-ray if no improvement after 4 weeks;
- Clinical Standards Advisory Group: suggests, consider X-ray after 6 weeks;
- Royal College of General Practitioners: X-ray may be indicated after 4 weeks;
- Royal College of Radiologists; X-ray is not indicated if there are no indicators of serious pathology.

The aim of this study is to compare the outcome of low back pain in those who have and those who do not have a lumbar spine X-ray. Over 400 patients from general practices in Nottingham, with low back pain for at least 10 weeks, were randomized to X-ray or no X-ray.

- At 3 months more patients in the X-ray group had pain compared with the control group.
- At 9 months the X-ray group were more satisfied with care than the control group.
- Most patients said that they would have liked to have an X-ray.

• Having an X-ray did not affect the outcome in terms of pain severity, patient functioning and health status.

X-rays increase doctors' workload. Patients need more education about the usefulness of X-rays in the management of low back pain.

FURTHER READING

Low back pain in general practice: reported management and reasons for not adhering to the guidelines in The Netherlands. Schers, H., Braspenning, J. Drivjeer, R., Wensing, M. *et al.*, Centre for Quality of Care Research, University of Nijmegen The Netherlands.
Br. J. Gen. Pract., **50**(457): 640-644, Aug. 2000.

Managing back pain in general practice-is osteopathy the new paradigm? Williams, N. General Practitioner and Osteopath, Health Centre, Llanfairechan, Wales, UK.
Br. J. Gen. Pract., **47**(423): 653-655, Oct. 1997.

BEREAVEMENT

- One study found that contact from the GP/surgery and an acknowledgement of the bereavement was found to be important in helping those left behind to deal with their loss.
- Patients with no spiritual beliefs are at increased risk of delayed or complicated recovery from grief following bereavement.

Spiritual beliefs may affect outcome of bereavement: prospective study. Walsh, K., King, M. and Jones, L. Department of Psychiatry and Behavioural Science, Royal Free Campus, Royal Free and University College Medical School, London, UK.
BMJ, 324(7353): 1551-1555, 29 June 2002.

This study examined whether or not spiritual belief affects the process of grieving. Standardised measures were used to assess the strength of spiritual belief and bereavement outcome in 129 relatives and close friends of patients undergoing palliative care at a Marie Curie centre. Measurements were taken prior to the patient's death, and at 9 months and 14 months following death. Participants were categorised as having no spiritual belief (16%), low strength of belief (41%) or high strength of belief (43%).

- Those with high intensity spiritual beliefs recovered from bereavement in a linear fashion, while those with low intensity beliefs had little improvement in the first 9 months, but recovered rapidly following this point. Those with no spiritual beliefs showed temporary improvement at 9 months, but symptoms of grief had increased by the final 14-month assessment.
- The effect of spiritual beliefs on recovery from grief was unaffected by age or sex, however social isolation and emotional closeness to the deceased reduced the effect of strength of spiritual belief.

The authors acknowledge that the sample size was small, however it may be appropriate for more attention to be given by palliative care services to spiritual beliefs of close relatives and friends of patients. While not suggesting a religious intervention for those without any spiritual belief, the authors conclude this may be a means of identifying people having difficulty in recovering from the loss of a relative or close friend.

Improving management of bereavement in general practice based on a survey of recently bereaved subjects to a single general practice. Main, J. Clinical Development Nurse (Research) Birmingham Specialist Community NHS Trust, Elderly Services Directorate, Moseley Hall Hospital, Birmingham, UK.
Br. J. Gen. Pract., 50(460): 863-866, November 2000.

The aim of this qualitative study was to evaluate the role of the GP in the care of the bereaved. It was carried out in a single general practice in Birmingham. Twenty three people participated in a semi-structured interview process. The findings were:

- poor communication and inadequate information (both prior and post bereavement) from the health professionals leads to distress and bereavement difficulties;
- patient satisfaction with the GPs particularly and the hospital is an important aspect of the bereavement process;
- contact from the GP/surgery and an acknowledgement of the bereavement was found to be important in helping those left behind to deal with their loss;
- the extent to which bereavement support is proactive or reactive appears to be related to the individual general practitioners interests, beliefs and knowledge of the individual patient and lacks a consistent approach.

Practical suggestions to develop this as a GP service include:
- a letter offering sympathy/support;
- a visit from GP/nurse;
- specific bereavement consultation;
- record of deaths and tagging of notes to allow the surgery staff to offer sympathy when appropriate

BREAST CANCER

> - The results of one study suggest that increased physical activity and reduced calorie intake may reduce the risk of breast cancer
> - Misinterpretation of symptoms is one of the reasons why women delay seeking medical help for symptoms of breast cancer
> - Breast self examination has no effect on breast cancer death rates

BACKGROUND

Breast cancer is the most common cause of cancer in women. Nearly 90% of deaths occur in women over the age of 50.

Screening

Breast cancer screening was introduced in 1988 after results of RCTs including the Swedish two counties study (*Lancet*, 1985) were published. In the Swedish study breast cancer mortality fell by 30%. The DOH set a target for the reduction in deaths from breast cancer of 25% by the year 2000. Screening in the under 50 age group is not thought to be beneficial. For screening to be effective, the number of cancers occurring between the 3 year screening interval should be kept lower than the background rate. A Manchester study involving 130 000 women (*BMJ*, Jan. 1995) found that the number of interval cancers after 2 years approaches the background incidence of breast cancer. A review of literature suggests that a decrease in interval cancers can be achieved by:

- using two radiological opinions;
- having a 2 year interval between mammographies;
- using two view mammography;
- increasing the optical density of films.

Mammographic screening has a response rate of 70% and this is expected to result in 1250 less deaths per year. However, some researchers would question whether screening has any effect at all on death rates. Quin *et al.* (*BMJ*, Nov. 95) reported that the observed reduction in mortality was more likely to be due to widespread use of tamoxifen.

Tamoxifen's effect on mortality from breast cancer is unclear. In 1996, the National Cancer Institute of America stopped a trial when it seemed that more than 5 years use was not likely to be beneficial. The American Food and Drug Administration looked at 14 trials (17 000 patients) and reported that tamoxifen use is associated with an excess of primary tumours in the ipsilateral arm. The State of California declared tamoxifen to be a carcinogen.

Tamoxifen is still widely used in the management of breast cancer. Studies show that long term adjuvant tamoxifen is associated with reduced deaths from MIs, reduced LDL levels and slightly increased risk of DVTs and PEs.

The combined oral contraceptive pill is associated with a slightly increased risk of breast cancer (odds ratio 1.24). Breast cancer in pill users tends to be less clinically advanced than those found in non-users (*BMJ*, July 1996)

Deprivation

The prevalence of breast cancer is highest in women from wealthier backgrounds and yet death rates are lowest in this group. A study by Carnon *et al.* (*BMJ*, Oct. 1994) involving 1300 patients found that tumour size, histological grade and lymph node status was not related to level of deprivation.

EDITORIAL – Breast self examination. Austoker, J. Director Cancer Research UK Primary Care Education Research Group, Division of Public Health and Primary Health Care, University of Oxford, Oxford, UK.
***BMJ*, 326**(7379): 1-2, 4 January 2003.

An extensive, well-conducted RCT in Shanghai has shown that teaching women to examine their breasts does not reduce breast cancer mortality. This study should end the longstanding confusion regarding whether breast self-examination should be carried out.

Breast examination has been recommended for 70 years, despite a lack of evidence proving its efficacy. Surveys have shown that even with high levels of awareness, only a small proportion of women regularly examine their breasts. Additionally, there have been no agreed standards for how to examine breasts, or how often this should be done.

The Shanghai trial involved over 266 000 women. Regular, intensive instruction and follow-up was given to the intervention group, while the control group received normal care. There was no difference in breast cancer deaths between the groups. The intervention group had more breast biopsies and benign lesions diagnosed.

The author emphasises the continued importance of women being aware of changes in their breasts, and reporting these to their GP. However, there is no longer any need to routinely train women to examine their breasts.

A qualitative study of delay among women reporting symptoms of breast cancer.
Burgess, C., Hunter, M.S. and Ramirez, A.J. ICRF Psychosocial Oncology Group, Adamson Centre for Mental Health, St Thomas's Hospital, London, UK.
***Br. J. Gen. Pract.*, 51**(473): 967-971, December 2001.

This is a qualitative study whose aim is to explore reasons why some women delay seeking treatment for symptoms of breast cancer. They interview a group of women (46 in total) who sought treatment immediately and a group who had waited at least 12 weeks. Some of the major themes that emerged were

Misinterpretation of symptoms
- Non-breast lump symptoms were often thought to be of no consequence.

Attitudes to attending general practice
- Those delaying treatment were likely to be non-regular attenders who did not like to 'bother' the GP with 'trivial' symptoms

Belief concerning the consequences of treatment
- Those who delayed, tended to have a negative view about the consequences of treatment

Competing priorities
- Those who delayed often cited family, work and other commitments e.g. holidays as reasons for delaying seeking treatment

Triggers to action
- Those who delayed often monitored their symptoms and sought help when something changed e.g. appearance of a lump.

EDUCATION AND DEBATE SECTION – Effect of sex and gender on psychosocial aspects of prostate and breast cancer. Kiss, A. and Meryn, S. Psychosomatic Division, Department of Internal Medicine, University Clinics Basel, Petersgraben 4, CH-4031 Basel, Switzerland.
BMJ, 323(7320): 1055-1058, 3 November 2001.

The article explores the similarities and differences between the psychosocial impacts of both prostate and breast cancer. Despite the similarities between the two cancers at an epidemiological and biological level, far more research has been performed on the psychosocial impact of breast cancer and mastectomy than has been performed on prostate cancer and the sequelae that follow its treatment (e.g. impotence).

In addition, owing to ideas that men themselves hold over what it is to be 'masculine' (e.g. to be self-sufficient, strong, powerful and successful) they may have less psychosocial support than their female counterparts.These gender differences manifest themselves even within support groups, those for breast cancer focus mainly on the 'emotions' of the women affected, whereas those for prostate cancer tend primarily to deal with the 'facts' about the disease.In general, doctors are poor at detecting psychological distress in cancer patients. Furthermore, the balance of interest in cancer's psychosocial impact on men compared to that on women needs to be addressed.

EVIDENCE BASED CASE REPORT: Advice about mammography for a young woman with a family history of breast cancer. Lucassen, A., Watson, E. and Eccles, D. Wessex Regional Genetics Service, Princess Anne Hospital, Southampton, UK.
BMJ, 322(7293): 1040-1042, 28 April 2001.

This is an evidence based case report of a 35 year old women with a family history of breast cancer. The question was, should she be offered mammography? There have been no RCTs conducted looking at the effectiveness of mammography in women under 50 with a family history of breast cancer. The studies that are available suggest that cancers may be detected earlier but there is no evidence to suggest that mortality is reduced. The negative points are that:

- in young people, because of the denser breast tissue, mammography has a lower sensitivity and specificity than in older women (high false positive and false negative rates);
- in addition there is a radiation risk from mammography which is cumulative, and women with a family history of breast cancer may be more sensitive to radiation than women without a family history.

It seems that the stronger the family history of breast cancer, the more likely one is to detect a cancer at mammography.

Many advise mammography if the risk of breast cancer (in someone under 50) is the same as for a women over the age of 50 (roughly a three fold increased risk). However, the final choice should be left to the woman.

Lifestyle, hormones and risk of breast cancer. Grazyna, Jasienska, Assistant Professor, Reproductive Biology, Institute of Public Health, Jagiellonian University, Krakow, Poland. *BMJ,* **322**(7286): 586-587, 10 March 2001.

This short paper looks at the links between nutrition, ovarian progesterone production and breast cancer. Salivary progesterone levels were measured daily in women from Bolivia, Congo, Nepal, Poland and the USA. Mid-luteal phase levels of progesterone were calculated.

- High mid-luteal phase levels were strongly associated with an increased incidence of breast cancer. USA had the highest levels of mid-luteal phase progesterone and breast cancer. The Congo had the lowest levels.
- Energy intake was also calculated. The lower the energy intake, the lower the incidence of breast cancer.

They postulate that low energy intake results in poor ovarian function which in turn reduces lifetime ovarian production of progesterone, which then reduces the risk of breast cancer. They suggest that increased physical activity and reduced calorie intake may reduce the risk of breast cancer.

EDITORIAL – How effective is screening for breast cancer? Lennarth, Nystrom, Senior Lecturer in Biostatistics, Department of Epidemiology, Public Health and Clinical Medicine, Umea, Sweden.
BMJ, **321**(7262): 647-648, 16 September 2000.

and

Effect of NHS breast screening programme on mortality from breast cancer in England and Wales. 1990–8: comparison of observed with predicted mortality. Blanks, R.G., Moss, S.M., McGalan, C.E., Quinn, M.J. and Babb, P.J., Cancer Screening Evaluation Unit, Institute of Cancer Research, Section of Epidemiology, Sutton, Surrey, UK.
BMJ, **321**(7262): 665-669, 1 August 2000.

The aim of this study was to look at the effect of the breast cancer screening programme, in England and Wales, on mortality from breast cancer. Estimating the effect of screening on mortality from breast cancer is difficult for the following reasons.
- Many of the deaths that occurred in the 1990s will have been in patients diagnosed with cancer before being invited for screening. These individuals are difficult to exclude from national mortality statistics (unlike RCTs).
- Although screening started in 1985, it did not reach full coverage until 1992.
- Breast cancer mortality started falling in 1990 and this may be due to better treatments e.g. tamoxifen, better NHS structure.

In this study, they use national mortality data and various mathematical models to make estimates.
- From 1990 to 1998 there has been a 21% reduction in death from breast cancer.
- Six to seven percent of this is estimated to be due to the screening programme.
- Around 15% is likely to be due to improvements in the management of breast cancer.

Because of the methodological difficulties, the accuracy of these estimates should be carefully scrutinized.

FURTHER READING

See 'Deprivation' for

Relation between socioeconomic status and tumour stage in patients with breast, colorectal, ovarian and lung cancer: results from four national, population based studies. Scottish Cancer Intelligence Unit, Information and Statistics Division, Trinity Park House, Edinburgh, UK.
BMJ, **322**(7290): 830-831, 7 April 2001.

Clonidine was effective for reducing tamoxifen associated hot flashes in postmenopausal women with breast cancer. Charles Loprinzi. Mayo Clinic Rochester, Minnesota, USA.
Evidence-based Medicine, **6**(1): 18, Jan./Feb. 2001.

How women with a family history of breast cancer and their general practitioners act on genetic advice in general practice: prospective longitudinal study. De Bock, G.H., Van Asperen, C.J., de Vries, J.M., Hageman, G.C.H. *et al.*, Department of Medical Decision Making, Leiden University Medical Centre Leiden, The Netherlands.
BMJ, **322**(7277): 26-27, 6 Jan. 2001.

Raising concerns about family history of breast cancer in primary care consultations: prospective, population based study. Women's Concerns Study Group.
BMJ, **322**(7277): 27-28, 6 Jan. 2001.

BURNOUT

- Unrealistic expectations of both doctors and patients contribute to the reasons why doctors are unhappy.
- GPs' own self care should underpin their care of patients
- Protected time for practice meetings, and strategies at partnership rather than individual level, are key to boosting GP morale

Morale among general practitioners: qualitative study exploring relations between partnership arrangements, personal style and workload. Huby, G., Gerry, M. and McKinstry, B.
BMJ, **325**(7356): 140-144, 20 July 2002.

This paper reports on qualitative results of a study of GP experiences working in South East Scotland. It involved 63 GP Principals, and consisted of three phases of interviews and focus groups with each phase building on the previous one.

- Partnership arrangements, workload and personal style were identified as the key factors whose dynamic interaction affected doctors' morale.
- Workload was given as the significant factor affecting morale.
- Partnership arrangements determined how workload and other issues were approached and resolved, successfully or otherwise; they also influenced the GP's personal functioning.
- The results indicate that GP morale may be boosted by implementing integrated solutions at partnership level, and at the level of policy and resource development, rather than focusing on individual coping strategies.
- Practices with equitable and inclusive partner and practice relationships were better able to manage their workload. Protected time and space is needed for partners and practice staff to meet, and in order that problem areas are identified and tackled prospectively rather than retrospectively.

The authors conclude that people working in primary care must be able to "express and deal with the complexity of primary care work", and that research is needed into approaches to developing partnership arrangements. They suggest that similar research be conducted with GP non-principals.

EDUCATION AND DEBATE SECTION – Unhappy doctors: what are the causes and what can be done? Edwards, N., Kornacki, M.J. and Silversin, J. NHS Confederation, London, UK.
***BMJ*, 324**(7341): 835–838, 6 April 2002.

This article addresses some of the reasons why doctors are unhappy. The article represents the views of senior doctors and managers from the UK and USA. Some of the points raised were as follows:
- Pay and workload. These could be improved, however, these two factors alone are insufficient to raise morale to a high level.
- Changes in patient's expectations. Patients want rapid access to services and longer opening times.
- Reduced autonomy coupled with increased accountability, with increased use of audit, protocols, inspection and regulation.
- Lack of respect for the medical profession, compounded by hostile media reports.
- Inadequate training to work in teams and dealing with organizations.
- Doctor's expectations. Dissonance between what doctors expect and what the job actually entails.

Some suggestions for improving the situation include:
- encouraging the government to use evidence to inform policy;
- better training for doctors, to enable them to work in teams;
- reorganise the relationship between doctors and the healthcare system i.e. set realistic targets.

Challenge of culture, conscience, and contract to general practitioner's care of their own health: qualitative study. Thompson, W.T., Cupples, M.E., Sibbett, C.H. and Skan, D.I. *et al.* Graduate School of Education, Queen's University of Belfast, Belfast, UK.
***BMJ*, 323**(7315): 728-731, 29 September 2001.

Questionnaire studies have revealed that general practitioners are exposed to a number of issues surrounding their own health: self prescription, working through illness, high stress and a high suicide rate to name a few. This qualitative study involved focus groups and in-depth interviews with 27 GPs from Northern Ireland and explored the GP's perceptions of how their profession and training has affected their attitudes to their own health and that of colleagues.
- GPs are concerned about the current level of illness in the profession and believe that medical education should strive to promote self-care.
- Medical knowledge makes GPs prone to swinging between panic and denial when they perceive themselves to be ill.
- GPs believe that their profession hinders their ability to acknowledge personal illness and participate in health screening. They perceive a need to portray a healthy image to both patients and colleagues, particularly in the case of psychiatric illness. Concerns over confidentiality are also an issue.

- The self-employed nature of GP's work means that they are likely to work through illness for reasons of conscience to patients and colleagues. They expect colleagues to do the same.
- GPs should underpin their knowledge and care of their patients with a sense of duty to look after their own health.

FURTHER READING

Stress in undergraduate medical education: 'the mask of relaxed brilliance'. Styles, W.M.
Br. J. Gen. Pract., **43**(367): 46-47, Feb. 1993.

CANNABIS

- One commentator concludes that 'currently available cannabinoids clearly lose the battle in both efficacy and safety with competitors of today'
- Cannabinoids, acting as 'mood enhancing adjuvants', may be used to control emetogenic chemotherapy in selected patients.
- Further trials are required before cannabinoids can be introduced into clinical practice for pain management
- Cannabis usage in adolescence increases the risk of schizophrenia symptoms in adulthood
- An Australian cohort study conducted in high school students found that frequent smoking of cannabis during adolescence increases the risk of developing anxiety or depression in early adulthood
- An editorial states that smoking cannabis is causally related to the development of depression and schizophrenia

Cannabis use in adolescence and risk for adult psychosis: longitudinal prospective study. Arseneault, L., Cannon, M. and Poulton, R. *et al.* SGDP Research Centre, Kings College, London, UK.
***BMJ,* 325**(7374): 1212-1213, 23 November 2002.

This study conducted in New Zealand looked at whether adolescent cannabis use is a risk factor for developing adult schizophrenia.

Around 1000 individuals (who were part of the Dunedin multi-disciplinary health and development study) were recruited with information of psychotic symptoms at age 11 and any drug use in the teenage years (age 15 and 18). Nearly 75% of these patients had records detailing any adult psychiatric illness as well. They were followed up at ages, 11, 15–18 and 26.

- Schizophrenia was more likely in those that had used cannabis by age 15 and 18 compared with controls.
- Cannabis users by age 15 were four times more likely to develop a psychotic disorder by the age of 26 than non-cannabis users.
- Even controlling for psychotic symptoms at age 11 the risk remains higher for cannabis users.

Early cannabis use is a greater risk for schizophrenia than later cannabis use. Use of cannabis should be strongly discouraged by teachers, parents and doctors particularly among vulnerable teenagers.

Cannabis use and mental health in young people: cohort study. Patton, G.C., Coffey, C. and Carlin, B.C. *et al.* Centre For Adolescent Health, Murdoch Childrens Research Institute, Parkville, Vic. 3052, Australia.
BMJ, **325**(7374): 1195, 23 November 2002.

Currently, the majority of young people in many Western countries, including the United Kingdom, use cannabis recreationally. The health risks associated with regular cannabis use remain uncertain, though it has been linked with increased rates of lung disease and mental illness. The current study aimed to examine the relationship between cannabis use in adolescence and development of anxiety and depression in adolescence, and also whether social factors and depressive or anxiety symptoms in adolescence predicted cannabis use (i.e. self medication). The authors performed a seven-wave cohort study on 60 000 high school students in Victoria, Australia. Subjects were assessed every 6 months over a 7-year period by a questionnaire to assess substance use (cannabis, alcohol and other illegal drugs) and depressive and anxiety symptoms. The study found:

• The prevalence of anxiety and depression increased with increasing cannabis use. Adolescent females using cannabis daily had a four-fold increase in depression and anxiety in early adulthood
• Adolescent depression or anxiety does not predict cannabis use, thus the association between cannabis and depression/anxiety is not one of self medication.

The authors argue for a direct link between cannabis use and depression/anxiety, operating via psychosocial effects or pharmacological effects of cannabis use.

EDITORIAL – Cannabis and mental health. Rey, J.M. Professor of Child And Adolescent Psychiatry and Tennant, C.C. Professor of Psychiatry University of Sydney, Royal North Shore Hospital, St Leonards, Australia.
BMJ, **325**(7374): 1183, 23 November 2002.

Throughout the 1990s cannabis use amongst young people increased considerably, reflecting increased availability of the drug, relaxation of laws and perception that cannabis is less harmful than alcohol or cigarettes. Current evidence now strongly suggests that the association between cannabis and mental health problems reflects a causal relationship and not self medication for prodromal symptoms. Studies in New Zealand, Sweden and Denmark have demonstrated that adolescent cannabis use predisposes to development of schizophrenia in early adulthood, and that a dose-response relationship for risk exists. Moreover, research from America, New Zealand and Australia has shown that adolescent cannabis use predicts depression in early adulthood and is especially associated with anhedonia and suicidal ideation. The authors conclude by suggesting that public health campaigns should seek to reduce the amount of cannabis smoked by individuals in an attempt to decrease incidence of schizophrenia in the population.

Cannabinoids for control of chemotherapy induced nausea and vomiting: quantitative systemic review. M.R., Carroll, D. and Campbell, F.A. *et al.* Division d'Anesthesiolgie, Departement Anesthesiologie, Pharmacologie Clinique et Soins Intensif de Chirurgie, Hoptiaux Universitaires, Geneve, Switzerland.
BMJ, **323**(7303): 16-21, 7 July 2001.

The aim of this systemic review was to investigate the anti-emetic efficacy and the adverse effects of cannabinoids when given with emetogenic chemotherapy. Thirty randomized control trials (nearly 1400 patients), comparing cannabinoids with placebo or conventional anti-emetics in this setting, were analyzed. Cannabinoids were found to be more effective anti-emetics in the first 24 hours of chemotherapy, than conventional anti-emetics e.g. prochlorperazine and metaclompramide (relative risk 1.38, NNT 6-8). Cannabinoids were associated with more 'potentially beneficial side effects', e.g. sensation of a "high" (relative risk 10.6, NNT 3). But also with more harmful side effects, e.g. dysphoria or depression (relative risk 8.06, NNT 8).

It is concluded that cannabinoids, acting as 'mood enhancing adjuvants', may be used to control emetogenic chemotherapy in selected patients. However, their widespread use will be limited due to their harmful side effects.

EDITORIAL – Cannabinoids for pain and nausea. Eija Kaslo, Eija Pain Clinic, Department of Anaesthesia and Intensive Care Medicine, Helsinki University Hospital, Finland.
BMJ, **323**(7303): 2-3, 7 July 2001.

New discoveries and questions on liberalising cannabinoids have fuelled the scientific community and society at large into an aggressive debate concerning the therapeutic use of cannabinoids. When considering new therapeutic indications, two factors need to be accounted for: adverse effects and effectiveness compared with existing alternatives. Two systemic reviews have added to this debate.

- Campbell *et al.* investigated nine randomised controlled trials (222 patients) and found that cannabinoids were no more effective than codeine in controlling pain and had side effects of depressing the central nervous system. Furthermore NSAIDs alone and in combination with opioids have been used successfully for cancer and post-operative pain.
- Tramer *et al.* investigated 30 randomised controlled trials (1366 patients) and found that cannabinoids were only effective in medium, but not high emetogenic setting, where serotonin receptor antagonists have shown the highest therapeutic index.

The author explains that the 'currently available cannabinoids clearly lose the battle in both efficacy and safety with competitors of today'. The only suggested use for cannabinoids is in clinical trials in conditions for which there is no effective treatment.

Are cannabinoids an effective and safe treatment option in the management of pain? A qualitative systematic review. Campbell, F.A., Tramer, M.R. and Carroll, C. *et al.* Pain Management Centre, Undercroft, South Block, Queen's Medical Centre, Nottingham, UK. ***BMJ,* 323**(7324): 13, 7 July 2001.

This paper is a systematic review of randomized controlled trials (RCTs) on the pain-relieving effects of cannabinoids. It aimed to establish if cannabinoids are both an effective and a safe treatment option in the management of pain. Nine trials met the inclusion criteria (222 patients). All evaluated cannabinoids rather than cannabis itself.

Cannabinoids were good at relieving post-operative pain and spasticity - having the same affect as 60 mg of codeine.

The side effects - which included mental clouding, ataxia and impaired memory - limited the dose that could be given

In acute pain, cannabinoids were no more effective than codeine.

The authors conclude that the widespread introduction of cannabinoids into clinical practice for pain management is undesirable - there is not significant efficacy compared to current pain-relieving medication and there are many side effects. Before cannabinoids can be considered for treating spasticity and neuropathic pain, further valid randomized controlled studies are needed. New and safe agonists at the cannabis receptor may be the way forward.

CERVICAL CANCER

- The debate about the usefulness of HPV testing with cervical smears continues
- HPV infection precedes cervical neoplasia and persistent infection predicts future high grade lesions.
- A discussion paper comments that limiting cervical screening to women aged 25–50 years would improve the efficacy of the screening programme by freeing resources to improve the quality of the programme.
- This prospective cohort study shows that exposure to a multifaceted prevention programme to general practices will improve implementation of the guidelines for cervical cancer screening.

BACKGROUND

Screening for cervical cancer began in 1964. In 1988 a call-recall system was introduced and coverage reached over 80% in 1993. Most deaths from cervical cancer occur in women who have never had a smear or who have had inadequate follow up of abnormal smears.

Several studies have found HPV 16 to be the main micro-organism linked to the development of cervical intraepithelial neoplasia (CIN). A study performed in The Netherlands found that CIN 2 was present in almost 90% of women who had HPV 16, 31 and 33 (*BMJ*, Jan. 1995). A Finnish study (*BMJ*, March 1996) followed a cohort of 18 000 women. Just over 70 went on to develop cervical cancer. The presence of HPV 16 at initial blood sampling was significantly associated with the development of cervical cancer. The mean time from blood test to diagnosis was 10 years.

A higher level of human papillomavirus 16 DNA was associated with an increased risk for cervical carcinoma in situ. Commentator, J. Melnikow, University of California, Davis Sacramento, CA, USA.
Evidence-Based Medicine, **6**(1): 29, Jan./Feb. 2001

Question: In women with a first normal cervical smear during screening, what is the association between human papillomavirus (HPV) DNA levels and development of cervical carcinoma in situ (CIS).

The following article is briefly presented
Viral load of human papillomavirus 16 as a determinant for development of cervical carcinoma in situ: a nested case–control study. Josefsson, A.M., Magnusson, P.K. and Ylitalo, N. *et al.*
Lancet, **355**: 2189–2193, 24 June 2000.
and

Persistently high loads of human papillomavirus 16 over time were associated with an increased risk for cervical cancer. Commentator, Melnikow J. Commentator, Nuovo J. University of California, Davis Sacramento, California, USA.
Evidence–based Medicine, **6:** 1, 30, Jan./Feb. 2001.

Question: In women with a first normal cervical smear, what is the temporal relation between human papillomavirus (HPV-16) infection and cervical carcinonma in situ (CIS)?

The following article is briefly presented
Consistent high viral load of human papillomavirus 16 and risk of cervical carcinoma in situ: a nested case–control study. Ylitalo, N., Søresensen, P. and Josefsson, A.M. *et al.*
Lancet, **355:** 2194–2198, 24 June 2000.

The Swedish case-control study involved nearly 500 women with CIS (whose first cervical smear was normal) and 5 controls for each case. They used DNA testing to analyse previous smears. The study was designed to answer the two questions given above.
• Just over 40% of women with CIS were HPV 16 positive.
• The higher the viral load the higher the risk of CIS.
• The average time from normal smear to developing CIS was around 20 years.

Commentary
The commentators point out that, more than half of the women with CIS were negative for HPV16. This would make it difficult to adequately use HPV as a triage tool to determine which women could be screened at less frequent intervals. HPV testing is unlikely to alter the fact that, most women who develop cervical cancer have never had a smear or have had inadequate follow up for an abnormal smear.

SCREENING

Adherence to guidelines on cervical cancer screening in general practice: programme elements of successful implementation. Hermens, R.P.M.G., Hak, E. and Marlies, E.J.L. *et al.* Centre for Quality of Care Research (WOK) University Medical Centre, Nijmegen, The Netherlands.
***Br. J. Gen. Pract.,* 51:** 897-903, November 2002.

This study evaluates which aspects of a nationwide multifaceted prevention programme are useful in the implementation of cervical screening guidelines in general practice. A third of all practices in the Netherlands (1586 out of 4758) were randomly selected to take part in this prospective cohort study, which was conducted over a 2 and a half year period. Questionnaires where used to measure baseline levels of adherence to cervical cancer screening guidelines and levels after exposure to the multifaceted prevention programme.

- After exposure to the prevention programme, all practices improved ($P < 0.001$) in their use of the guidelines for effective cervical screening in practice.
- The most important elements of the programme were: facilitating software modules (computer software used to aid patient selection and monitoring of attendance and follow up); two or more 'practice visits' by outreach visitors (which consisted of educational sessions for practice assistants).
- Practice characteristics were not a major indicator of successful implementation of the programme.

The authors conclude that successful adherence of national guidelines for cervical screening in general practice is associated a multifaceted prevention programme, whose important elements include, software modules, outreach visits and educational sessions.

Type specific persistence of high risk human papillomavirus (HPV) as indicator of high grade cervical squamous intraepithelial lesions in young women: population based prospective follow up study. Kjaer, S.K., van den Brule, A.J.C. and Paull, G. *et al.* Danish Cancer Society, Institute of Cancer Epidemiology, Copenhagen, Denmark. ***Drug and Therapeutics Bulletin,* 325**(7364): 572-578, 14 September 2002.

This study investigated the role of HPV in development of cervical neoplasia. Nearly 11 000 women with normal cervical cytology (from Copenhagen) were examined at enrolment and again 2 years later. The prevalence of HPV in cytologically normal women was 14%. HPV type 16 was most prevalent across the entire study population.

- HPV prevalence was significantly higher in those with high grade lesions.
- Women who were HPV positive at enrolment were more likely to have atypical cells, low-grade lesions or high-grade lesions (odds ratios 3.2, 7.5 and 25.8, respectively).
- HPV positive women at follow up were much more likely to have low and high grade lesions (odds ratios 34.3, and 60.7, respectively).
- The risk of having a high grade lesion was greatly increased if the woman was positive for the same type of HPV (compared with a women who were negative at both examinations). This was particularly so in the 25–29 year age group (OR 813.0).

They conclude that HPV infection is common in young women and can precede cervical neoplasia. It is an accurate predictor of future high grade lesions, especially where there is persistent infection with the same HPV type.

DISCUSSION – How can we develop a cost-effective quality cervical screening programme? Wilson, S. and Lester, H. Department of primary care and general practice, Division of Primary Care, Public and Occupational Health, University of Birmingham, Birmingham, UK. *Br. J. Gen. Pract.*, **52**(472): 485-490, June 2002.

The cervical cancer screening programme costs around £130 million per annum, and has been shown to reduce deaths from cervical cancer. However, a significant proportion of invasive lesions are still undetected, and well publicised incidences of false negative tests occur. This paper discusses ways of altering the screening programme to increase its effectiveness. The authors suggest that the current policy of screening all women aged 20–64 every 3 years should be altered to a programme where women aged 25–50 are screened every 5 years. These proposals are justified as follows:

- Women under 25 are extremely unlikely to have invasive cancer, and the pre-clinical lesions which are present can not be detected by smear tests.
- The incidence of invasive lesions in post-menopausal women is also very low, an abnormal smear having a positive predictive value of under 3%.
- A smear should be taken every 5 years as there is little difference in prevention of invasive disease compared with screening every 3 years.

The benefits of such an approach may be:

- Freeing resources to improve the quality of the programme; e.g a lower workload may increase the accuracy of cytologists readings of smears.

EDITORIAL – HPV testing for clarifying borderline cervical smear results. Michele Manos, M. Division of Research, The Permanente Medical Group, Oakland GA, USA. *BMJ,* **322**(7291): 878-879, 14 April 2001.

and

Human papillomavirus testing and management of women with mildly abnormal cervical smears: an observational study. Rebello, G., Hallam, N., Smart, G. and Farquharson, D. *et al.* Colposcopy Clinic, Royal Infirmary of Edinburgh, Lothian University Hospitals NHS trust, Edinburgh, UK. *BMJ,* **322**(7291): 893-894, 14 April 2001.

Two large American studies have suggested that HPV testing is useful for identifying women with abnormal smears who may have high grade cervical intraepithelial neoplasia. Indeed many organizations now routinely use HPV testing alongside routine cervical smears.

The UK study by Rebello advises a certain amount of caution. The study involved around 330 women with persistently abnormal smears. The results report lower levels of sensitivity, specificity and predictive values compared with the American studies.

The editorial goes on to discuss possible reasons for the conflicting results.

CHILDREN

- Childhood headache is related to 'psychosocial adversity and learned illness behaviour from parents'. In later life it is strongly associated with increased risk of adult headache, multiple physical symptoms and psychiatric morbidity
- A Chinese RCT showed that, babies with diarrhoea who were given small frequent feeds recovered faster than those receiving larger less frequent feeds
- Racecadotril is superior to oral rehydration solution alone for the treatment of watery diarrhoea in children
- Slow intrauterine growth increases vulnerability of men to the effects of poor living conditions on coronary heart disease.
- The emergence of widespread drug resistance in human head lice means that experiments conducted to assess the effectiveness of head lice treatments, can no longer be considered useful.
- The Effective Health Care bulletin distributed in 1992 may have helped to reduce the number of grommet operations providing a saving of £27m.
- Confirmed permanent childhood hearing impairment in the United Kingdom among children aged 9–16 years is higher than previous estimates
- An 18 month longitudinal study found that childhood psychopathology is likely to be persistent.
- The use of babywalkers should be discouraged.
- The incidence of Kawasaki disease in Britain has doubled since 1991; better monitoring is needed to detect further changes in its incidence.
- "off label" prescribing in paediatrics is a problem that needs to be tackled.
- Unlicensed and "off label" prescriptions for children are too common in general practice.

DIARRHOEA

Racecadotril was effective for severe watery diarrhoea in children. Commentator, Manjula Datta, Tamil Nadu Dr MGR Medical University, Chennai, Tamil Nadu, India. *Evidence–based Medicine,* **6**(3): 87, May/June 2001.

Question: In children with severe watery diarrhoea, is racecadotril (acetorphan, an enkephalinase inhibitor), as an adjunct to oral rehydration therapy, more effective than oral rehydration alone?

The following article is briefly presented
Racecadotril in the treatment of acute watery diarrhoea in children. Salazar–Lindo, E. and Santisteben–Ponce, J. *et al.*
N. Eng. J. Med., **343:** 463–467, 17 Aug. 2000.

This was a RCT involving 135 boys aged 3–35 months with at least a 5 day history of watery diarrhoea. Boys received either placebo or racecadotril. All received oral rehydration fluids.

- At 5 days, the racecadotril group were more likely to be cured than the placebo group, with decreased stool production and reduced intake of oral rehydration solution.

Commentary

This was a well planned study. Racecadotril acts by inhibiting the inactivation of endogenous encaphalins and reduces water secretion into the gut. It controls symptoms within 1–2 days. It is superior to oral rehydration solution alone.

OTHERS

Impact of effective health care bulletin on treatment of persistent glue ear in children: time series analysis. Mason, J., Freemantle, N. and Browning, G. Centre for Services Research, University of Newcastle upon Tyne, Newcastle upon Tyne, UK.
***BMJ,* 323**(7321): 1096-1097, 10 November 2001.

In 1992 an Effective Health Care bulletin advising on the treatment of persistent glue ear was distributed nationally in the NHS. The aim of this retrospective study was to investigate surgery rates before and after distribution of the bulletin. The number of "grommet" procedures performed in children under 15 was obtained from 1989 to 1996 from 14 regions.
- The small increase in the number of procedures in the 3 years before the bulletin, became a decrease in the 4 years after publication.
- The changing trend in surgery provided a theoretical saving of £27m at 1992–1993 prices.

The author concludes that distributing 'printed recommendations to decision makers may influence surgery rates', as the number of operations reduced after publishing this bulletin.

EDITORIAL – Treatment of head lice: Choice of treatment will depend on local patterns of resistance. Dodd, C. School of Biosciences, Cardiff University, Cardiff, UK.
***Br. J. Gen. Pract.,* 323**(7321): 1084, 10 November 2001.

The author highlights a number of points
- Resistance to synthetic pyrethroids has been reported in France, the Czech Republic, Israel and England along with organophosphates. Resistance may vary geographically.
- Headlice are essentially harmless. They may remain on the scalp for up to 3 months before they are noticed, usually due to sensitization to louse saliva.
- Often the main problems related to lice infestation are psychological. Infestation is often seen as a sign on uncleanliness although this has never been proven.

EDITORIAL – Legacy of bacterial meningitis in infancy. Grimwood, K. Professor of Paediatrics Wellington School of Medicine and Health Sciences, New Zealand.
BMJ, 323(7312): 523-524, 8 September 2001.

The global burden of childhood bacterial meningitis is substantial, but there are few reports of the long-term complications of bacterial meningitis. Bedford *et al.* (in the same issue of the *BMJ*) report the results of a questionnaire survey of the parents and GPs of just over 1700 children aged 5 years, who had had meningitis during infancy, together with matched controls.

- Those who had had meningitis were at significantly greater risk of disability across all health, developmental, and behavioural categories tested, but especially in the domains of learning and neuromotor function. Simple educational interventions may help compensate for these deficits, improving academic performance, behaviour, and self esteem.
- Strategies required to reduce neonatal meningitis include improved antenatal care, aseptic techniques during labour and delivery, and promotion of breast feeding and domestic hygiene.
- This study provides future opportunities for comprehensive neuropsychometric assessments during school years and into adolescence and adulthood, which should help in understanding critical phases of postnatal brain development.

Measuring the prevalence of permanent childhood hearing impairment. Russ, S. Assistant Professor of Pediatrics Department of Primary Care Pediatrics, Cedars-Sinai Medical Center, Los Angeles, USA.
BMJ, 323(7312): 525-526, 8 September 2001.

A neonatal hearing programme was introduced in June 200. There is currently only one existing controlled trial of this approach. A UK study has recently been completed, whose aim was to determine the prevalence of permanent childhood hearing impairment in all children born in 1980-1995

The study has two important findings with implications for service providers.

- The observed prevalence of confirmed permanent childhood hearing impairment increased with age.
- The prevalence of confirmed permanent childhood hearing impairment in the United Kingdom among children aged 9-16 years is higher than previous estimates, being at least 1.65/1000 for impairments >40 dB in the better ear and possibly as high as 2/1000.

Bug busting (wet combing) was less effective than malathion lotion for eliminating head lice in children. Commentator, William Feldman, University of Toronto, Toronto, Ontario, Canada.
Evidence–based Medicine, 6(3): 93, May/June 2001.

Question: Is bug busting (wet combing with a fine toothed comb) as effective as malathion lotion for removing head lice in children?

The following article is briefly presented
Comparison of wet combing with malathion for treatment of head lice in the UK: a pragmatic randomised controlled trial. Roberts, R.J. and Casey, D. *et al.*
Lancet, **356:** 540–544, 12 Aug. 2000.

This study involved 81 children from primary schools in Wales and the UK. Around half were assigned to bug busting and the other half to malathion lotion.
  • Seven days post treatment, significantly more of the bug busting children had live head lice compared with the malathion group.

Commentator
Malathion was twice as effective as bug busting. The authors of the article suggest that malathion should be used in favour of bug busting. Feldman points out that as 40% of children were cured with bug busting, a more reasonable approach would be to use bug busting first and malathion second, if bug busting failed. This would be cheaper and reduces the rate of development of resistance to malathion.

Relation between headache in childhood and physical psychiatric symptoms in adulthood: national birth cohort study. Fearon, P. and Hotopf, M. Institute of Psychiatry and Guy's, King's and St.Thomas's School of Medicine, London, UK.
BMJ, **322**(7295): 1145-1148, 12 May 2001.

The data from this study comes from the perinatal mortality survey. Data was collected from over 17 000 births in 1958. Follow-ups occurred at regular intervals. In 1991 when the subjects were aged 33, data was collected from nearly 10 000 of the cohort. The aim of this study was to assess the relationship between childhood headaches and later morbidity.
  • Headache in childhood was strongly associated with increased risk of adult headache, multiple physical symptoms and psychiatric morbidity.
  • Headache was associated with manual social class, and separation from mother for periods of time greater than 1 week.
  • Headache was also associated with chronic physical illness in the mother, or mental illness in a family member.
The authors suggest that childhood headache is related to 'psychosocial adversity and learned illness behaviour from parents'. Headache is one of the commonest childhood complaints. Intervention at an early stage may reduce later morbidity.

Mental health problems of children In the community: 18 month follow up.
Goodman, R., Ford, T. and Meltzer, H. Department of Child and Adolescent Psychiatry, Institute of Psychiatry, King's College London, London, UK.
BMJ, 324(7352): 1496-1497, 22 June 2002.

A previous study by Meltzer et al. found that 9% cohort of 10 500 British children aged 10-15 had a psychiatric disorder. This study examined the persistence of mental disorders in this cohort 18 months after diagnosis. A questionnaire was sent to parents of all children with mental disorders (936) and to 3029 parents of children without psychopathology (response rate 73%). They assessed scores both symptoms and the impact of those symptoms on the child. At 18 months they found that:

- There was no change in both scores for conduct disorders.
- Symptoms changed significantly for hyperkinetic disorders symptoms. There was no change in impact scores.
- For emotional disorders both symptom and impact scores fell significantly.

The authors used elevated symptom scores (>14) and impact scores (>2) to define whether a child was a psychiatric case or not, and concluded:

- At 18 months 3% of children with no initial psychopathology and 62% of children with initial disorders met the criteria of a psychiatric case.
- At 18 months 36% of emotional disorders and 73% of conduct or hyperkinetic disorders were still present.

Locomotor milestones and babywalkers: cross sectional study. Garrett, M., McElroy, A. and Staines, A. University College Dublin School of Physiotherapy, Mater Hospital, Dublin 7, Ireland.
BMJ, 324(7352): 1494, 22 June 2002.

This cross-sectional survey of nearly 200 normal healthy infants attending day centres compared the age at which infants using babywalkers and those who did not reached locomotor developmental milestones. Previous investigations, although not exclusively, suggest that babywalker users achieve independent walking at a later age than non-users. Anonymous questionnaires determined the age of locomotor developmental milestones; raising the head when prone, rolling over, sitting with support and alone, crawling, standing with support and alone, walking with support and alone. Just over half of the infants used babywalkers - the median duration of use was 26 weeks.

- There was a strong association between babywalker use and the extent of developmental delay.
- Each aggregated 24 hours of babywalker use was associated with a delay of just over 3 days in walking, and nearly 4 days in standing alone.

Rising incidence of Kawasaki disease in England: analysis of hospital admission data. Harnden, M., Alves, B. and Sheikh, A. Department of Primary Health Care, Institute of Health Sciences, University of Oxford, Oxford, UK.
***BMJ,* 324**(7351): 1424-1425, 15 June 2002.

The leading cause of acquired heart disease in children in the developed world is Kawasaki disease, which is thought to be caused by an infectious agent. This study used hospital data to look at emergency inpatient admissions for children less than 17 years old, where the primary diagnosis was Kawasaki disease, in the period 1 April 1999-31 March 2000.
   • There was a significant increase in admissions due to Kawasaki disease with 143 in 1991-1992 rising to 308 in 1999-2000.
This may indicate an increased incidence, as is the case in Japan, (perhaps due to changes in the infectious agent or increased susceptibility to infection amongst the population) or to better recognition, particularly following a period of heightened awareness in 1991. The authors conclude that better monitoring of this disease is needed to identify further changes in its incidence, and to detect altered patterns of severity and complication rates in patients with this illness.

EDITORIAL - Off label prescribing in children. Banner, W. Medical Director The Children's Hospital At Saint Francis, Tulsa, Oklahoma 74136 USA.
***BMJ,* 324**(7349): 1290-1291, 1 June 2002.

During the drug licensing process the efficacy of a drug for treatment of a defined disease is assessed. Conventionally the drug is only studied in adult males. However, once licensed a drug may be utilised in populations, and diseases, not studied during licensing. The term "off label" describes prescribing medication to populations, or for diseases, not listed on the drug's packaging. Thus, many drugs routinely prescribed in paediatrics are "off label". The author describes American attempts to solve this problem:
   • In 1994 regulations were established permitting the Food and Drugs Administration (FDA) to approve drugs for paediatric use on the basis of literature demonstrating the product's efficacy.
   • The1997 FDA Modernization Act granted pharmaceutical companies 6-month extensions to drug patents in exchange for performing studies leading to approval of the drug for paediatric use.
   • In 1999 FDA rules were implemented allowing the FDA to mandate paediatric studies if a product is to be widely used in children.
Problems with these measures are:
   • Patent extension can be profitable, manufacturers will only seek paediatric labelling for profitable products.

Unlicensed and off label prescription of drugs to children: population based cohort study. Jong, G.T., Eland, I.A. and Sturkenboom, M.C.J.M. *et al.* Department of Paediatrics, Sophia Children's Hospital, Erasmus Medical Centre, Rotterdam, Netherlands.
***BMJ*, 324**(7349): 1313-1314, 1 June 2002.

Many drugs prescribed to children are either unlicensed for use in children, or are prescribed outside the terms of the product license ("off label"). This study examines the prevalence of such prescribing in general practice. Patient records from 150 general practices in the Netherlands were analysed. The following data were recorded from a 1-year period of children's records: number of GP consultations; number of prescriptions; and license status of prescriptions.

- 28.9% of all prescriptions were either unlicensed for children or off label.

The authors consider this situation to be "highly unsatisfactory", and suggest that effort to minimise unlicensed and off label prescribing are needed. The risk of adverse drug reactions to such prescriptions is high, due to inadequate information on appropriate dosing schemes.

Size at birth and resilience to effects of poor living conditions in adult life: longitudinal study. Barker, D.J.P., Forsen, T., Uutela, A., Osmond, C. and Eriksson, J.G. Environmental Epidemiology Unit, University of Southampton, Southampton General Hospital, Southampton, UK.
***BMJ*, 323**(7324): 1-5, 1 December 2001.

Males who experience a period of retarded growth *in utero* have an increased risk of developing coronary heart disease later in life. This study examines the interaction between retarded intrauterine growth and poor social circumstances as risk factors for coronary heart disease.

Information about nearly 3700 Finnish males was studied using data from various sources including child welfare clinic records, school health records, census statistics and hospital records. Subjects were classified according to various indices of socioeconomic status and to "ponderal index" (kg/m^3) at birth. Coronary heart disease hazard ratios were calculated for each group.

- Men who were thin at birth were at higher risk of coronary heart disease, and this risk was further increased by poor living standards in adult life.
- Men who were not thin at birth were less affected by poor living standards.

Effect of seeing tobacco use in films on trying smoking among adolescents: cross sectional study. Sargent, J.D., Beach, M.L. and Dalton, M. *et al*, Department of Pediatrics, Dartmouth Medical School, USA.
***BMJ,* 323**(7326): 1394-1397, 15 December 2001.

This was a study to assess the relationship between seeing smoking in films and smoking amongst 9-15 year olds. Letters were sent to 30 randomly selected schools (~ 4900 children).
- Exposure to smoking in films was significantly related to presence of smoking especially in adolescents.
- The higher the rating for tobacco use in the film, the higher the likelihood of smoking amongst the children.
- These associations remained even after confounding factors such as sociodemographic variables were taken into account.

EDITORIAL – Fabricated or induced illness in children. Wilson, R., Kingston NHS Trust, Kingston, UK.
***BMJ,* 323**(7308): 296-297, 11 August 2001.

This editorial highlights the name change from 'Munchausen by proxy' to "fabricated or induced illness in children by carers". Parents have the ability to do great harm to their children. Health professionals may also have a part to play by over-investigation and treatment. The Department of Health have issued guidance on how to deal with fabricated or induced illness in children. Some measures include long term therapy and support for the child as well as therapy aimed at helping the parent. This may warrant separation of child and carer. Health professionals should not shy away from early referrals to social services on the grounds of need. He concludes by saying "We need to have open minds and develop our skills to understand the complex origin of children's symptoms and illnesses and protect those at risk of being harmed".

FURTHER READING

Prevalence of breastfeeding at four months in general practices in south London. Sikorski, J., Boyd, F., Dezateaux Wade, A. *et al.,* Department of General Practice and Primary Care, Guy's, King's and St. Thomas's School of Medicine London.
***Br. J. Gen. Pract.,* 51**(467): 445-450, June 2001.

See 'Diabetes mellitus' for

EDITORIAL - Type 2 diabetes in children. Division of Diabetes Translation, National Center for Chronic Diseasae Prevention and Health Promotion, Centers for Disease Control and Prevention, Atlanta, GA, USA.
***BMJ,* 322**(7283): 377-378, 1 Feb. 2001.

See 'Respiratory infections' for

The natural history of acute cough in children aged 0-4 years in primary care: a systematic review. Division of Primary Health Care, University of Bristol, Cotham Hill, Bristol, UK.
Br. J. Gen. Pract., **52**(478): 401-409, May 2002.

CHLAMYDIA

- Opportunistic testing from a practice in Yorkshire found a chlamydia prevalence of nearly 11%
- A prospective cohort study conducted in the Netherlands found no reinfection 1 year after screening and treatment for asymptomatic cases of *Chlamydia trachomatis*
- A cross sectional study found that self administered vaginal swabs and first-pass urine analysis with the ligase chain reaction is a viable method of screening pregnant women in the community for *C. trachomatis* infection

BACKGROUND

Between 1998 and 1999, several studies evaluated the usefulness of home urine testing. Danish studies found that more people responded to home sampling than conventional testing. In 1999 the Expert Advisory Group (EAG) to the Chief Medical Officer concluded that home sampling was a feasible method of screening.

Detection of *Chlamydia trachomatis* infection in early pregnancy using self administered vaginal swabs and first pass urines: A cross sectional community based survey. Oakeshott, P., Hay, P. and Hay, S. *et al.* Department of General Practice and Primary Care, St Georges Medical School, London, UK.
***Br. J. Gen. Pract.*, 483**(52): 830-833, 1 October 2002.

This cross sectional study aimed to assess the prevalence of *C. trachomatis* infection in pregnant women in the community, and to evaluate self-administered vaginal swabs and first pass urines analyzed by ligase chain reaction for the detection of *C. trachomatis*. Almost 1000 pregnant women, at under 10 weeks gestation, were recruited from 32 General Practices and five family planning clinics in South London. The subjects were asked to take the appropriate samples, and complete a questionnaire at 16 weeks gestation. The samples were then analyzed for *C. trachomatis* by ligase chain reaction. The authors found:

- Overall prevalence of *C. trachomatis* in newly pregnant women was 2.4%, with a prevalence of 2% in General Practices and 6.7% in family planning clinics.
- Infection rate was higher in younger patients; 8.6% in women under 25 and 14% in teenagers.
- Being younger than age 25 and being of black ethnicity were both independently associated with *C. trachomatis* infection.

• The use of urine analysis was more popular than use of vaginal swabs.

The authors conclude that the use of self administered vaginal swabs and urine testing is a feasible method of screening for *C. trachomatis* infection in pregnant women in the community.

Partner notification among asymptomatic Chlamydia trachomatis cases, by means of mailed specimens. van Valkengoed, I.G.M., Morre, S.A, van den Brule, A.J.C. and Meijer, C.J.L.M. Institute for Research in Extramural Medicine, Vrije Universiteit, Amsterdam, The Netherlands. *Br. J. Gen. Pract.,* **52**(481): 652-654, 1 August 2002.

Partner notification is an important aspect of the control of *Chlamydia trachomatis* infection. This study examined a simple mailing strategy, in which partners of infected patients were mailed a package containing an information leaflet, a coded sterile urine sample container, and a pre-stamped addressed envelope. Upon receipt of urine samples, a simple diagnostic test for Chlamydia infection was performed.

Ninety three index cases from one general practice participated.
• For 62% of index cases, one or more partner participated.
• Amongst participating partners, the infection rate was 48%.

The authors concluded that the mailing strategy was an effective method for partner notification. They suggested that the high prevalence of infections in partners of index cases highlights the need for the screening of sexual partners.

Follow-up, treatment, and reinfection rates among asymptomatic Chlamydia trachomatis cases in general practice. van Valkengoed, I.G.M., Morre, S.A. and van der Brule, A.J.C. *et al.* Institute for Research in Extramural Medicine, Vrije Universiteit, Amsterdam, The Netherlands. *Br. J. Gen. Pract.,* **52**(481): 623-627, 1 August 2002.

This study aimed to evaluate the success of a screening programme for *Chlamydia trachomatis* by investigating the rates of diagnostic confirmation, successful treatment and reinfection of *C. trachomatis* infection 1 year after being detected in the screening programme. This was a prospective cohort study consisting of 15 general practices in the Netherlands. Between January 1997 and December 1998, 124 men and women aged between 15 and 40 years were screened and tested positive for an asymptomatic *C. trachomatis* infection. They were asked to provide a urethral swab and urine specimen to allow diagnostic confirmation. One year after the initial screening, all the patients were invited for a second screening.
• Out of the 110 patients who attended diagnostic confirmation, 84 percent were confirmed positive and received treatment.
• At the second screening 56 patients who received treatment attended, and none of them were found to be reinfected.

Due to the zero reinfection rate after diagnostic confirmation and treatment as shown in the study, the author comments that this 'underlines the effectiveness of the screening and treatment strategy'.

Chlamydia trachomatis: **opportunistic screening in primary care.** Tobin, C., Aggarwal, R. and Clarke, J. *et al.* Consultant in Genitourinary Medicine, Wakefield. *Br. J. Gen. Pract.,* **51**(468): 565-566, July 2001

This study was conducted in a surgery situated in an ex-mining village in Yorkshire. The aim of the study was to assess the prevalence of chlamydia infection using opportunistic screening using urine tests. All sexually active women between age 13 and 24 years were invited to participate. Sixty percent of those targeted chose not to submit a sample.

- In those who submitted a sample the prevalence of chlamydia was nearly 11%.

Qualitative analysis of psychosocial impact of diagnosis of *Chlamydia trachomatis:* **implications for screening.** Duncan, B., Hart, G., Scoular, A. and Bigrigg, A. *et al.* MRC Social and Public Health Sciences Unit, University of Glasgow, Glasgow, UK. *BMJ,* **322**(7280): 195-199, 27 January 2001.

This study is in response to the Chief Medical Officer's EAG's proposed pilot studies which involve screening for chlamydia. It is a qualitative study, conducted in Glasgow, whose aim as to assess women's reactions to and the implications of a diagnosis of chlamydia. Seventeen women with a diagnosis of chlamydia identified at family planning clinics and genito-urinary medicine clinics were interviewed. Three main themes emerging from the interviews were:

- stigma associated with the disease;
- worry and uncertainty about future fertility;
- anxiety about telling partners.

The themes were related to stereotypical views about who is most at risk from chlamydia. The women tended to believe that certain 'types' of women catch chlamydia, and they themselves were invulnerable. Hence, a diagnosis of chlamydia was associated with degrees of self-disgust and a reluctance to tell people who under normal circumstances would act as support givers.

The authors point out that a national programme of screening will need to destigmatize chlamydia and provide advice and support for those who take part in the programme.

CHRONIC DISEASE

- The goal in chronic disease management is not cure but "maintenance of pleasurable and independent living"
- Effective care in chronic illness is reliant on a co-ordinated and multidisciplinary approach.
- For any chronic disease management strategy the patient should always be the focus of care.
- Standardized assessments tools and databases offer a means of building the necessary evidence to inform decisions concerning interventions in the elderly
- Integrated care and integrated care pathways are key factors in the NHS modernization agenda.
- Clinicians and their patients require effective teaching on chronic disease management
- System changes can improve care of chronic illnesses
- Poor patient-clinician partnerships may prevent optimal health care for minority groups
- A discussion paper explores self management of oral anticoagulation as an alternative to the traditional model of clinic-based INR testing
- A meeting of health care leaders at the WHO headquarters in May 2001 concluded that, no nation will escape the impact of chronic disease unless it acts to reform services.
- In Singapore, the increasing prevalence of chronic disease has led health care providers to seek new, more effective means of delivering services for those suffering chronic ill health.
- The disease management model for chronic diseases is a viable alternative to the current shared care model, as demonstrated in diabetes care in the Netherlands.

EDITORIAL – Meeting the needs of chronically ill people. Wagner, E.H. MacColl Institute for Healthcare Innovation, Center for Health Studies, Group Health Cooperative of Puget Sound, Seattle, USA.
BMJ, 323(7319): 945-946, 27 October 2001.

Providing optimal care for patients with chronic illnesses is an increasingly difficult task. Evidence-based treatment strategies continue to become more complex, while the need for supportive self-management and monitoring of chronic conditions is an ongoing demand.

A number of points are raised.

- Patients with disabilities, other concurrent illnesses, and patients of ethnic minorities are all less likely to receive optimal care for chronic illnesses.
- Specialist education improves evidence-based healthcare. Specialist doctors are more likely to adhere to practice guidelines for conditions associated with their specialty.
- It has been suggested that for healthcare to be optimised, systems must be changed.

- Recently, a group of Danish general practices have achieved an improvement in control of diabetic patients through introducing a system involving education and prompts for the doctors, and routine appointments for the patients.
- Similar system changes can be employed to improve the care of other chronic illnesses.

EDITORIAL – Disparities in outcomes from chronic disease. Krishnan, J.A., Diette, G.B. and Rand, C.S. Division of Pulmonary and Critical Care Medicine, Department of Medicine, John Hopkins University School of Medicine, Baltimore, USA.
BMJ, 323(7319): 950, 27 October 2001.

Minority groups, such as those with low socio-economic status, and ethnic minorities, experience increased morbidity and earlier death. This editorial suggests that barriers between the patient and clinician prevent these minority groups from receiving optimal health care. A number of factors are proposed to cause such barriers, including:
- Patient-related factors, such as low expectancy for treatments to work, lack of knowledge about treatments, and a perception of inability to carry out prescribed therapy (self efficacy).
- Clinician-related factors, such as the perception of an inability to teach minority patients about management of their conditions, and poor availability during urgent consultations.

EDUCATION AND DEBATE SECTION – Recommendations for patients undertaking self management of oral anticoagulation. Fitzmaurice, D.A. and Machin, S.J. on behalf of the British Society of Haematology Task Force for Haemostasis and Thrombosis. Department of Primary Care and General Practice, Medical School, University of Birmingham, Birmingham, UK.
BMJ, 323(7319): 985-911, 27 October 2001.

Self-management of oral anticoagulation involves patients measuring their international normalised ratios (INRs) at home, and adjusting their medication appropriately. This article explores self-management as an alternative to the traditional model of clinic-based INR testing. The following points are made:
- The United Kingdom Medical Devices Agency Coagulation Centre has evaluated three portable prothrombin time coagulometers. All gave accurate, reliable INR readings.
- Evidence suggests that 6 hours of training is sufficient for most patients to become competent in self-management. However, such formal training programmes are not widely available in Britain at present.
- Studies carried out in Germany and America have shown improved control of INR with self management over physician-based models. However, physician-led management in the United Kingdom achieves greater control than these countries, and it is unknown whether self-management might allow any further improvement.

- If self-management is proven to be therapeutically effective, further studies will be needed to determine the cost effectiveness, optimum frequency of testing, requirements for patient training, and appropriate criteria for patient selection.

The authors make a number of recommendations for clinicians including advice regarding patient selection and the monitoring of self-management plans.

EDITORIAL – the challenge of chronic conditions: WHO responds. Epping-Jordan, J., Bengoa, R. and Kawar, R. *et al.* Department of Management of Noncommunicable Diseases, World Health Organisation, Geneva, Switzerland.
BMJ, **323**(7319): 947-948, 27 October 2001.

Chronic disease is expected to be the major cause of death by 2020, and will account for two thirds of the global cost of healthcare. These diseases included diabetes, chest and heart disease, mental health disorders and HIV and AIDS. This article proposed changes that may be implemented by individuals and teams involved in providing healthcare.

Healthcare workers:

- Patient education to promote better self-management and better adherence to treatment. Reports suggest that in the developed world, 50% of patients with chronic conditions do not take their medicines. This figure is thought to higher in developing countries.
- It has been suggested that increasing adherence will have a greater impact than improved biomedical treatment.

Policymakers:

- Move away from treatment systems that focus on episodic care of acute illness.
- Redesign healthcare provision to better use of resources to meet peoples long-term needs.

Conclusions: A meeting of healthcare leaders at the WHO headquarters in May 2001 made the following conclusions. No nation will escape the impact of chronic disease unless it acts to reform services. The prevalence of all chronic disease is increasing and will require a coordinated system to cope. The burden of these conditions falls most heavily on the poor. Unidimensional solutions will not address this complex problem and any future solutions must not be delayed.

EDUCATION AND DEBATE SECTION – Chronic disease management: a Singapore perspective. Cheah, J. Department of Community, Occupational and Family Medicine, National University of Singapore, Singapore.
BMJ, **323**(7319): 990-993, 27 October 2001.

The increasing prevalence of chronic disease in Asian populations has led health care providers in these states to seek new, more effective means of delivering services for those suffering chronic ill health. This paper outlines the chronic disease management approaches in Singapore.

- Care is delivered through a multidisciplinary team of physicians, nurses, physiotherapists etc.
- For each condition, details of the core components of the management plan (e.g. patient education) and evidence based treatment protocols are disseminated by the Ministry of Health to facilitate optimal care nationwide.
- There is constant evaluation of clinical and financial outcomes to ensure that the disease management programmes are appropriately designed.

Benefits of these programmes
- Clinicians from multiple institutions meet to develop the management plans therefore the multidisciplinary care team gains understanding of the process of care as a whole.
- Increased sharing of patient information.
- Reduced costs - investigations are not duplicated, treatment protocols ensure the most cost effective therapeutics are utilized.

EDUCATION AND DEBATE SECTION – Adoption of disease management model for diabetes in region of Maastricht. Vrijhoef, H.J.M., Spreeuwenberg, C. and Eijkelberg, I.M.J.G. *et al.* Department of Health Care Studies, Faculty of Health Sciences, University of Maastricht, Maastricht, Netherlands.
BMJ, 323(7319): 983-985, 27 October 2001.

Chronic diseases and associated conditions pose many challenges to current health systems. Despite their benefits, new health care models are not adopted soon enough. Since 1997, the disease management model gradually superseded the integrated and shared care models for type 2 diabetes mellitus care in a region of Maastricht. This successful experience demonstrated that:
- Diabetes care evolved from shared care, which was shown to be more viable than traditional practices, from a management perspective. Consequently, shared care met the conditions for the development of disease management model.
- Redefining the roles of diabetes caregivers to suit the new model and prioritising patients according to disease intensity have produced desirable results.
- Nurse specialists assumed a greater role in diabetes care. Patients were segregated according to care intensity and preference. These changes allowed doctors to focus on complicated conditions.
- The lack of evidence is a barrier to the widespread use of disease management models, especially evidence concerning impact on daily practice and cost.
- Evidence from health technology assessments alone may not be sufficient to promote the expansion of the disease management models.

The role of patient care teams in chronic disease management. Wagner, E.H. and MacColl, W.A. Institute for Healthcare Innovation, Center for Health Studies, Group Health Cooperative of Puget Sound, 1730, Minor Avenue, Seattle, USA.
***BMJ,* 320**(7234): 569-572, 1 February 2000.

This article examines teamwork in the context of chronic disease. Evidence is from the USA health care systems. Effective care in chronic illness is reliant on a co-ordinated and multidisciplinary approach. A patient care team consists of a diverse group of clinicians who participate in and are in regular communication about the care of a defined group. A successful team may involve professionals from one practice, more than one practice or across practices and organization boundaries. The trained staff which may include nurse care managers, medical specialists, clinical pharmacists, social workers and lay or community health workers, complement the doctor in the provision of holistic care. Patient care teams are associated with better outcomes and improve professional adherence to guidelines, patient satisfaction, clinical and health status, and the use of the health services.

Management of chronic disease by practitioners and patients; are we teaching the wrong things. Clark, N.M. and Gong, M. University of Michigan School of Public Health, Michigan, USA.
***BMJ,* 320**(7234): 572-575, 26 February 2000.

In this article the authors examine the standard of education available to patients and practitioners who manage chronic disease. Using asthma as an example, the authors attempt to demonstrate that patients and their clinicians are not being adequately prepared for optimum chronic disease management. The aim of asthma treatment as with any chronic disease is to control symptoms, bring about full physical and psychosocial functioning, ameliorate effects on social relationships and improve quality of life. To achieve this, there are some fundamental management techniques that are required. In addition to these common fundamental management techniques, individuals have their own personal style of coping with their disease management tasks. These tasks are time related and dependant on the particular disease features, personal characteristics and lifestyle choices. Managing a chronic disease like asthma is a continuously changing process and so the patient needs to make constant adjustments. This needs some degree of autonomy by the patient in his/her decision making, as well as, obtaining guidance from the doctor's guidelines. The clinician and patient need to work in partnership to achieve their common goal of disease management. The patient's behaviour and practitioner's performance thus plays a role in chronic disease management. To achieve effective disease control and prepare patients for the part they must play, the authors argue in favour of adopting and modifying current beneficial educational programmes. They view management as a process rooted in the patient's ability to self

regulate (autoregulation). Effective learning is reinforced through this process of self-regulation. **"Self regulation is defined as the means by which patients determine what they will do, given their own specific goals, social context and their own perceptions of their own ability."**
Education programmes:

- should be underpinned by an empirical understanding of human behaviour, motivating factors and an acknowledgement of the principles of learning;
- must incorporate things that enable the patient to manage his/her disease;
- should be capacity building and encourage self-regulation;
- should develop self efficacy and empower the patient.

Tensions exist between practitioner's objective measurements of success and the patient subjective focus. Management goals need to be patient centred. From the practitioners point of view the range of clinical education is somewhat limited. In asthma, there is a marked emphasis on drug regimes and monitoring devices but patchy evidence on the effect of education on patient's health or patient views about doctor's efficiency. Barriers to effective communication have been identified and an RCT has demonstrated the advantages of improving communication and patient education techniques in chronic disease. Adopting effective and proven communication principles will add benefit, improve patient health status, promote self-regulation and may reduce hospital admissions.

EDITORIAL – Patients as partners in managing chronic disease. Holman, H. and Loring, K. Stanford University School of Medicine, Palo Alto, USA.
***BMJ,* 320**(7234): 526, 26 February 2000.

This editorial describes three programmes which put the patient at the centre of chronic disease management programmes.

Self management education: Here the patient learns to manage their disease in the context of social, workplace and emotional variations.

Group visits: Here groups of patients visit their lead clinician and the agenda is largely set by the patient.

Remote medical management: Management is facilitated by use of telephone and email.

The goal in chronic disease management is not cure but "maintenance of pleasurable and independent living". This requires a greater understanding of the trends in illness patterns. Ultimately, these trends are best understood by the patient.

EDITORIAL – Advances in managing chronic disease. Davis, R.M., Wagner, E.G. and Groves, T.
***BMJ,* 320**(7234): 525, 26 February 2000.

As the health burden of chronic disease continues to rise chronic disease management is beginning to evolve as an important component of health care in its own right. Chronic illnesses can no longer be considered or managed in isolation, as similar strategies can be effective for treating differing conditions such as asthma, diabetes, arthritis. However, research, quality improvement and performance management are key areas for continued progress. High quality research into innovative methods for treatment of chronic illness will help to clarify the organizational changes required to achieve better outcomes at lower costs. These include:

- greater emphasis on supporting patient self management;
- optimizing drug treatment;
- more intensive and systematic follow up;
- clear delegation of tasks by primary care doctors.

To achieve success the patient must:

- be the focus of care;
- be well informed about the disease;
- be knowledgeable about where to access care;
- be involved as partners in their care;
- have a greater control over treatment.

There also needs to be a recognition of the emotional dimensions of the disease. In the treatment of chronic disease, performance indicators will help demonstrate the quality of care, stimulate improvement efforts and evaluate effectiveness. The debate continues over who should deliver care for the chronically ill and what kind of treatment should be on offer.

EDITORIAL – Building evidence on chronic disease in old age. Carpenter, G. I., Bernabei, R. and Hirdes, J. P. *et al*, Centre for Health Services Studies, University of Kent, Canterbury, UK. *BMJ,* **320**(7234): 528-529, 26 February 2000.

This editorial examines alternative methods of gathering evidence on which to base interventions in older people. Most older people have features which exclude them from participating in randomized controlled trials. Without the relevant data we stand to exclude frail elderly people from quality standards. Standardized assessments tools and databases offer a means of building the evidence base. These assessment measures might consist of diagnosis, physical, and psychosocial function of the older person. The use of databases and standardized assessment tools in not widespread in the UK. The US, Canada and Iceland have introduced the **minimum data set resident assessment instrument**- (a uniform comprehensive standardised assessment of long term routine care of older people) - and early reports found improvements in care. Standardized assessment scales using the same set of scales as the minimum data set resident assessment instrument have been developed for community care, mental health, acute and post acute care of older people. Systematic evaluations of these instruments are ongoing in many countries through the Inter RAI collaborative research network.

EDITORIAL – Disease management: has it a future? Hunter, D., Professor of Health Policy and Management, University of Durham, Durham, UK.
BMJ, 320(7234): 530, 26 February 2000.

The editor states that "disease management has a compelling logic but needs to be tested in practice". Disease management puts the patient as the focus around which health care is organised. The traditional divisions in health care e.g. between primary and secondary care are lost and instead the divisions are between diseases. Hence, an integrated organization conducts prevention, screening, diagnosis, treatment and follow up for a particular disease.Integrated care and integrated care pathways are key factors in the NHS modernization agenda. It combines patient education, practice guidelines, appropriate consultation, and supplies of drugs and services; which will hopefully lead to more effective use of resources. These systems will need evaluation to show cost savings and improved outcomes and performance.Some concerns are:

- the clinician may lose autonomy in their decision making;
- reduced patient/user involvement;
- reduced choice of treatment.

There are also concerns about the increasing use of the public-private partnerships. Some worry that these may not be sufficiently critical about care, but rather they may concentrate more on commercial issues.

CHRONIC FATIGUE SYNDROME

- A UK study found that patients diagnosed with chronic fatigue syndrome (CFS) consulted their GP nearly twice as often as controls in the 15 years prior to diagnosis of the condition
- A UK study found that counselling was as good as cognitive behavioural therapy for the treatment of CFS
- An educational programme to encourage graded exercise was better than standard care for the management of CFS
- A systematic review found that infectious mononucleosis can lead to a distinct fatigue syndrome, and that onset of this syndrome is predicted by low pre-morbid physical activity and poor physical functioning
- Six out of seven RCTs confirm the benefit of rehabilitation programmes for the management of CFS

BACKGROUND

Aetiology

The fact that CFS was previously known by so many other names (myalgic encephalitis, 'yuppie flu', post-viral fatigue syndrome) is evidence that the aetiology of CFS is poorly understood. The Royal Colleges of Physicians, Psychiatrists and General Practice published a report concerning CFS in 1996. CFS is the preferred term for the condition as the other terms are less accurate. It is thought that an acute viral illness can trigger the condition but this is not always the case. An Irish study (*BJGP*, Oct. 1997) found that it affected all social classes and hence the term 'yuppie flu' which indicates a preference for the higher social classes, is not an appropriate term. There is a higher prevalence in women than men. Studies suggest that the hypothalamic-pituitary-gonadal axis may be dysfunctional. High serotonin levels (which affect the sleep centres) have also been implicated (*BMJ*, July 1997).

Management

The report by the Royal Colleges suggests that a biopsychosocial approach to treatment should be used, recognizing the social, behavioural and emotional aspects of the illness. Treatments that have been studied in recent years include:

- cognitive behavioural therapy;
- exercise.

Numerous studies have shown that CBT is superior to standard care (*BMJ*, Jan. 1996, *EBM* July/Aug. 1997). An RCT performed at the National Sports Medicine Institute in London found that a graded exercise programme was better than relaxation and flexibility. They reported that their results were as good as those found with CBT, although the exercise study had excluded all those with psychiatric illness.

Children can be affected by CFS (editorial *BMJ*, June 1997). This has the potential to cause severe disruption to school life. Management in children should be a multidisciplinary effort, involving the family, school, GP, psychologist, psychiatrist and physiotherapist.

Recovery from infectious mononucleosis: a case for more than symptomatic therapy? Candy, B., Chalder, T. and Cleare, A.J. *et al.* Department of Psychological Medicine, Guys, Kings And St Thomas School of Medicine, London, UK.
Br. J. Gen. Pract., **483**(52): 844-850, 1 October 2002.

In a typical general practice of 10 000 patients, seven new cases of infectious mononucleosis (IM) will be seen every year. A proportion of these patients will progress to chronic IM, a syndrome consisting chiefly of fatigue persisting for longer than 3 months. This systematic review aimed to assess how frequently IM becomes chronic, what the risk factors for chronicity are and if any treatments can prevent chronicity. The authors found:

- At 6 months post-acute phase 1.5–56% of IM patients complained of fatigue compared with 15% of controls who suffered an upper respiratory tract infection (URTI).
- Hypersomnia was present in 22% of IM patients 6 months post acute phase, compared with 2% of patients with an URTI.
- IM is a risk factor both for a discrete acute fatigue syndrome and chronic fatigue syndrome.
- No single clinical/psychological factor was consistently associated with poor recovery, but poor pre-morbid physical functioning predicted long disease duration.
- No drug intervention (aciclovir or prednisolone) was shown to reduce recovery time in uncomplicated IM.

Patient education to encourage graded exercise improved physical functioning in chronic fatigue syndrome. Sharpe, M. Commentator University of Edinburgh, Edinburgh, UK. ***Evidence-based Medicine,*** **6**(5): 156, Sept./Oct. 2001.

and

Cognitive behaviour therapy reduced fatigue severity and functional impairment in chronic fatigue syndrome. Sharpe, M. Commentator University of Edinburgh, Edinburgh, UK. ***Evidence-based Medicine,*** **6**(5): 156, Sept./Oct. 2001.

Question: In patients with chronic fatigue syndrome (CFS) how effective is an education programme in encouraging graded exercise and in improving physical function?

The following articles are briefly presented
Randomised controlled trial of patient education to encourage graded exercise in chronic fatigue syndrome. Powell, P., Bentall, R.P., Nye, F.J.

and Edwards, R.H.T. Regional Infectious Diseases Unit, University Hospital, Aintree, Liverpool, UK.
BMJ **322(7283):** 387-390, 17 Feb. 2001.

and

Question: In patients with the chronic fatigue syndrome (CFS) how effective is cognitive behaviour therapy (CBT) in reducing fatigue and functional improvement?

Cognitive behaviour therapy for chronic fatigue syndrome: a multicentre randomised controlled trial. Prins, J.B., Bleijenberg, G., Bazelmans, E. *et al.*
Lancet **357:** 841-847, 17 March 2001.

The study by Prins et al. is an RCT involving around 280 patients aged 18–60 years with a diagnosis of CFS and attending mental health centres in the Netherlands. They were allocated to either CBT, guided support groups or no treatment.
- At 8 months follow up, CBT was better than the other treatments.
- There was no difference between no treatment and guided support.

Commentary for both studies
A total of seven RCTs have now been performed which have assessed the efficacy of rehabilitative programmes either psychological or physical for the management of CFS. Six of these have shown evidence of benefit. However, Sharpe notes that the numbers in all of these studies were small and many patients continued to report fatigue even though functioning was improved.

Frequency of attendance in general practice and symptoms before development of chronic fatigue syndrome: a case–control study. Hamilton, W.T., Hall, G.H. and Round, A.P. North and East Devon Health Authority.
Br. J. Gen. Pract., **51**(468): 553-558, 1 July 2001.

This study examines the consulting behaviour of patients suffering from CFS in the 15 years before they are diagnosed with the condition. They use 49 patients with CFS and 49 matched controls from 11 practices in Devon.
- CFS patients consulted nearly twice as much as controls for the 15 years prior to diagnosis.
- They consulted for a wider range of illnesses than controls with lethargy and URTIs being the most common reasons for attendance.

They conclude that behavioural factors may have a role to play in the development of CFS.

Randomised controlled trial of patient education to encourage graded exercise in chronic fatigue syndrome. Powell, P., Bentall, R.P., Nye, F.J. and Edwards, R.H.T. Regional Infectious Diseases Unit, University Hospital, Aintree, Liverpool, UK.
BMJ, 322(7283): 387-390, 17 February 2001.

This was an RCT involving around 150 patients with CFS. The aim of the study was to assess the efficacy of an educational programme to encourage graded exercise. Subjects received either standard care or interventions designed to educate the patient and encourage exercise (three interventions ranged from minimal contact with the patient, to intensive patient contact). At 1 year follow up:

- two out of 34 control patients were clinically improved compared with more than half of those in the three intervention groups;
- there was no difference between the intervention groups;
- physical functioning, fatigue, sleep and mood were all improved in the intervention group;
- a third of patients in the intervention group still complained of fatigue despite improvements in physical function.

The NNT for the intervention groups was 1.6. Other studies have shown CBT to be beneficial with an NNT of two. An educational programme requiring less skilled staff may be highly appropriate for the management of CFS.

Chronic fatigue in general practice: is counselling as good as cognitive behaviour therapy? A UK randomised trial. Ridsdale, L., Godfrey, E., Chalder, T. and Seed, P. *et al.,* Guy's, King's and St. Thomas's School of Medicine, King's College, London, UK.
Br. J. Gen. Pract., **51**(462): 19-24, 1 January 2001.

and

Chronic fatigue in general practice: economic evaluation of counselling versus cognitive behaviour therapy. Chisholm, D., Godfrey, E., Ridsdale, L. and Chalder, T. *et al.,* Centre for the Economics of Mental Health.
Br. J. Gen. Pract., **51**(462): 15-18, Jan. 2001.

The randomized trial was conducted in 10 general practices in London and involved 160 patients with chronic fatigue. The aim of the study was to compare counselling with cognitive behavioural therapy (CBT). Patients were randomized to one of the two therapies. There was no 'standard medical care' control group.

- At 6 months there was no difference between the two groups in terms of anxiety, depression and social functioning.
- GP consultations and use of antidepressants fell in both groups.
- Using 'controls' from previous studies (historical controls) suggests that counselling and CBT were better than usual care; with an NNT of five for counselling and CBT.
- The cost analysis showed the cost of counselling to be £109 and the cost of CBT to be £164 per person.

CHRONIC OBSTRUCTIVE PULMONARY DISEASE

- A systematic review found that physical activity (e.g. swimming) improves exercise tolerance in mild to moderate COPD
- A pilot study found that it is possible to deliver efficacious pulmonary rehabilitation programmes in primary care
- General practice should be central in providing up to date and long term care to COPD patients, but this can only be achieved with new resources

Effects of physical activity in mild to moderate COPD: A systematic review.
Chavannes, N., Vollenberg, J.J.H., Schayck, C.P. and Wouters, E.F.M. Department of General Practice, University of Maastricht, Maastricht, The Netherlands.
Br. J. Gen. Pract., 52: 547-579, 1 July 2002.

The efficacy of pulmonary rehabilitation for severe COPD is widely accepted. However, the evidence that physical exercise, such as walking and swimming, benefits patients with mild-moderate COPD is less clear. The authors thus performed a systematic review of the literature to assess the benefits of exercise on quality of life, dyspnoea, and exercise tolerance in mild-moderate COPD. Five original papers met the inclusion criteria, and were analyzed. The authors found:
- Physical activity significantly improves exercise tolerance in mild-moderate COPD.
- The effects of exercise on quality of life are inconclusive, one paper finding no significant improvement while the other did.

The review concludes:
- Physical activity can improve exercise tolerance in patients with mild-moderate COPD, but more research is needed to resolve whether there is an improvement in dyspnoea and quality of life.

A pilot study of pulmonary rehabilitation in primary care. Jones, R.C.M., Cooper, S., Riley, O. and Dobbs, F. Department of Primary Health Care and General Practice, University of Plymouth, Plymouth, UK.
Br. J. Gen. Pract., 52: 567-568, 1 July 2002.

Pulmonary rehabilitation programmes are proven to benefit patients with chronic obstructive pulmonary disease (COPD). Pulmonary rehabilitation improves quality of life and exercise tolerance in COPD patients. These programmes are usually delivered in secondary care, and are costly. This study, in a single general practice, aimed to examine the feasibility of delivering rehabilitation in a general practice setting. Thirteen patients with COPD participated in the study. Rehabilitation was delivered by a multi-disciplinary team, and consisted of seven sessions, each session featuring 1 hour of exercise and 1 hour education. The effect of rehabilitation was assessed by comparing results of shuttle walking test, Chronic Respiratory Disease Questionnaire (CRDQ) and Hospital Anxiety and Depression Questionnaire (HAD) before and 3 and 12 months after intervention.

The authors found:

- The programme produced a mean increase in the score on the shuttle walking test of 37%, falling to baseline after 12 months.
- Sustained improvements occurred in health status measurements: for CRDQ the mean total score improved by 47% and the HADS depression score fell by 13%.
- Cost per patient was £220.10, compared with £200-£400 for hospital programmes.

Conclusion:

- Primary care based rehabilitation can give outcomes similar to that produced by hospital based programmes.

EDITORIAL – Chronic obstructive pulmonary disease and primary care. Elkington, H. and White, P. Department of General Practice and Primary Care, Guy's, King's and St Thomas' School of Medicine, London, UK.
***Br. J. Gen. Pract., 52**(480): 532-533, 1 July 2002.*

Chronic obstructive pulmonary disease (COPD) accounted for 26000 deaths in 1999 in England and Wales. However, this condition may also be under-diagnosed. Management of COPD patients focuses on controlling symptoms, exacerbations and improving quality of life. Smoking cessation is the only intervention that can arrest declining lung function. Pulmonary rehabilitation is a "multidisciplinary programme of care for patients with chronic respiratory impairment that is individually tailored" and includes exercise training. This programme has shown improvements in walking ability, general and disease-specific health status compared to standard medical management in a 200 patient RCT. The author suggests that rehabilitation and exercise advice are indicated for symptomatic patients. With such large numbers of eligible patients, demand may exceed resources. COPD patients often also suffer from depression, however, few receive further assessment and treatment. Health care for these patients has been described as "ad hoc and reactive" and illustrates how their needs are not being met. GPs are "central" to service provision of COPD patients with each patient requiring long-term surveillance. The author comments that there is a need to define the size of the problem and identify the infrastructure support that will be needed, otherwise those with COPD will remain "disadvantaged, socially isolated and largely silent".

COMPLEMENTARY MEDICINE

- Complementary medicine is becoming more accepted and integrated with conventional medicine, but issues of safety need to be addressed
- A large double blind placebo controlled trial found that *Ginkgo biloba* was no more effective than placebo for the treatment of tinnitus
- Will the integrated care of today be the orthodox medicine of the millennium?
- Agnus castus was superior to placebo for the management of PMS
- Two acupuncture studies have reported very low adverse event rates, with no serious adverse events being reported.
- A Swiss study has found that the herbal remedy Butterbur is a reasonable treatment for seasonal allergic rhinitis and should be used instead of cetirizine when the sedative action is to be avoided.
- A study has found no overall difference between placebo and homeopathic immunotherapy for the treatment of house dust mite allergy in asthma sufferers. However, some intermediate differences were found that were unexplainable.

COMPLEMENTARY MEDICINE

Access to complementary medicine via general practice. Thomas, K., Nicholl, J. and Fall, M. Medical Care Research Unit, University of Sheffield, UK.
Br. J. Gen. Pract., 51(462): 25-30, January 2001.

This study looks at the provision of, and access to complementary therapies in general practice in 1995. A sample of partnerships in England were analysed via postal questionnaire. This involved around 1200 individual GPs. The response rate was 79%.

- Nearly 40% of partnerships provided access to complementary therapies.
- Just over 20% offered the service via a member of the primary health care team.
- Around 25% made NHS-funded referrals.
- A therapist working within the practice provided therapy in 1 in 16 practices.
- Provision of complementary therapies was more common in fundholding practices.
- About one quarter of in-house services were funded either fully or in part by patients.
- Patients in practices that were fundholding were less likely to have to pay for their services than patients in non-fundholding practices.
- The most commonly provided therapies were acupuncture and homeopathy.

The authors discuss the future role of primary care trusts in the provision of complementary therapies within individual practices.

EDITORIALS.
BMJ, 322(7279): January 2001.

Integrated medicine. Lesley Rees, Director of Education, Royal College of Physicians, London.Pages 119–120.

Enhancing human healing. David, Reilly, Consultant Physician, Glasgow Homeopathic Hospital, Glasgow.Pages 120–121.

Complementary medicine and medical education. Brian, Berman, Professor of Family Medicine and Director, Complementary Medicine Program, University of Maryland School of Medicine, Baltimore, USA.Pages 121–122.

EDUCATION AND DEBATE SECTION ARTICLES.
BMJ, 322(7279): January 2001.

Can doctors respond to patients' increasing interest in complementary and alternative medicine? Owen, D.K., Lewith, G. and Stephens, C.R. Winchester Homeopathic Practice, Winchester, Hants. Pages 154–158.

Regulation in complementary and alternative medicine. Simon, Mills. Complementary Health Studies Programme, Department of Lifelong Learning, School of Education, Exeter. Pages 158–160.

Research into complementary and alternative medicine: problems and potential. Nahin, R. and Straus, S. Division of Extramural Research, Training and Review, National Center for Complementary and Alternative Medicine, National Institutes of Health, Bethesda, USA. Pages 161–164.

Much of the *BMJ* of the 20th of January 2001 relates to integrated, orthodox and complementary and alternative medicine (CAM). The editorials and three out of four of the 'Education and Debate' section articles have been combined in the summary below. HRH Prince Charles also writes in the 'personal view' section of this issue.

Integrated medicine is focused more on 'health and healing rather than diagnosis and treatment'. It approaches the patient holistically rather than from a 'system' point of view.

Critics of CAM sight lack of evidence to support its use. Indeed writing in the *Times*, HRH the Prince of Wales noted that in 1999, UK charities spent 0.05% on research into CAM. In America the response to increasing interest has been to set up the National Center for Complementary and Alternative Medicine (NNCAM) as part of the National Institutes of

Health. They have a planned programme of research including looking at the following:

- *Hypericum* for the treatment of depression;
- *G. biloba* for Alzheimer's disease;
- *Serenoa repens* (saw palmetto) for BPH;
- Glucosamine and chondroitin suphate for osteoarthritis.

These trials will look at an individual aspect/intervention of a specific therapy. The challenge is to develop high quality trials which can test the whole modality. Trials which compare intervention with placebo may not always be the most appropriate. Indeed for therapies such as acupuncture attempts at using a placebo would be particularly difficult.

If GPs are to continue in their role as 'gatekeepers' in medicine, they need to familiarize themselves with CAM so that they can advise patients appropriately. Some medical schools offer modules in CAM which usually give an overview of the spectrum of therapies, but do not teach actual clinical skills. Those who practise CAM need both support and regulation. The House of Lords select committee on science and technology have acknowledged the increased interest and use in CAM and have recommended tighter regulation. They have put CAMs into three groups and made recommendations based on these. Briefly these groups are:

- Group 1: acupuncture, chiropractic, herbal medicine, homeopathy and osteopathy;
- Group 2: includes aromatherapy, hypnotherapy, reflexology and others;
- Group 3: includes Chinese herbal medicine, iridology, crystal therapy and others.

The increasing public use of CAM is due to a frustration with conventional medicine. Time constraints and an overemphasis on technology forces patients into the arms of CAM practitioners who spend more time and place more of an emphasis on self care.

Prince Charles as founder and president of The Foundation for Integrated Medicine, encourages the re-balancing of the Leaning Tower of Pisa i.e. the dominance of orthodox over CAM. Indeed in 1982 when president of the BMA, he concluded that the alternative medicine of today would be the orthodox medicine of tomorrow. The Leaning Tower of Pisa may yet be re-aligned.

HERBAL/PLANT REMEDIES

Randomised controlled trial of butterbur and cetirizine for treating seasonal allergic rhinitis. Schapowal, A. on behalf of Petasites Study Group. Allergy Clinic and Hochwangstrasse, S. CH-7302 Landquart, Switzerland.
BMJ, 324(7330): 144-146, 19 January 2002.

The aim of this randomised double blind placebo controlled trial was to compare the efficacy of the antihistamine, cetirizine with the herbal remedy Butterbur for the treatment of seasonal allergic rhinitis. Butterbur (or butter dock, bog rhubarb, exwort) is an Asteraceae herbaceous plant containing petasines, which inhibit leukotrienes. Patients (125) came from outpatient departments in Switzerland and Germany. One half were given butterbur one tablet four times a day and the other half were given cetirizine one tablet daily, both for 2 weeks.

- Outcomes were similar for both drugs.
- Cetirizine was associated with sedating adverse effects.

They conclude that Butterbur is a reasonable treatment for seasonal allergic rhinitis and should be used instead of cetirizine when the sedative action is to be avoided.

Treatment for the premenstrual syndrome with agnus castus fruit extract: prospective randomised placebo controlled study. Schellenberg, R. for the study group, Institute for Health Care and Science, Hüttenberg, Germany.
***BMJ,* 322**(7279): 134-137, 20 January 2001.

This RCT involved 178 women suffering from premenstrual sydrome (PMS) and took place in general medical outpatient clinics. Patients were randomized to receive either agnus castus one tablet per day or placebo for three menstrual cycles.

- Agnus castus was better than placebo at treating irritability, mood alteration, anger, headache and breast fullness. There was no difference between the groups for bloating.
- Over 50% of women in the agnus castus group responded to treatment compared with 24% in the placebo group.
- There was no difference in adverse events between the two groups.

They conclude that agnus castus should be used as a therapeutic option in women with PMS.

Effectiveness of *Ginkgo biloba* in treating tinnitus: double blind, placebo controlled trial. Drew, S. and Davies, E. Pharmacology Department, Division of Neuroscience, University of Birmingham, Birmingham, UK.
***BMJ,* 322**(7278): 73-75, 13 January 2001.

This UK study involved over 1100 subjects with tinnitus and was a double blind placebo controlled trial. Subjects were recruited from advertisements or from the British Tinnitus Association. The study was conducted entirely by telephone or mail (questionnaire). Subjects received either *Ginkgo biloba* extract LI 1370 (the most popular brand used in the UK) 50 mg three times a day or placebo for 12 weeks.

- There was no difference between the two groups at any stage of follow up.
- Adverse effects were similar between the two groups.
- Beneficial effects e.g. feeling of wellbeing, circulation and hearing were significantly more frequent in the *Ginkgo* group.

HOMEOPATHY

Use of ultramolecular potencies of allergen to treat asthmatic people allergic to house dust mite: double blind randomised controlled clinical trial. Lewith, G.T., Watkins, A.D. and Hyland, M.E. Medical Specialties Southampton General Hospital, Southampton, UK.
BMJ, **324**(7336): 520-523, 2 March 2002.

This aim of this RCT was to compare homeopathic immunotherapy with placebo for the management of asthmatic people with house dust mite allergy. Two hundred and forty two people from 38 general practices in Hampshire and Dorset took part in the study and were followed up over 4 months.
- There was no difference in outcomes between the two groups.
- They did find differences for three outcome variables (mood, morning peak flow rates and asthma visual analogue scales), but they were unable to explain these differences.

ACUPUNCTURE

Adverse events following acupuncture: prospective survey of 32 000 consultations with doctors and physiotherapists. White, A., Hayhoe, S, Hart, A. and Ernst, E. Department of Complementary Medicine, School of Postgraduate Medicine and Health Sciences, University of Exeter, UK.
BMJ, **323**(7311): 485-486, 1 September 2001.

This was a prospective study of 78 doctors and physiotherapists who also practiced acupuncture. Data was collected over a period of 21 months.
- Fourteen "significant" events per 10 000 consultations were reported, none of which could be classed as serious.
- Minor adverse effects were reported as 671 per 10 000.
- The most common adverse events were bleeding, needling pain and aggravation of symptoms.
- Seventy percent of those reporting aggravation of symptoms had a subsequent improvement in their symptoms.

The York acupuncture safety study: prospective survey of 34 000 treatment by traditional acupuncturists. MacPherson, H., Thomas, K., Walters, S. and Fitter, M. Foundation for Traditional Chinese Medicine, York, UK.
BMJ, **323**(7311): 486-487, 1 September 2001.

This was a prospective study of professional acupuncturists who were members of the British Acupuncture Council. Data was collected over a period of 4 weeks. Of around 1850 acupuncturists, 31% took part in the study (around 570 professionals).
- No serious events were reported.

- The minor adverse event rate was 1.3 per 1000 treatments.
- The most common adverse events were nausea, fainting, bleeding. Some avoidable events were moxibustion skin burns and needles being left in.

OTHERS

Complementary medicine use in children: extent and reasons. A population-based study. Simpson, N. and Roman, K. Child Health Department, Bath NHS House, Newbridge Hill, Bath, UK.
Br. J. Gen. Pract., **51**(472): 914-916, 1 November 2001.

The authors state that this is the 'first population survey of complementary medicine in children in the UK'. They survey a random sample of 1230 children aged 16 and under in the Bath area of England and just under 900 responded (80%)
- Just under 18% had tried complementary medicine.
- Around 7% had visited a complementary medicine practitioner
- Complementary medicine was said to have helped the child in 85% of cases.
- Reasons for complementary medicine use included dissatisfaction with conventional medicine and fewer side effects.
- The most common types of complementary medicine used were homeopathy, aromatherapy and herbal medicine.
- Two thirds of those using complementary medicine had not told their doctor.Health professionals need to be aware of complementary medicine use in their patients and be alert to side effects and possible interactions with conventional medicines.

FURTHER READING

EDITORIAL - Randomised controlled trials for homeopathy.
BMJ, **324**(7336): 498-499, Jan. 2002.

CONTINUING PROFESSIONAL DEVELOPMENT (CPD)

- Insufficient studies exist which evaluate the cost-effectiveness of continuing professional development activities
- Competency based assessment is unsuitable for medical education; there are some advantages however, that merit its inclusion in some areas
- If we are to see a reduction in the increasing number of reports of failed care by doctors, all practitioners to accept responsibility
- Insufficient studies exist which evaluate the cost-effectiveness of continuing professional development activities
- The Good CPD guide, details 46 formal and informal methods of needs assessment.
- The workplace climate affects a physicians methods of learning at work
- Case method learning in general practice resulted in a beneficial change in clinical practice.

Learning in practice section: Postal survey of approaches to learning among Ontario physicians: implications for continuing medical education. Delva, M., Kirby, J. and Knapper, C. *et al.* Department of Family Medicine, Ontario, Canada. **BMJ, 325**(7374): 1218-1223 , 23 November 2002.

This survey conducted in Canada amongst 800 physicians, looked at the approaches to learning to enable continuing medical education (CME).

The questionnaire used included questions asking physicians to rate their most useful CME activities and any barriers or motivations they felt towards CME. Around 350 surveys were returned. They found that:

- Physicians were more likely to learn by a deep learning approach or a surface rational approach. The deep learning approach involves an integrative approach whereby new ideas are related to situations where they might be applicable. The surface rational approach involves a need for order and routine and places importance on learning important facts.
- Those who adopted a deep approach were more likely to feel in control at work and have supportive reception environments.
- Over worked, young, primary care physicians, working in rural situations were more likely to be disorganised in their learning.
- Those who had learned using problem based learning as undergraduates were also more likely to be disorganised in their learning.
- A deep approach was associated with internal motivation.
- A disorganised approach was associated with external motivation for learning.

Learning to practice: Efficacy of case method learning in general practice for secondary prevention in patients with coronary artery disease: randomised controlled study. Kiessling, A. and Henriksson, P. Department of Medicine, Karolinska Institute, Stockholm, Sweden.
***BMJ,* 325**(7369): 877-880, 19 October 2002.

Lipid lowering has been shown to reduce coronary artery disease but there is a gulf in what is achieved in clinical practice and what should be achieved for therapeutic effectiveness based on scientific evidence.

A study was conducted in Sweden to see whether Case method learning improved clinical practice. Case method learning involves a case, which is a description of a particular situation and allows the learner to take the role of being the decision maker. The aim was to see whether case method learning had an effect on patients cholesterol concentrations.

Around 250 patients with coronary artery disease were chosen and split into groups depending on whether their specialist or GP played the major role in their care. The GP patients were then further randomised into control and intervention groups. The GPs looking after patients in the intervention group were offered case method learning seminars.

The seminars included case presentations and discussions of factors that influence patient decisions. The main study variable measured was the change in the LDL cholesterol concentration in the intervention group compared to the control group.

- LDL cholesterol concentrations decreased by 10% in the intervention group but showed no change in the control group.
- In the Specialist group LDL levels dropped by over 12%.
- GPs in the intervention group felt they had a higher perceived knowledge of scientific evidence and practice guidelines than controls.

Case method learning for GPs reduced LDL cholesterol concentrations to a level that would be expected to decrease mortality and morbidity in coronary artery disease.

Learning in practice: Competency based medical training: review. Wai-Ching, L. Medicine, Health Policy and Practice, University of East Anglia, Norwich, UK.
***BMJ,* 325**(7366): 693-695, 28 September 2002.

Competency based approaches to assessment are widely used at key stages of medical training. Occupational roles are converted into outcomes, which candidates must achieve in order to pass.

This form of assessment is objective, and allows for flexible training using transparent standards. However, assessing competency remains a subjective task, and it is difficult to adequately represent the range of competencies needed for an occupational role, as discrete units for assessment. Using checklists to pass or fail candidates is demotivating, and the author argues this simplistic approach is unsuitable for higher education.

Medical education has traditionally been assessed with a focus on understanding of basic concepts, with skills assessed globally. Competency based approaches are now beginning to take over, though there is little evidence to suggest it is more effective than its predecessor, and in some cases may be less effective.

Competency based assessment allows candidates to learn at their own pace, however the length of medical training is currently fixed in the UK. This approach also ignores the learning process, which is vital for lifelong learning.

The author concludes that competency based medical education provides an opportunity for personalised, flexible training. However, there is a danger of focusing on minimum standards rather than excellence and of reducing the efficacy of education, particularly where well defined learning outcomes are absent.

This approach is just one of many that may be useful at different stages of medical training.

EDITORIAL – Managing alleged performance problems are we ready? Wilson, T. RCGP Quality Unit, Royal College of GPs, London, UK. *Br. J. Gen. Pract.,* **52**(482): 707-708, 1 September 2002.

Failure of one person to take responsibility and act when they observe something wrong with a patients management has led to cases of failed care and criminal action, many of which receive significant media attention.

Very few doctors intentionally provide sub-standard care. However, until doctors begin to accept some responsibility for dealing with poor performance the complaints, criticisms and suboptimal care will continue.

Steps to target the problems include the introduction of the National Clinical Assessment Authority. However, the vast and constant restructuring of health service provision has only meant shifts in the burden of responsibility with little implementation.

Furthermore, the systems in place for dealing with medical practitioners deemed to be practising poorly do not reflect the fact that a complaint against a practitioner is a significant personal and professional life event.

The process of assessing and investigating cases of questioned care is difficult, as many failures are not due to one person or one incident alone yet the legal system continues to seek someone to blame.

The introduction of an occupational health service for GPs is one reflection of the significance of this problem. The GMCs new guidelines for GPs have made a significant first step in encouraging GPs to take responsibility for their own actions in the pursuit of a higher standard of care.

Learning in practice section: Problem based learning in continuing medical education: a review of controlled evaluation studies. Smits, P.B.A. and Verbeek, J.H.A.M. Netherlands School of Occupational Health, Amsterdam, Netherlands.
***BMJ,* 324**(7330): 153-156, 19 January 2002.

This study was a systematic review whose aim was to assess the efficacy of problem- based learning. Six studies met their inclusion criteria. However, no study looked at the stated outcomes of performance or patient health.
- They could find "no consistent evidence that problem based learning in continuing medical education was superior to other educational strategies"

They admit that overall studies were not of sufficient relevance to answer the question being asked.

Learning in practice section: Learning needs assessment: assessing the need. Grant, J. Open University Centre for Education in Medicine, Milton Keynes, UK.
***BMJ,* 324**(7330): 156-159, 19 January 2002.

One of the reasons the PGEA system was thought to have failed was because needs assessment was not part of educational planning. A change in behaviour is more likely to occur if needs assessment is conducted before hand. The type of needs assessment should correspond to the defined purpose of the need eg curriculum planning, accountability, diagnosing conditions. Methods of needs assessment are multiple. The **Good CPD guide** (Grant, J., Chambers, G. and Jackson, G. (eds.) *The Good CPD guide.* Sutton: Reed Healthcare, 1999), details 46 formal and informal methods of needs assessment, under the following headings:
- **Clinicians own experiences** e.g. diaries;
- **Interactions within the clinical team and department** e.g. clinical meetings, mentoring;
- **Formal approaches to quality management and risk assessment** e.g. audit, patient satisfaction surveys;
- **Specific activities directed at needs assessment** e.g. gap analysis, revalidation;
- **Peer review** e.g. internal, external;
- **Non-clinical activities** e.g. conferences, journal articles.

The article chooses seven methods to describe in more detail.
- **Gap or discrepancy analysis.** This involves comparing performance with a stated standard.
- **Reflection.** May involve use of video or audiotapes. PUNS (patient unmet need) and DENS (doctors educational needs) is also an example of this.
- **Self-assessment.** Use of diaries is limited by poor motivation and compliance.
- **Observation.** Doctors may be watched performing a skill.
- **Critical incident analysis and significant event auditing.** An incident can be analysed to identify areas of need.

• **Practice review.** A routine review of notes or prescribing can be made.

Needs assessment needs to be different from assessment. We also need to make sure that the resulting learning goals do not become too narrow. We must also accept that doctors use different methods of learning.

Learning in practice section: Cost effectiveness of continuing professional development in health care: a critical review of the evidence. Field, S.J., Brown, C.A. and Belfield, C.R. Centre for Research in Medical and Dental Education, School of Education, University of Birmingham, Birmingham, UK.
***BMJ,* 324**(7338): 652-655, 16 March 2002.

Defined in this paper as 'post-registration acquisition of skills or knowledge by healthcare professionals', continuing professional development (CPD) is an important but expensive tool for improving health. The NHS spent £1bn on CPD in 1999–2000. Efficient use of resources is essential to ensure maximum benefits from participating in CPD so good quality economic evaluation of such activities is necessary.

This Department of Health-funded study set out to assess the evidence on the cost-effectiveness of such interventions. A widespread database search identified only nine studies. None fulfilled all the criteria for appropriate use of economic methods specifically designed to assess health technologies and there were inconsistencies in approach, making a full systematic review impossible.

The authors comment that more high quality studies are needed to benefit both the public, and the policy makers who allocate resources.

Model for directly assessing and improving clinical competence and performance in revalidation of clinicians. Mckinley, R.E., Fraser, R.C. and Baker, R. Department of General Practice and Primary Health Care, University of Leicester, Leicester General Hospital, Leicester, UK.
***BMJ,* 322**(7288): 712-715, 24 March 2001.

Proposals for revalidation include the following:
- review of patient's case notes;
- professional values;
- patient satisfaction;
- professional relationship with patients;
- keeping up-to-date and monitoring performance;
- complaints procedure;
- good clinical care;
- record keeping;
- accessibility;
- team work;
- effective use or resources.

None of the above involve direct observation of the clinician during the consultation. The consultation is said to be the cornerstone of clinical

practice, especially as everything we do stems from it. This article discusses methods to directly assess the consultation. These may include:
- covert or overt methods;
- live or recorded methods;
- real or simulated surgeries,
- use of involve lay or professional assessors.

They discuss the relative merits of each of the points above. They point out that an assessment of competence will not guarantee that the doctor will actually use his/her skills. Ensuring that doctors put their skills into practice requires vigilance from patients and fellow professionals. Those deemed to be incompetent require focused feedback and remedial training. Repeated incompetence may mean that some doctors are withdrawn from practice. Decisions will need to be made regarding who bears the cost of this process.

FURTHER READING

A continuous curriculum for general practice? Proposals for under-graduate-postgraduate collaboration. Jones, R. and Oswald, N., Guy's, King's and St. Thomas's School of Medicine, London.
Br. J. Gen. Pract., **51**(463): 135-138, Feb. 2001.

CONTRACEPTION

- Analysing data from the General Practice Research Database, Farmer *et al.*, found that compared with older pills, 3rd generation pills **were not** associated with a doubling of the risk of venous thromboembolism. However, Jick *et al.*, analysing the same data, found that 3rd generation pills **were** associated with a doubled risk of venous thromboembolism
- Family history is a poor tool for identifying those at risk of a venous thromboembolism during oral contraceptive pill use
- A meta-analysis of mainly case-control studies has found that oral contraceptive pill use is associated with a slightly increased risk of ischaemic stroke
- The Courts judgment concerning 3rd generation pills was hampered by the use and interpretation of statistics alongside evidence from witnesses
- Younger women and women from deprived backgrounds prefer to risk pregnancy rather than face the stigmatism attached to emergency contraception

BACKGROUND

- Third generation pills (containing desogestrol and gestodene) are associated with venous thromboembolism in 30 per 100 000 users.
- Second generation pills (containing levonorgestrol and norethisterone) are associated with venous thromboembolism in 15 per 100 000 users.
- The background risk is five per 100 000.
- The risk in pregnancy is 60 per 100 000.
- Mortality from venous thromboembolism is low at 1–2%, which is equivalent to 2–3 per million users.

Two large British cohort studies are responsible for much of our data concerning the oral contraceptive pill. The RCGP Oral Contraceptive Study involved 14 000 GPs and 46 000 women (half using the pill and half not). The second study by the Oxford Family Planning Association involved 17 family planning clinics and 17 000 women (over half of whom were using the pill and rest were using a diaphragm or intrauterine device). From these and other case-control studies we know the following concerning the combined pill.

Positive points:
- high efficacy and acceptability;
- it suppresses menstrual disorders;
- decreased risk of iron deficiency anaemia;
- decreased risk of pelvic inflammatory disease;
- suppresses functional ovarian cysts;
- decreased risk of ovarian and endometrial cancer by 50%.

Negative points:
- increased risk of venous thromboembolism;
- increased risk of stroke;
- increased risk of MI;

- increased risk of breast cancer by 25% (not detectable after 10 years of stopping the pill);
- increased risk of cervical cancer;
- increased risk of gall bladder disease;
- increased risk of chronic inflammatory bowel disease;
- increased risk of liver tumours (very rare).

The arterial effects are confined to those who smoke and measuring blood pressure before and during pill use can decrease this risk.

The limitations of these two studies are that they concern pills containing 50 μg of oestrogen. Recent studies also suggest that the type of progestogen used may be important as far as venous thromboembolism is concerned.

THROMBOEMBOLISM

EDITORIAL – Oral contraceptives, venous thromboembolism, and the courts. Skegg, David C.G. Department of Preventative and Social Medicine, University of Otago, New Zealand. **BMJ, 325**(7363): 504-505, 7 September 2002.

This article examines the validity of a recent court judgement in which women claimed they had been harmed by third generation oral contraceptives, and challenged three drug companies in court. The author doubts the judicial process is helpful in reaching sensible conclusions.

He points to the sophisticated statistics around which much of the arguments focused, and the judges elementary ability with such concepts. Additionally, it was apparent that expert witnesses had exchanged documentation relating to their analyses, prior to the trial.

Skegg comments also that the judges decision was based on his impression of witnesses surely not a practice to be encouraged when examining complex scientific data.

The judgement was based on evidence from one witness in particular; this was notable since this witnesss analytical methods were not especially suited to this scenario.

The judge also reached a conclusion based on the totality of evidence; that women using third generation pills had a 70% greater risk of venous thromboembolism. It was also noted that pharmaceutical funded studies found much lower relative risks than other studies, but little significance was given to this.

The author concludes that a system of no-fault compensation may be fairer on consumers, and that little scientific agreement is likely to be reached in court.

Value of family history in identifying women at risk of venous thromboembolism during oral contraception: observational study. Cosmi, B., Legnani, C. and Bernardi, F. *et al.* Cardiovascular Department, Division of Angiology, Unità ricerca Clinica sulla Trombofilia "M Golinelli", University Hospital, Sorsola-Malpighi, Bologna, Italy.
***BMJ,* 322**(7203): 28 April 2001.

The aim of this Italian cohort study was to evaluate the sensitivity and predictive values of family history as a screening tool for identifying those at risk of venous thromboembolism whilst using the oral contraceptive pill. Over 300 women attending family planning clinics were analysed by questionnaire regarding family history, and blood tests for clotting abnormalities.

- The sensitivity of family history amongst first and second degree relatives was 16% and the predictive value 9%.

These values are not satisfactory to identify those with a clotting disorder and hence at increased risk of venous thromboembolism during pill use. Large numbers of at risk women could be missed using this strategy.

Risk of venous thromboembolism among users of third generation oral contraceptives compared with users of oral contraceptives with levonorgestrel before and after 1995: cohort and case–control analysis. Jick, H., Kaye, J.A., Vasilakis-Scaramozza, C. and Jick, S.S. Boston Collaborative Drug Surveillance Program, Boston University School of Medicine, Lexington MA, USA.
***BMJ,* 321**(7270): 1190-1195, 11 November 2000.

In this study Jick *et al.* counter the findings of Farmer *et al.* (summarized below). Using data from the same source (General Practice Research Database) they perform both cohort and case-control analyses on the data to look at the relative risk of venous thromboembolism (VT) before and after October 1995.

- They estimate that a decrease occurred in VT after the pill scare.
- The relative risk of VT in 3rd generation pill users compared with levonorgestrel pill users was found to be 1.9 (confidence interval 1.3-2.8), for the cohort analysis and 2.3 (CI: 1.3-3.9) for the case-control study.

They discuss why their findings differ from those found by Farmer *et al.* below

- In the Jick study, attempts are made to confirm the diagnosis and exclude non-pill causes of VT. This was not done in the Farmer study.
- The Jick study confines itself to a comparison of 3rd generation pills with levonorgestrel pills. Including **all** pills in the analysis (as was done by the Farmer group) could have skewed the results. For example cyproterone acetate pills were prescribed more often after the pill scare and these pills have been associated with an increased risk of VT compared with other pills.
- The Jick study controls for confounding including smoking and body mass index. This was not done in the Farmer study.

They conclude that the newer generation pills **do** double the risk of VT compared with levonorgestrel pills.

Effect of 1995 pill scare on rates of venous thromboembolism among women taking combined oral contraceptives: analysis of General Practice Research Database. Farmer, R.D.T., Williams, T.J., Simpson, E.L. and Nightingale, A.L. Pharmacoepidemiology and Public Health Postgraduate Medical School, University of Surrey, Guildford, UK.
***BMJ,* 321**(7259): 477-479, 19 August 2000.

In 1995 the UK Committee on Safety of Medicines stated that 3rd generation pills were associated with a doubling of the risk of VT compared with older pills. This present study examines the impact of this report and the 'pill scare' on rates of VT.
- After October 1995, the prescribing of 3rd generation pills fell from 53% to 14%.
- The VT rates did not change appreciably after October 1995.

They conclude that there is no evidence that desogestrel and gestodene containing pills double the risk of VT.

GENERAL HEALTH

Review: Current oral contraceptive use increases the risk for ischaemic stroke. Commentator, James Douketis, St Joseph's Hospital, Hamilton, Ontario, Canada.
***Evidence–based Medicine,* 6**(2): 60, Mar./Apr. 2001.

Question: Is oral contraceptive use associated with an increased risk for ischaemic stroke?

The following article is briefly presented
Ischaemic stroke risk with oral contraceptives. A meta–analysis. Gillum, La, Mamidipudi, S.K. and Johnston, S.C.
JAMA, **284:** 72–78, 5 July 2000.

Sixteen studies, which were mainly case-control studies, were analysed in this MA.
- For low dose oestrogen pills, the risk of stroke was increased by a factor of nearly two, which represents four additional cases of stroke per 100 000 pill users.

They conclude that oral contraceptive pill use is associated with a slightly increased risk of ischaemic stroke.

Commentary
The commentator states that when risk factors are controlled for the increased risk of stroke is reduced to about one and a half times increased risk. In addition half of the seven studies looking at low dose oestrogen found no association between pill use and risk of stroke. He suggests that these findings should not change our clinical practice.

EMERGENCY CONTRACEPTION

Young womens accounts of factors influencing their use and non-use of emergency contraception: in-depth interview study. Free, C., Lee, R.M. and Ogden, J. Department of General Practice and Primary Care, Guys, Kings College and St Thomass School of Medicine, London, UK.
BMJ, **325**(7377): 1393-1397, 14 December 2002.

This qualitative study examined the factors influencing the use and non-use of emergency contraception following problems with normal contraception. Thirty women from the London area, aged between 16 and 25 years, were interviewed regarding their experience of emergency contraception.

- Emergency contraception was generally used when no contraception had been used, or when there was uncertainty regarding whether condoms had been used properly, and in one case because of a problem with the contraceptive pill.
- Women who were concerned about becoming pregnant used it more often, however younger women reported a feeling of personal failure associated with its use.
- Younger and more deprived women preferred to ignore the risk of pregnancy rather than face any stigmatism connected to using emergency contraception.
- Some women avoided using emergency contraception due to concern about side effects. Requesting emergency contraception from a healthcare professional was difficult; especially when consultations focused on the risks the woman had taken.

The reasons for non-use given above should be taken into account when addressing the poor use of emergency contraception. Educational interventions should promote the attitudes and personal skills required to obtain emergency contraception.

DEPRIVATION

- A study looking at treated chronic disease and deprivation found that for all diseases analysed there is a strong deprivation gradient, with people in deprived areas being the least well treated
- A complex web of factors prevent people from using services for CHD
- One study found that lone motherhood and ethnic minority status is associated with poor health outcomes.
- New data suggests that there is no correlation between income inequality and health. There is however a positive relationship between individual income and health.
- In a discussion paper, N. Beale comments that "good health and deprivation do not share a duvet"
- A Scottish study found that men and women in the lowest socio-economic category (and aged under 65) had double the mortality of those in the highest socio-economic group.

BACKGROUND

'Inequalitites in health' continue to receive a steady stream of attention. The gap between rich and poor is widening and wealth is more important than smoking as a factor affecting world-wide health.

Psychosocial stressors acting throughout life can have adverse effects on morbidity and mortality. In adult life some of the main stressors seem to be:
- perceived financial strain;
- job insecurity;
- low control and monotony at work;
- stressful life events;
- poor social networks;
- low self esteem;
- fatalism.

The metabolic syndrome (central obesity, insulin resistance, glucose intolerance, lipid disturbances, decreased fibrinolysis) may reflect the effects of psychosocial stress on the hypothalamic-pituitary-adrenal axis. Stress is known to be associated with abnormal functioning of the immune system. Studies have found that low autonomy and decision-making latitude at work can predict coronary heart disease. However, highlighting these mechanisms should not detract from the central role of social organization in the generation of health inequalities.

DATA ANALYSIS

The Jarman Index is the most popular way of assessing deprivation in GP populations. However, it was initially developed as a tool to detect increased workload rather than deprivation. It uses Census data, which are collected at 10 year intervals and hence can be inaccurate. Alternative methods have been proposed.

Prescription data
One study (Lloyd, *BMJ* 1995) used Prescription Pricing Authority data to give a new index of deprivation. The index was good when used to look at Health Authority populations but poor at the general practice level because of differences in individual prescribing. However, the value of these data is that they can be updated annually or even quarterly.

Unemployment rates
Another study (Pringle, *Br. J. Gen. Pract.* 1994) found that unemployment rates were more closely correlated with prescribing variables than the Jarman Index. Perhaps this provides more evidence that deprivation and health are related. This index can also be updated annually.

Using enumeration districts rather than wards
Census data deal with populations from electoral wards. This can be inaccurate because wards are large and insensitive. They may also under-represent refugees and homeless people. Enumeration districts representing around 500 people are smaller and more homogeneous than electoral wards. Jarman in his original article suggested the use of enumeration districts.

Increasing the number of deprivation categories
Another way to make the deprivation payments more equitable would be to increase the number of deprivation categories (at present there are three). The linear increase in workload with decreasing socio-economic status of the population is not reflected in the deprivation scale payments which have sharp cut-off points.

Using person-based data
This would be even more accurate than using populations and would eliminate the assumption that all people living in deprived areas are deprived (the ecological fallacy).

Barriers to uptake of services for coronary heart disease: qualitative study.
Tod, A.M., Read, C., Lacey, A. and Abbot, J. Public Health, Rotherham Health Authority, Bevan House, Rotherham, UK.
***BMJ,* 323**(7306): 2147, 28 July 2001.

This qualitative study evaluates the barriers to the uptake of services for CHD in the South Yorkshire mining area. Fourteen patients, seven GPs, one health visitor and a pharmacist are interviewed. The following factors affected uptake of services.

Structural
- Poor transport links to GP services.
- Inconvenient surgery hours.
- No drop-in services. Patients preferred a no-appointment system.

Personal factors
- Fear and denial of illness.

Social and cultural
- The South Yorkshire culture of stoicism and independence prevented people from talking about their illness or coming forward at an early stage.

Past experiences and expectations
- Negative attitudes of health professionals. Mining communities had low expectations for their health. Chronic ill health from a young age was expected.

Diagnostic confusion
- Mining communities often attributed symptoms to lung rather than heart disease.

Knowledge and awareness
- The culture of not talking about illness means that the community has a poor understanding of heart disease.

Many of these barriers are in operation before the patient reaches the GP. A community development approach is required which recognizes the social, economic and environmental causes of ill health.

Inequalities in treated heart disease and mental illness in England and Wales, 1994–1998. Moser, K. Senior Research Officer, Office for National Statistics, London, UK. **Br. J. Gen. Pract., 51**(467): 438-444, 1 June 2001.

This study uses data from the General Practice Research Database (211 practices in England and Wales). The aim of the study is to evaluate the relationship between deprivation and prevalence of treated chronic disease (type 2 diabetes mellitus, heart disease, mental illness).
- They found that for all diseases analysed there is a strong deprivation gradient.
- The highest prevalence of untreated disease was found in the most deprived areas.
- These differentials were larger for females heart disease and diabetes.
- The differentials tended to be larger for the middle age group (rather than children and elderly people).

They conclude that the existence of a deprivation gradient suggests that optimum treatment goals are not being reached for the majority of the population with chronic disease.

Relation between socioeconomic status and tumour stage in patients with breast, colorectal, ovarian and lung cancer: results from four national, population based studies. Brewster, D.H., Thomson, C.S., Hole, D.J. and Black, R.J. *et al.* Scottish Cancer Intelligence Unit, Information and Statistics Division, Trinity Park House, Edinburgh, UK.
BMJ, 322(7290): 830-831, 7 April 2001.

The aim of this Scottish study was to determine whether tumour stage at presentation was related to socio-economic status. Data was extracted from the Scottish Cancer Registry and medical records. Medical records were analysed, from around 2500 patients with breast cancer, 2800 patients with colorectal cancer, 1400 with ovarian cancer and 3800 with lung cancer.

- For breast and colorectal cancer there was no evidence of a socio-economic status/tumour stage difference. These results conflict with results from another Scottish study.
- There was a trend towards deprived patients with ovarian cancer presenting with more advanced disease.
- Deprived patients with lung cancer were more likely to present earlier than 'wealthier' patients. For this analysis medical records were more likely to be missing in the deprived group. This may have affected the results. Alternatively, the deprived group are more likely to be smokers and are more likely to have co-morbid diseases which may result in a lower threshold for investigation.

MORBIDITY AND MORTALITY

Inequalities in morbidity and consulting behaviour for socially vulnerable groups. Baker, D., Mead, N. and Campbell, S. National Primary Care Research and Development Centre, Manchester, UK.
Br. J. Gen. Pract., **52**(475): 124-130, 1 February 2002.

This questionnaire study looks at the relationship between social vulnerability and use of primary care services. Socially vulnerable groups were, lone mothers, ethnic minorities, unemployed and elderly living alone. A random sample of 200 patients from each of 10 practices in the six health authorities were sent questionnaires (response rate 38%).

They found that, of the group studied, lone motherhood and ethnic minorities, were associated with poor health outcomes.

- Lone motherhood was associated with a higher prevalence of anxiety and sleep problems.
- Being a member of an ethnic minority group was associated with an increased prevalence of diabetes, migraine, cold/flu, anxiety and depression.
- Being a member of an ethnic minority group was associated with increased consultation rates especially for back pain, indigestion, migraine and minor respiratory symptoms

EDITORIAL – Income inequality and population health. Mackenbach, Johan P. Professor of Public Health, Department of Public Health, Erasmus University Rotterdam, Rotterdam, Netherlands. *BMJ,* **324**(7328): 1-2, 5 January 2002.

This editorial is a comment on four papers published in the same issue (see **Further reading**), which are concerned with the relationship between income inequality and health. In 1992, a landmark paper suggested that income inequality was negatively correlated with life expectancy. Data and articles emerging since then refute this finding. Three of the articles in this issue look at income inequality in different populations (Denmark, USA and Japan). All of these studies found no correlation between income inequality and health. What they do find however is a positive correlation between **individual** income and health, with those on higher incomes living longer than those on lower incomes. The fourth paper is a meta-regression analysis which showed that educational attainment is a more powerful predictor of mortality than income inequality.

DISCUSSION PAPER: Unequal to the task: deprivation, health and UK general practice at the millennium. Beale, N. General Practitioner Northlands R&D Practice, Northlands Surgery, Calne, Wiltshire, UK. *Br. J. Gen. Pract.,* **51**(467): 478-485, 1 June 2001.

This discussion paper analyses how deprivation and health impact upon general practice. Beale states that the inequalities in health and wealth have been increasing over the last 20 years. Social (status) and material (things) deprivation may be equally important. Also we must not forget to include such groups as those with learning difficulties, the homeless, asylum seekers and drug addicts amongst the deprived. Over the years there have been attempts to develop markers of deprivation (e.g. Townsend, Carstairs and Morris) many are flawed by one or more confounders. What is clear is that good health and deprivation do not share a duvet. Even when the better off smoke more and have worse diets than the deprived, the former still live longer. Working in deprived areas is harder than working in advantaged areas. Jarman, in 1981, surveyed GPs for their views on which patients caused the most work (under-Privileged Area 8 score). The politicians of the day used this untested list to make deprivation payments. Beale suggests that we need an index which takes account of the socio-economic status of individuals or households so that the socio-economic footprint of each UK practice can be determined and resources allocated according.

Relation between socio-economic deprivation and death from a first myocardial infarction in Scotland: population based analysis. Macintyre, K., Stewart, S. and Chalmers, J. *et al.* Department of Public Health, University of Glasgow, Glasgow, UK.
BMJ, **322**(7295): 1152-1153, 12 May 2001.

This study examines the relationship between socio-economic deprivation and death from MI. They analyse data from Scotland over a 10 year period between 1986 and 1995.

• They found that those in the lowest socio-economic category (and aged under 65) had double the mortality of those in the highest socio-economic group.

• The effect was greatest amongst women.

They conclude that trying to address these figures will require attention to primary prevention strategies which begin in utero and extend throughout adult life.

FURTHER READING

See 'Doctor-patient relationship' for

Deprivation, psychological distress and consultation length in general practice. Department of General Practice, University of Glasgow, Glasgow, UK.
Br. J. Gen. Pract., **51** (467): 456-460, June 2001.

Relations of income inequality and family income to chronic medical conditions and mental health disorders: national survey. Sturm, R. and Gresenz, C.R., RAND 1700 Main Street, Santa Monica, CA, USA.
BMJ, **324** (7328): 20, 5 Jan. 2002.

Education, income inequality, and mortality: a multiple regression analysis. Muller, A., Department of Health Services Administration, University of Arkansas at Little Rock, Little Rock, AR, USA.
BMJ, **324** (7328): 23, 5 Jan. 2002.

DIABETES MELLITUS

- Glycaemic control is more important than intensive therapy for reducing the risk of diabetes-related end points (UKPDS 35)
- UKPDS 36: Over the 10 year period, risk of all complications (except cataracts) and death was strongly associated with the updated mean systolic blood pressure
- AT1 receptor blockers combined with ACE inhibitors are better than either single therapy for reducing blood pressure and urinary albumin excretion in type 2 diabetics
- A study performed in The Netherlands found that insulin therapy improved glycaemic control with no increase in hypoglycaemic events in type 2 diabetics who were not controlled on oral medication
- There is a worrying increase in the prevalence of type 2 diabetes in children around the world
- Amongst the offspring of type 2 diabetics knowledge of risk factors and complications of the disease is poor
- Lifestyle changes such as weight loss and increasing physical activity should be recommended to pre-diabetics as they may benefit most from this intervention.
- As type 2 diabetes reaches epidemic proportions, weight loss maybe the key in preventing diabetes and slowing progression to established diabetes.
- Lowering cholesterol and blood pressure protects type II diabetics from cardiovascular disease
- Both lifestyle interventions or metformin can delay onset of Type 2 diabetes in people at risk.
- A review has found that tight blood pressure control is more important than class of drug when treating hypertensive diabetics
- Most practices adequately identify diabetics in their practice but many practices feel lacking in education when it comes to diabetes care
- A Finnish RCT (NEJM 2001) has shown that lifestyle changes can reduce the risk of progression to type 2 diabetes by nearly 60% over 4 years
- HBA_{1c} seems to be an additional risk factor for cardiovascular disease even in non-diabetic individuals
- Several studies have shown that ACE inhibitors have a more favourable effect on cardio-vascular outcomes, in hypertensive diabetic patients, than calcium channel blockers
- The DCCT (Diabetes Control and Complications Trial; *N. Engl. J. Med.*, 1993) showed that tight blood glucose control reduced microvascular complications in type 1 diabetics; the UKPDS now shows the same to be true in type 2 diabetics
- Integrated care for diabetics was as good as conventional care in terms of glycaemic control and patient education
- A meta-analysis has shown that dietary strategies alone cause the greatest reduction in weight in NIDDM, compared with anorectic drug treatment, behavioural and exercise therapies
- Baseline urinary albumin excretion is the most important predictor of the development of incipient or overt diabetic nephropathy
- A meta-analysis has shown that microalbuminuria is a risk factor for overall mortality and cardiovascular mortality and morbidity

- New health service framework for diabetes is impractical for use in a clinical setting.
- A qualitative and quantitative study concludes that General Practitioners have a poor awareness of the clinical significance and management of impaired glucose tolerance.
- A meta-analysis has shown that glycaemic control is better with insulin infusion therapy compared with insulin injections, but the difference in control is small
- It is unclear which factors in the general practice setting are important for ensuring optimal care for diabetic patients.

BACKGROUND

UKPDS BMJ 1995 - Drug treatment is better than diet

UKPDS 23 BMJ 1998 - six risk factors in type 2 diabetics

UKPDS 38 BMJ 1998 - Tight blood pressure control is associated with:
- a 24% reduced risk of diabetic end points; and
- a 32% reduced risk of diabetes related deaths.

Intensive blood glucose control results in a 12% reduced risk of diabetic end points.

HOT (Hypertension Optimal Treatment) Lancet 1998 - Intensive blood pressure control was more effective at reducing cardiovascular end points in diabetic than non-diabetic patients (it also looked at effect of low dose aspirin in treated hypertensives).

UKPDS 33 Lancet 1998 - Intensive blood glucose control is associated with fewer diabetic end points than less intense control. But no difference in mortality.

UKPDS 34 Lancet 1998 - In the obese, metformin should be used as a first-line agent unless contraindicated.

DCCT (Diabetes Control and Complications Trial) NEJM 1993 - Tight blood glucose control reduced microvascular complications in type 1 diabetics.

UKPDS 35 BMJ Aug 2000 - Compare this with UKPDS 33. A re-analysis of the data from an epidemiological point of view found that glycaemic control is more important than the intensive nature of the therapy. Even small reductions in HbA_{1c} will prevent diabetes-related complications and death.

UKPDS 36 BMJ Aug 2000 - Another re-analysis. A 10 mmHg reduction in blood pressure is associated with up to a 20% reduction in risk of micro/macrovascular complications. Antihypertensives have an effect over and above their blood pressure lowering effect.

CALM BMJ 2000 - Multicentre RCT, 200 people with type 2 diabetes Dual blockage of the renin-angiotensin system with both ACEI and AT1 blocker worked better than either therapy on its own, with few drop outs.

TYPE 1 DIABETES

Microalbuminuria (30-300 mg/24 h)

Thirty to forty per cent of insulin-dependent diabetics will go on to develop nephropathy (recognized by persistent proteinuria (>500 mg/

24 h)). Urinary albumin excretion is increased before reaching this stage (microalbuminuria). Poor glycaemic control (glycated haemoglobin >10%) and raised initial albumin excretion are associated with the development of persistent micro-albuminuria.

All-cause mortality is associated with:
• urinary albumin excretion;
• poor glycaemic control (one study found that a 1% increase in HBA_{1c} was associated with an 11% increase in the risk of dying).

Predictors of cardiovascular mortality include:
• microalbuminuria;
• overt nephropathy;
• arterial hypertension;
• smoking;
• age.

Intensive insulin therapy

Intensive insulin therapy has been shown to decrease the risk of developing microalbuminuria by 56%. However, in those who already have microalbuminuria, intensive therapy does not delay the onset of clinical albuminuria. In this situation the main determinant of progression to albuminuria is arterial blood pressure. Intensive insulin therapy has also been shown to prevent or delay progression to neuropathy. Intensive insulin therapy is associated with increased episodes of hypoglycaemia. Although hypoglycaemia is both unpleasant and dangerous, studies have failed to find any long-term adverse effects from receiving intensive insulin therapy.

TYPE 2 DIABETES

Drinking 2-4 alcohol-containing drinks per day is associated with a decreased risk of developing diabetes.

UKPDS (*BMJ*, Jan. 1995) found that drug treatment was better than diet alone at maintaining glycaemic control. Tighter glycaemic control was associated with more side effects. Sulphonylureas and insulin induced weight gain and hypoglycaemic episodes (chlorpropamide induced fewer hypoglycaemic episodes than glibenclamide).

Microalbuminuria

All-cause mortality and cardiovascular mortality are positively associated with microalbuminuria.

TYPE 2 DIABETES

EDITORIAL – Targeting people with pre-diabetes. Lifestyle interventions should also be aimed at people with pre-diabetes. Narayan, K.M.V., Imperatore, G. and Benjamin, S.M. *et al.* Division of Diabetes Translation, National, Centre for Chronic Disease Prevention and Health Promotion, Centres for Disease Control and Prevention, Altanta GA, USA.
***BMJ,* 325**(7361): 403-404, 24 August 2002.

Three major randomised controlled trials have confirm that effective lifestyle intervention can prevent or delay progression to type 2 diabetes in groups at high risk, such as overweight people with impaired glucose tolerance. In response to this evidence, the American Diabetes Association has recommended screening to detect people with impaired glucose tolerance or impaired fasting glucose of people aged 45 years with a body mass index of 25 or more. Those detected with impaired glucose tolerance (pre-diabetics), will be counselled on weight loss and increasing physical activity. It could be argued that the lifestyle factors targeted to prevent diabetes should be aimed at the population at large, but the author suggests that our energy should be focused on high risk groups because of the following reasons.

- There is a non-linear relation between glycaemia and diabetes with the risk threshold coinciding the onset of pre-diabetes.
- Approximately 17 million people in the United States about as many as have diabetes have pre-diabetes.
- Clinical trials have only shown benefit for people with pre-diabetes.
- All those with diabetes go through the pre-diabetes stage, therefore targeting these people will be to target future diabetics.
- The health belief model suggests that for people to comply with preventative interventions they need to perceive both risk and potential benefit.

The author suggests that success in preventing or postponing type 2 diabetics could be a catalyst for promoting lifestyle changes across society.

EDITORIAL – Prevention and cure of type 2 diabetes. Weight loss is the key to controlling the diabetes epidemic. Pinkey, J. University Department of Medicine, Diabetes and Endocrinology Research Group, University Hospital Aintree, Liverpool, UK.
***BMJ,* 325**(7358): 232-233, 3 August 2002.

Type 2 diabetes is now reaching epidemic proportions. Obesity has been causally linked to type 2 diabetes. Recent data suggest that weight management may prevent diabetes and have an impact on those with established diabetes. Obesity is defined as a body mass index above 30 kg/m 2. The prevalence of diabetes in the United States is 15% in people over 60 years of age, driven by epidemic obesity. In urban Manchester (United Kingdom), 20% of Europeans, 22% of Afro-Caribbeans, and 33% of Pakistanis had type 2 diabetes. Obesity and physical inactivity were the prinicpal associated factors.

- In a prospective study of approximately 85 000 female nurses followed for 16 years, a combination of dietary behaviour, physical activity, weight, and cigarette smoking was associated with a 91% reduction in diabetes.
- A Finnish study showed that weight loss of 3-4 kg over 4 years led to a 58% reduction in incident diabetes.

The author suggests that much could be done to prevent diabetes in individuals at high risk and that substantially greater awareness of the risk factors such as obesity is needed. The author comments that prevention of diabetes requires sustained cultural change. In those with new diabetes who are overweight, weight loss of at least 5-10% would be a logical goal alongside glycaemic and cardiovascular targets.

Review: interventions that lower cholesterol concentrations or blood pressure in diabetic patients prevent cardiovascular disease. Ganda, M.D. Joslin Diabetic Center, Boston, MA, USA.
Evidence-based Medicine, 7(4): 107, July/Aug. 2002.

Question: In patients with type 2 diabetes mellitus, do medications for intensive reduction of cholesterol and glucose concentrations and blood pressure prevent cardiovascular disease (CVD)?

The following article is briefly presented
The effect of interventions to prevent cardiovascular disease in patients with type 2 diabetes mellitus. Huang, E.S., Meigs, J.B., Singer, D.E. University of Chicago, Chicago, Illinois, USA.
Am. J. Med. **111:** 633-642, 1 Dec. 2001

This was a review of RCTs and quasi-RCTs examining the effects of intensive risk factor reduction in on the development of cardiovascular disease in type II diabetics. Eighteen trials met the inclusion criteria.
- Lowering cholesterol and blood pressure reduced cardiac event rates. Further analysis showed that this was true for secondary but not primary prevention.
- Lowering blood glucose concentrations did not reduce cardiac event rates

Commentary
Ganda comments that these results should be interpreted with caution, given various differences in the RCTs. In addition, the finding that lowering blood glucose did not reduce cardiac event rates contradicts epidemiological evidence, which suggests the opposite.

A lifestyle intervention or metformin prevented or delayed the onset of type 2 diabetes in people at risk. Motori, V.W. Mayo Clinic, Rochester, MN, USA.
Evidence-based Medicine, 7(5): 139, Sept./Oct. 2002.

Question: In overweight people with increased fasting and postload plasma glucose concentrations, does an intensive lifestyle intervention or treatment with metformin plus standard lifestlye recommendations prevent or delay onset of type 2 diabetes?

The following paper is briefly presented.
Reduction in the incidence of type 2 diabetes with lifestyle intervention or metformin. Diabetes Prevention Programme Research Group.
N. Engl. J. Med. **346:** 393-403, Feb. 2002

This double blind RCT enrolled just over 3000 patients at risk of type 2 diabetes (overweight, elevated blood glucose fasting/postload) from 27 centres in the US. The intervention arm was split into two groups: (1) Intensive lifestyle modification programme including diet and exercise; (2) Metformin glucose control. Main results:
- At 3 years diabetes was lower in the lifestyle (incidence = 4.8 patients per 100 person years) and metformin (incidence 7.8) groups than placebo group (incidence 11.0).

Commentary
They conclude that lifestyle intervention and metformin are better than placebo at reducing the risk of developing type 2 diabetes. If the ultimate goal is preventing cardiovascular disease then lifestyle modification is theoretically preferred over metformin. However, the use of metformin may be more practical as patients may not adhere to lifestyle modifications and implimenting lifestyle modification programmes requires expertise.

Insulin therapy in poorly controlled type 2 diabetic patients: does it affect quality of life? de Grauw, W.J.C., van de Lisdonk, E.H., van Gerwen, W.H.E.M., van den Hoogen, H.J.M. and van Weel, C. Department of General Practice and Social Medicine, University of Nijmegen, The Netherlands.
Br. J. Gen. Pract., **51**(468): 527-532, July 2001.

This study undertaken in The Netherlands looks at the effects of insulin therapy in type 2 diabetes. In particular they look at glycaemic control and quality of life. Patients were selected if they were poorly controlled on oral medication. Of the 38 patients starting the study, three dropped out and seven did not switch to insulin therapy.
- Glycaemic control improved significantly in those who switched over to insulin.
- There was no increase in hypoglycaemic events in those who switched over to insulin.
- Quality of life was not affected in those switching to insulin.

They conclude that GPs need not be overly concerned about switching their poorly controlled type 2 diabetics to insulin if oral therapy and diet fail.

EDITORIAL – Prevention of type 2 diabetes. Narayan, K.M., Bowman, B.A. and Engelgau, M.E. Division of Diabetes Translation, National Center for Chronic Disease Prevention and Health Promotion, Centers for Disease Control and Prevention, Altanta, GA, USA.
BMJ, **323**(7304): 63-64, 14 July 2001.

A Finnish RCT (NEJM 2001) has shown that lifestyle changes can reduce the risk of progression to type 2 diabetes by nearly 60% over 4 years. The study involved just over 500 subjects who were overweight and had impaired glucose tolerance. The subjects were advised about their weight and encouraged to exercise. They were also encouraged to reduce their intake of saturated fat, and increase their intake of dietary fibre. They estimate that 22 subjects would need to be treated for 1 year to prevent one case of diabetes. The results of the Finnish study confirm earlier results from less well designed Swedish and Chinese studies. They comment that lifestyle interventions not only prevent disease but also promote health and well being and empower people to be positive about their health, rather than fostering a reliance on medicine.

EDUCATION AND DEBATE SECTION – Should we screen for type 2 diabetes? Evaluation against National Screening Committee criteria. Warehma, N. and Griffin, S.J. Department of Public Health and Primary Care, Institute of Public Health, University of Cambridge, Cambridge, UK.
BMJ, **322**(7292): 986-988, 21 April 2001.

This article evaluates the case for a national screening programme for type 2 diabetes according to the National Screening Committee's criteria. Diabetes is an important public health problem which is associated with high morbidity and mortality. Approximately 50% of diabetes is undiagnosed. At diagnosis one quarter of people already have micro-vascular complications. The article discusses the difficulties that arise when trying to decide whom to invite for screening. For example, when using blood glucose as the test (2 hours after a glucose challenge), the risk of microvascular complications increases sharply at around 11 mmol/l. However, the risk of cardiovascular disease increases gradually over the whole range of glycaemia. The effectiveness of treatment for diabetes is related to the prevalence of undiagnosed diabetes and the background risk of cardiovascular disease. It may be better to screen high risk subgroups than to screen the whole population. One of the criteria for screening is that there should be optimal management of the condition. There is still room for improvement in the management of already diagnosed diabetes. If screening were to throw up many more cases, the current system may not be able to cope with the strain. They conclude that universal screening cannot be justified.

Risk and prevention of type II diabetes: offspring's views. Pierce, M., Harding, D. and Ridout, D. *et al.* Department of Primary Health Care and General Practice, Imperial College School of Medicine, London, UK.
Br. J. Gen. Pract., **51**(464): 194-199, March 2001.

This study was performed in order to evaluate the knowledge of diabetes amongst the offspring of type 2 diabetics. The study was performed in south London and the offspring of 152 type 2 diabetics were approached. Around 70% completed questionnaires.

- Nearly 70% thought that their risk of developing diabetes was low.
- Between 30 and 70% underestimated their risk of developing diabetes.
- Just over 50% felt that prevention was possible, but few recognized being overweight or lack of physical activity as possible risk factors.
- Knowledge of the relationship between cardiovascular disease and diabetes was poor.

In order for offspring of type 2 diabetics to reduce their risk of developing diabetes, they need to gain a better understanding of the disease.

EDITORIAL – Type 2 diabetes in children. Fagot-Campagna, A. and Narayan, K.M.V. Division of Diabetes Translation, National Center for Chronic Disease Prevention and Health Promotion, Centers for Disease Control and Prevention, Atlanta, GA, USA.
BMJ, **322**(7283): 377-378, 17 February 2001.

There is a worrying increase in the prevalence of type 2 diabetes in children around the world. The increase goes hand in hand with a rise in the prevalence of obesity and inactivity amongst children. In America the average age at diagnosis is 12–14 years and the disease affects girls more than boys. Other risk factors are:

- non-European origin;
- family history of type 2 diabetes;
- exposure to diabetes in utero;
- signs of insulin resistance.

Haemoglobin A1c tends to be in the range between 10 and 13% and these children may also have hypertension, high triglyceride levels, albuminuria, sleep apnoea and depression. Management is particularly difficult as many of the drugs used to treat adults are not licensed for children. Type 2 diabetes is poorly managed in adults and the situation is likely to be worse in children. They conclude that tackling type 2 diabetes in children will require a global strategy.

Randomised controlled trial of dual blockade of renin–angiotensin system in patients with hypertension, microalbuminuria, and non–insulin dependent diabetes: the candesartan and lisinopril microalbuminuria (CALM) study. Department of Medicine, M, Kommunehospitalet, University Hospital, Denmark.
BMJ, 321(7274): 1440–1444, 9 December 2000.

ACE inhibitors block the renin-angiotensin system. Angiotensin II type 1 (AT1) receptor blockers provide an alternative mechanism for blocking the renin-angiotension system. CALM is a multicentre RCT involving 200 people, from four countries (Australia, Denmark, Israel and Finland) which compares an ACE inhibitor (lisinopril) with an AT1 blocker (candesartan) and a combination of the two. They look at the effect on blood pressure (BP) and urinary albumin excretion in patients with type 2 diabetes, hypertension and microalbuminuria.

- Both single treatments reduced BP and urinary albumin excretion.
- The combination therapy was better than either single therapy at reducing BP and urinary albumin excretion.
- The drop out rates due to adverse effects were low.

The combined therapy effect on BP (~ 8 mmHg reduction in BP) is more than would be expected from higher doses of a single agent.

Association of glycaemia with macrovascular and microvascular complications of type 2 diabetes (UKPDS 35): prospective observational study. Stratton, I.M., Adler, A.I., Neil, H.A.W. and Matthews, D.R. et al. on behalf of the UK Prospective Diabetes Study Group.
BMJ, 321(7258): 405-412, 12 August 2000.

UKPDS 35 is an observational study involving around 3600 patients (White, Asian Indian and Afro-Caribbean). The aim of this study was to assess the effect of hyperglycaemia (HbA_{1c}) on microvascular and macrovascular complications. HbA_{1c} averaged over the 10 years is reported as the 'updated mean HbA_{1c}'.

- Microvascular and macrovascular and all cause mortality were strongly associated with the updated mean HbA_{1c}.
- With increasing hyperglycaemia, the risk of microvascular complications increased more steeply than macrovascular complications. Although, at near normal concentrations of HbA_{1c}, the risk of MI was 2-3 times higher than the risk of microvascular complication.
- Every 1% reduction in HbA_{1c} was associated with:
  - 43% reduction in peripheral vascular disease;
  - 37% reduction in amputation;
  - 16% reduction in heart failure;
  - 14% reduction in MI;
  - 12% reduction in stroke.
  - In general terms, a 1% reduction in HbA_{1c} was associated with a 37% reduction in microvascular complications and a 21% reduction in any diabetes-related end point.

- There was no evidence of a lower threshold for glycaemia, beyond which there was no risk of complications. Hence the lower the HbA_{1c}, and the closer to normal it is, the better.

Previous UKPDS results have suggested that intensive control of blood glucose, with sulphonyl ureas and insulin, was the reason for the decrease in risk of complications. This present analysis suggests that the reduction in risk is due to a lowering of the HbA_{1c} and not the intensive nature of the therapy.

Previously UKPDS reported a 16% reduction in risk of MI for the intensive therapy group. This figure is very similar to the 14% reduction seen in the present analysis and the former is likely to be due to glycaemic control and not intensive therapy.

They conclude that even small reductions in HbA_{1c} will prevent diabetes-related complications and death.

Association of systolic blood pressure with microvascular and microvascular complications of type 2 diabetes (UKPDS 36): prospective observational study.

Adler, A., Stratton, I.M., Neil, H.A.W. and Yudkin, J.S. *et al.* on behalf of the UK Prospective Diabetes Study Group.
BMJ, **321**(7258): 412-419, 12 August 2000.

UKPDS 36, like 35 uses complementary epidemiological data from the clinical trial. This provides an epidemiological analysis of the association between systolic blood pressure over time and complications of type 2 diabetes. Patients were just over 4800 White, Asian Indian and Afro-Caribbean diabetics.

- Over the 10 year period, risk of all complications (except cataracts) and death was strongly associated with the updated mean systolic blood pressure.
- The risk of MI and microvascular complications, both showed a strong association, but the risk of MI was twice as high as the risk of microvascular complications.
- A 10 mmHg reduction in systolic blood pressure was associated with a reduction in macrovascular and microvascular complications by between 12 and 19%.
- There was no threshold below which there was no decrease in risk. Hence, the closer to normal the systolic blood pressure the better.
- Compared with the actual clinical trial, tight blood pressure control had a stronger effect on heart failure, stroke and diabetes-related death. Analysis suggests that the antihypertensive drugs had an effect on risk that was in addition to their blood pressure lowering effects. (For example, ACE inhibitors may prevent heart failure and hence reduce the risk of stroke and death).
- The results from the clinical trial did not show an effect on MI. However when the size of the effect from the clinical trial is translated to the epidemiological setting, a reduced risk of MI is in fact an appropriate finding.

The early assessment and management of blood pressure in diabetics is of paramount importance, to prevent complications and death.

EDITORIAL – Thiazolidinediones for type 2 diabetes. Krentz, A.J., Bailey, C.J. and Melander, A.
BMJ, **321**(7256): 252-253, 29 July 2000.

Troglitazone was introduced briefly in 1997. Like metformin it sensitizes target tissue to insulin. Troglitazone and other glitazones (thiazolidine-diones):
- reduce glucose concentrations and circulating non-esterified fatty acids;
- increase HDL.

Weight gain is common but there seems to be a redistribution from central obesity.

Troglitazone was withdrawn after a few weeks because of reports from the USA of deaths associated with hepatotoxicity. Rosiglitazone has recently been introduced in the UK. It and pioglitazone will be licensed for the following:
- as an add-on to metformin in obese patients;
- as an add-on to sulphonyl ureas if metformin is contraindicated or not tolerated.

Combinations of glitazones with insulin are contraindicated because of an increased risk of cardiac failure. Contraindications to the use of glitazones are hepatic failure or if the alanine aminotransferase is more than 2.5 times normal, and cardiac failure.

Glitazones induce the cytochrome P450 and hence may reduce the efficacy of the oral contraceptive pill.

Survey of diabetes care in general practice in England and Wales. Pierce, M., Agarwal, G. and Ridout, D. Department of General Practice and Primary Health Care, Imperial College School of Medicine, London, UK.
Br. J. Gen. Pract., **50**(456): 542-545, July 2000.

In 1997 the following key features were recommended by the British Diabetic Association (BDA) and Primary Care Diabetes (PCD) UK, as prerequisites for providing effective care for diabetics in general practice.
- Protected time for diabetes care.
- Written management protocols agreed with local diabetologists.
- Disease register.
- Practice nurses with some knowledge of diabetes.

This study is the first national survey of diabetes care in general practice. It was a postal questionnaire completed by a random sample of around 1300 practices (response rate 70%).
- Most (96%) practices had a diabetic register.
- Most ($\sim$70%) had diabetic clinics.
- Most of these ($\sim$60%) were run by a GP and a nurse. Around a third were run solely by nurses.

- The prevalence of diabetes in those with a register was just under 2%, which is in line with published prevalence rates (range 1.5–2.1%).
- Just over half of practices had a shared care protocol with the secondary care team.
- Most practices felt that they needed further diabetes training. Nearly 50% of practices had only received a half-day training session in diabetes in the preceding 3 years.

CLINICAL REVIEW – Intensive blood glucose control reduced type 2 diabetes mellitus–related end–points.

and

Metformin reduced diabetes–related end–points and all–cause mortality in overweight patients with type 2 diabetes. Commentator, Gerstein, H.C. McMaster University Health Sciences Centre, Hamilton, Ont., Canada.
Evidence-based Medicine, 4(1): 11, Jan./Feb. 1999.

The following articles were briefly presented
Intensive blood–glucose control with sulphonylureas or insulin compared with conventional treatment and risk of complication in patients with type 2 diabetes (UKPDS 33).
Lancet, **352:** 837–853, 12 Sept. 1998.

This UKPDS study involved 10 years of follow up and 23 hospital-based diabetic clinics in the UK, representing around 3870 patients with newly diagnosed type 2 diabetes. Around 2730 patients were allocated to intensive treatment, aiming at a fasting plasma glucose of <6 mmol/l. Intensive therapy included diet and oral agents (chlorpropamide, glipizide, glibenclamide or metformin) or insulin. Around 1140 patients were allocated to conventional dietary therapy aiming for a fasting plasma glucose of <15 mmol/l.
- The authors found that, for the intensive treatment group,
  - glycated haemoglobin was lower than in the conventional therapy group;
  - there were fewer diabetic-related clinical end-points;
  - there was less microvascular disease;
  - there were more episodes of major hypoglycaemia;
  - there was more weight gain.
- There was no difference for macrovascular disease, diabetes-related deaths and all-cause mortality.

Effect of intensive blood–glucose control with metformin on complications in overweight patients with type 2 diabetes (UKPDS 34).
Lancet, **352**(854–865): 12 Sept. 1998.

This UKPDS study involved nearly 11 years of follow-up, 15 hospital-based clinics, representing around 1700 patients who were newly diagnosed diabetics with a body weight of ≥120% of ideal. Patients were allocated to intensive blood glucose control with metformin, chlorpropamide, glibenclamide or insulin, aiming for fasting plasma glucose levels of <6 mmol/l or to conventional dietary therapy aiming for a normal body weight and fasting plasma glucose levels of <15 mmol/l.

- Compared with the conventional therapy group, metformin
  - reduced diabetes-related end-points;
  - reduced diabetes-related deaths;
  - reduced all-cause mortality.
- Compared with other intensive therapies, metformin
  - reduced diabetes-related end-points;
  - reduced all-cause mortality;
  - resulted in fewer hypoglycaemic episodes.

Commentary

The DCCT (Diabetes Control and Complications Trial; *N. Engl. J. Med.*, 1993) showed that tight blood glucose control reduced microvascular complications in type 1 diabetics. The UKPDS now shows the same to be true in type 2 diabetics (with a trend towards a decline in risk of MI as well). Caution should be exercised when using metformin in all groups (obese and non-obese). Further analysis has shown that diabetes-related deaths and all-cause mortality may be increased.

- Reducing blood glucose should now be a major aim in the management of type 2 diabetes.
- Because of the adverse effects, insulin should be used as second-line behind other oral agents.
- In the obese, metformin should be used as a first-line agent unless contraindicated.

TYPE 2 DIABETES: RISK FACTORS

PRIMARY CARE SECTION – Impaired glucose tolerance: qualitative and quantitative study of general practitioners knowledge and perceptions. Wylie, G., Hungin, A.P.S. and Neely, J. Centre for Integrated Health Care Research, Wolfson Research Institute, University of Durham, Stockton-on Tees, UK.
BMJ, 324(7347): 1190-1192, 18 May 2002.

The recently published Diabetes NSF recommends that, in order to reduce the incidence of Type 2 diabetes, those with impaired glucose tolerance should be identified and managed. The NSF highlights the fact that impaired glucose tolerance is also associated with an increase risk of cardiovascular disease.

Twenty-six GPs completed questionnaires and participated in four focus group discussions, while eight GPs participated in semi-structured interviews.

The author highlights a number of points:

- GPs perceive the need for considerable extra resources in order to implement the new Diabetes NSF.

- Awareness of the existence of impaired glucose tolerance is good, but awareness of the prevalence, clinical significance and management is poor.
- In the UK, the prevalence of impaired glucose tolerance in the 35-65 year age group is around 17%, however, only a small proportion of patients with impaired glucose tolerance are known to practices.
- GPs are unwilling to screen and intervene in this condition being reluctant to divert resources away from other areas.
- GPs have major reservations about the appropriateness and effectiveness of giving lifestyle advice to patients with impaired glucose tolerance.
- There is concern amongst GPs that screening and treating impaired glucose tolerance medicalises an essentially social problem.
- GPs expressed positive attitudes towards a health educational approach to the problem, promoting fruit at school, exercise and government led health promotion.

TYPE 2 : MANAGEMENT

EDUCATION AND DEBATE SECTION – Effective diabetes care: a need for realistic targets. Winocour, Peter H. Department of Diabetes and Endocrinology, Queen Elizabeth II Hospital, Welwyn Garden City, Herts, UK.
BMJ, **324**(7373): 1577-1580, 29 June 2002.

A national service framework for the optimal care of diabetes has recently been published. Discussion focuses on type 2 diabetes. Current evidence suggests that strict control of blood sugar and blood pressure can reduce adverse vascular outcomes, and that treatment of dyslipidaemia and use of anti-platelet medication can prevent secondary macrovascular disease. However, the main drawbacks of the framework are that:
- Only 50–70 of patients can attain the targets set for glycaemia, lipids and blood pressure.
- Patients are unwilling to comply with their prescribed polypharmacology; up to a tenth of patients will require three hypoglycaemic agents, three anti-hypertensive agents, two hypolipidaemia agents and aspirin.

It is for these reasons that it is argued these guidelines are impractical, and that treatment programmes tailored to each individual patient are more effective in routine clinical practice.

TYPE 1 DIABETES

Glycaemic control with subcutaneous insulin infusion compared with intensive insulin injections in patients with type 1 diabetes: meta-analysis of randomised controlled trials. Pickup, J., Mattock, M. and Kerry, S. Department of Chemical Pathology, Guys, Kings and St Thomas's School of Medicine, London, UK.
BMJ, **324**(7339): 705-708, 23 March 2002.

This aim of this meta-analysis (MA) was to compare glycaemic control using insulin infusion with glycaemic control using insulin injections in type 1 diabetics. Thirteen trials met the inclusion criteria, (~300 subjects).

- Glycaemic control was with infusions rather than injections. The blood glucose concentration on average was 1 mmol/l lower in those receiving continuous insulin infusion subcutaneously as opposed to insulin injections.
- Patients using insulin infusion had, on average, 0.5% lower levels of HbA1 compared to the insulin injection patients.
- Patients on insulin infusion therapy were also found to have a much reduced variability in blood glucose concentrations.
- The improved glycaemic control achieved by insulin infusion also resulted in an average dosage reduction of 14% in the amount of insulin required.

They conclude that, glycaemic control is better with insulin infusion therapy but the difference in control is small. This can reduce the risk of microvascular complications but the cost effectiveness for this degree of benefit needs to be assessed.

OTHERS

Review: intensive blood pressure control and drugs reduce morbidity and mortality in hypertension and diabetes mellitus. Commentator, Victor Montori, Mayo Clinic, Rochester, Minnesota, USA.
Evidence–based Medicine, **6**(2): 44, March/April 2001.

Question: In patients with hypertension and diabetes mellitus, what is the effectiveness of various antihypertensive treatments?

The following article is briefly presented
High blood pressure and diabetes mellitus. Are all antihypertensives drugs created equal? Grossman, E., Messerli, F.H. and Goldbourt, U.
Arch. Intern. Med., **160**: 2447–2452, 11 Sept. 2000.

The aim of this review was to assess the effectiveness of antihypertensives in reducing morbidity and mortality in hypertensive diabetic patients. Eight studies (around 5200 patients) are analysed. The studies compared drug treatment with placebo. Follow up ranged from 2 to 8 years.

- They found that intensive blood pressure control was more important than the class of antihypertensive (diuretic, β-blocker, ACE inhibitor, calcium antagonist).

Commentary

These studies compared drug with placebo. All drugs were effective but this does not tell us how they compare with one another. The question still remains as to which drug should be used as first line in diabetics with hypertension. Ramipril reduces cardiovascular risk by 25% in hypertensive diabetics. This effect is over and above a purely antihypertensive effect. Montori suggests that ACE inhibitors should still be considered as first line, but tight blood pressure control is also important.

EDITORIAL – The management of diabetes. Griffin, S.J. Department of Public Health And Primary Care, Institute of Public Health, Cambridge University, Cambridge, UK. **BMJ, 323**(7319): 946-947, 27 October 2001.

The management of diabetic patients has, in recent years, been steadily moving from specialist hospital clinics to the general practice setting. It is, however, unclear which sector gives the best outcomes. This editorial summarises recent evidence on diabetes care in general practice:
- Giving extra training to GPs and improving the recall and review system for diabetic patients in primary care can reduce the morbidity and mortality associated with Type 2 diabetes.
- With appropriate training and facilities, the standard of diabetes management in primary care compares favourably with that in hospital practice.
- Personalised diabetes management plans may be associated with improved outcome in Type 2 diabetes.

The author suggests potential difficulties in future primary care diabetes management:
- The effect on overall costs of care is uncertain.
- GPs not specifically motivated towards diabetes management may not provide adequate levels of care; with the projected increase in diabetics there may be insufficient GPs to manage diabetes in primary care.
- It is unclear which factors in the general practice setting are important for ensuring optimal patient care.

Glycated haemoglobin, diabetes and mortality in men in Norfolk cohort of European Prospective Investigation of Cancer and Nutrition (EPIC–Norfolk). Khaw, K.T., Wareham, N. and Luben, R. *et al.* Department of Public Health and Primary Care, Institute of Public Health, University of Cambridge School of Clinical Medicine.
BMJ, **322**(7277): 15-18, 6 January 2001.

This study looked at the association between population HBA_{1c}, diabetes and mortality. Subjects were taken from the Norfolk cohort of European Prospective Investigation of Cancer and Nutrition, which consists of around 26 000 men and women aged 45–79, resident in Norfolk. Baseline data were collected between 1993 and 1997. The study represents follow up data on men until December 1999.

- Men with diabetes or undiagnosed diabetes had the greatest risk of dying. A 1% increase in HBA_{1c} was associated with a roughly 30% increase in all cause mortality and a 40% increase in mortality from cardiovascular mortality.
- When men with diabetes or heart disease were removed, increasing HBA_{1c} concentrations were still associated with increased risk of death and there seemed to be no lower cut off point.
- The majority of the population had a HBA_{1c} between 5 and 6.9%. When the population was taken as a whole more than 80% of the excess mortality was found in this group. The 5% of the population who had diabetes were responsible for less than 20% of excess mortality.
- They estimate that in the non-diabetic population, 12% of the excess deaths could be prevented by lowering the population mean HBA_{1c} by 0.1%, which would reduce deaths by 5%.

HBA_{1c} seems to be an additional risk factor for cardiovascular disease even in non-diabetic individuals. Population lifestyle changes may be helpful in reducing population levels of HBA_{1c}.

FURTHER READING

Cost effectiveness of an intensive blood glucose control policy in patients with type 2 diabetes: economic analysis alongside randomised controlled trial (UKPDS 41). Gray, A., Raikon, M., McGuire, A., Fenn, P. *et al.*, on behalf of the United Kingdom Prospective Diabetes Study Group.
BMJ, **320**(7246): 1373-1378, 20 May 2000.

Seeing what you want to see in randomised controlled trials: versions and perversions of UKPDS data. McCormack, J. and Greenhalgh, T.
BMJ, **320**(7251): 1720-1723, 24 June 2000.

Reducing long-term complication of type 2 diabetes.
Drug and Therapeutics Bulletin, **37**(11): 84-87, Nov. 1999.

DIET

> - Eating seafood regularly prior to 20 weeks of pregnancy may have a positive effect on intrauterine growth.
> - Folate deficiency is associated with depression and dementia, and may also be related to ageing.

EDUCATION AND DEBATE SECTION – Folic acid, ageing, depression and dementia. Reynolds, E.H. Institute of Epileptology, King's College, London, UK. **Br. J. Gen. Pract., 324**(7352): 1512-1515, 22 June 2002.

This paper aimed to review the evidence relating folate deficiency to depression and dementia, especially in the ageing nervous system. The evidence discussed has shown important correlations, including:
- A number of different reasons for deficiency are observed; some related to ageing, some secondary to mental illness, and some primary causes.
- There is a definite aetiological link between folate deficiency and specific effects on mood, drive, initiative, alertness, concentration, psychomotor speed and social activity.
- The duration of folate deficiency is important, along with degree of deficiency and predisposing factors, e.g. genetic factors.

Large-scale community-based studies of folate deficiency may provide evidence for the prophylaxis of vascular disease, and prevention, or at least reduction of depression and dementia.

Low consumption of seafood in early pregnancy as a risk factor for pre-term delivery: prospective cohort study. Olsen, S.F. and Secher, N.J. Danish Epidemiology Science Centre, Statens Serum Institut, Copenhagen, Denmark. **BMJ, 324**(7335): 447-450, 23 February 2002.

This prospective cohort study involved around 8700 pregnant women in Denmark. They were grouped according to seafood consumption during pregnancy, determined by a questionnaire at weeks 16 and 30 of pregnancy. The aim of the study was to evaluate the relationship between eating seafood during pregnancy, and the risk of pre-term delivery and low birth weight.
- Increasing fish intake in pregnancy decreased incidence of pre-term delivery, retarded intrauterine growth, and low birth weight.
- Duration of gestation and mean birth weight increased with increasing fish intake during pregnancy.

Olsen acknowledges the risk of confounding factors influencing these results. This and other studies suggest that fish oil intake influences intrauterine growth prior to weeks 16-20. However, other retrospective studies have reported contradictory findings.

FURTHER READING

See 'Lipids' for

Dietary fat intake and prevention of cardiovascular disease: systematic review. Manchester Dental and Education Centre (MANDEC). University Dental Hospital of Manchester, Manchester.
BMJ, **322**(7289): 757-763, 31 March 2001.

DOCTOR–PATIENT RELATIONSHIP

- A Northumbrian retrospective study found that frequent attendance is a function of chronic health problems
- A west of Scotland study found that increasing deprivation was associated with shorter consultations i.e. evidence of Tudor Hart's inverse care law (*Lancet*, 1971)
- Self management booklets do not reduce GP attendance rates
- A questionnaire survey found that the most common reason for removing a patient from the practice list was violent, threatening or abusive behaviour. A large proportion of GPs said they might consider removing patients who effectively cost the practice money
- A cohort study based in primary care shows that correcting for age and sex variations in consulting patterns is vital for defining populations of patients who are "frequent attenders" at GP clinics.
- Communication skills are effectively learned using ongoing feedback from real consultations, and by attending relevant courses
- One study found that the longest consultations are with women in urban areas, regarding issues perceived as psychosocial by the doctor and patient and consultation time varies between different countries
- A quantitative study conducted by postal questionnaire, concludes that patients with serious medical conditions place considerable value on continuity of care
- The use of depersonalized metaphors by the doctor may be a reassuring reinterpretation of the patients vivid descriptions
- A study by P. Little has shown that high attenders in general practice are more likely to suffer with MUPS.
- A study by P. Little et al. has shown that high consultation rates in children can largely be explained by parental factors and parental anxiety/depression.
- Different aspects of the patient centred approach are associated with patient outcomes in primary care
- New types of decision support systems (usually interactive and computer based) are being developed which will enable patients to take a more active role in the decision making process
- Clinical treatments must not be viewed in isolation but in the context of a doctor-patient relationship, which has the ability to modify therapeutic effectiveness.
- A valuable first step in involving patients in shared decision making is to ask them how much they want to be involved in this process.
- Patients seem to prefer smaller practices even though consultation lengths tend to be shorter in such practices.
- One of the recommendations by the Select Committee on Public Administration is that GPs should not be allowed to remove patients without a reason or without getting permission from the Health Authority. In one study most GPs (81%) agreed that GPs should not have to comply with such recommendations.
- An observational study concludes that patients at risk of atrial fibrillation consider stroke avoidance more important than the increased risk of bleeding associated with anticoagulants.

- A study found that the recording of health experiences, such as pain or fatigue, is associated with poor patient compliance when paper diaries are used.
- GPs need longer consultations with their patients.
- Identifying and empathising with patients emotions is vital for good
- Further research confirms that frequent attenders are more likely to be female and to be referred to psychiatric services.

BACKGROUND

Frequent attenders (FA) can account for up to 6% of practice workload. Studies have analysed the characteristics of a frequent attender. Some of these are:
- mainly female;
- elderly;
- chronic or multiple health problems;
- associated with depression. Patients with symptoms of depression are 17 times more likely than controls to be FAs.

FAs tend to see their consultations as a dynamic process having three stages. These involve:
- developing the relationship with their GP;
- validating the relationship, by gathering information that supports their view;
- consolidation of the relationship, by testing and setting boundaries of power, knowledge and personal interaction.

Some might argue that we are failing to cater for the needs of our FAs.

There may be a certain amount of overlap between FAs and **heart sink (HS) patients.** O'Dowd first used the term heart sink in 1988 to describe the negative reaction the doctor has to the patient. Heart sinks however tend to be a product of the doctor as well as the patient (*BJGP*, June 1995). GPs with high numbers of HS patients tend to have:
- lower job satisfaction;
- greater perceived workload;
- lack of training in counselling/communication;
- lack of appropriate qualifications.

The HS views the doctor as a source of their 'salvation'. The doctor, however, wants to spend as little time as possible with the patient. The unfulfilled nature of the doctor-patient interactions in these situations, may simply encourage the patient to seek further consultations until 'salvation' is encountered.

Randomised controlled trial of self management leaflets and booklets for minor illness provided by post. Little, P., Somerville, J. and Williamson, I. *et al.* Southampton, UK. *BMJ,* **322**(7296): 1214-1217, 19 May 2001.

This Southampton study analyses whether giving information booklets or summary cards to patients will reduce general practice attendance rates. Around 4000 patients from six general practices are randomly allocated to receive either a card detailing surgery times, a booklet containing details of 42 common complaints entitled 'What should I do?' or a two-sided summary card of respiratory and other common ailments. Questionnaires were sent out initially and at 12 months.

- There was a 4% reduction in those attending frequently for minor ailments in the two intervention groups compared with control group.
- However, compared with the previous year, there were only small and non-significant reductions in attendance rates for minor illnesses in the intervention groups.
- Most found the interventions useful and said that having the booklets and summary cards increased their confidence about managing common ailments. However, this did not alter their willingness to wait any longer before seeing their GP.

They conclude that it may not be cost effective to send booklets and summary cards to patients.

Assessment of impact of information booklets on use of healthcare services: randomised controlled trial. Heaney, D., Wyke, S. and Wilson, R. *et al.* Department of Community Health Sciences-General Practice, University of Edinburgh, Edinburgh, UK. *BMJ,* **322**(7296): 1218-1221, 19 May 2001.

This Scottish study evaluated the effect of information booklets sent to patients on general practice attendance rates. It was an RCT involving around 9000 patients and 20 general practices. Patients were randomized to one of three groups: (1) controls, who received no information; (2) intervention group 1, who received the information booklet 'What should I do?'; (3) intervention group 2 who received the 'Health Care Manual'. They analyzed use of health services 12 months after receiving the information.

- Use of health services did not change after receiving the booklet or manual, for minor illnesses or for out of hours consultations.
- The Health Care Manual was associated with relatively reduced health service use compared with 'What should I do?', but this did not effect overall health service use.

General practitioners' reasons for removing patients from their lists: postal survey in England and Wales. Pickin, M., Sampson, F., Munro, J. and Nicholl, J. Medical Care Research Unit, University of Sheffield, Sheffield, UK.
BMJ, 322(7295): 1158-1159, 12 May 2001.

This questionnaire survey involved 1000 GPs from a random sample of practices. It examines reasons for removal of patients from practice lists. The response rate was 76%. Three hundred practices (40%) had removed patients in the preceding 6 months.
- The most common reason was violent, threatening or abusive behaviour (59%).
- Less common reasons were failure to comply with childhood immunizations or cervical smear testing (1% and 7% respectively).
- Around 50% of GPs said that financial incentives might influence potential removal from the list e.g. smear/immunization targets, out-of-hours payments and drug budgets.

Preferences of patients for patient centred approach to consultation in primary care: observational study. Little, P., Everitt, H. and Williamson, I. *et al.* Primary Medical Care Group, Community Clinical Sciences Division, University of Southampton, Aldermoor Health Centre, Southampton, UK.
BMJ, 322(7284): 468-472, 24 February 2001.

A theoretical model of the 'patient-centred' approach to the consultation has been advocated. It has five main components:
1. exploring patient's experience of the disease, their ideas, concerns and expectations;
2. understanding the whole person, including the emotional and social context;
3. partnership; encompassing the roles of the doctor and patient, goals of treatment and priorities of treatment;
4. health promotion;
5. enhancing the doctor-patient relationship through sharing and caring and hence promoting the healing relationship.

An additional component is 'efficient use of time'.

This study explores the patient's desire for a patient centred consultation. Over 800 patients from three practices filled in a questionnaire before and after their consultation.
- Three main domains were identified from the patient's point of view:
  1. communication - including listening, the doctor exploring the patient's concerns, as well as giving clear explanations and information;
  2. partnership including mutual agreement;
  3. health promotion.
- Patients wanting this approach were more likely to be out of work, unwell, frequent attenders and worried about their condition.

The patient perceived model does not marry up entirely with the theoretical model. Doctors need to be sensitive towards those people who may require this approach, namely those who are disadvantaged socio-economically or those suffering with ill health.

THE CONSULTATION

Consultation length in general practice: cross sectional study in six European countries. Deveugele, M., Derese, A. and van den Brink-Muinen, A. *et al.* Department of General Practice and Primary Health Care, Ghent University, Ghent, Belgium.
***BMJ,* 325**(7362): 472-476, 13 August 2002.

This study evaluated the determinants of consultation length in general practice particularly focusing on the effects of psychosocial problems. Data was gathered using patient questionnaires, and by videotaping some 3674 consultations, by 190 GPs from six European countries. The GP sample group had lower than average workloads, hence the authors caution against generalization of their results.
- Mean consultation length (10.7 minutes) was determined by variables relating to patients (55%), doctors (22%), and the doctors country (23%)
- The authors attribute differences in consultation length in different countries, to differences in primary healthcare organisation and doctors renumeration arrangements. They suggest that further research be carried out in this area.
- Consultations concerning a new problem, those in urban practices, and with older or female patients were generally longer. Doctors age and sex, and the patients level of education, had no bearing on consultation length. Consultation time decreased slightly with increasing GP workload.
- Patients reasons for consulting did not increase the consultation time. However psychosocial and other issues identified by the GP, but not mentioned by patients, increased consultation length.

Evolving general practice consultation in Britain: issues of length and context. Freeman, G.K., Horder, J.P. and Howie, J.G.R. *et al.* Centre for Primary Care and Social Medicine, Imperial College of Science, Technology and Medicine, London, UK.
***BMJ,* 324**(7342): 880-882, 13 April 2002.

This paper systematically reviewed current opinion and 14 relevant papers, regarding the length of General Practitioners consultations with patients.
- The best consultations are those that directly address the patients concerns, in the context that these problems affect their lives.
- Longer consultations allow the GP to deal more effectively with psychosocial aspects of the presenting complaint, and so are of benefit

to the patient. They are also associated with reduced rates of prescribing.

- Shorter consultations may be more appropriate for trivial complaints requiring a Doctors signature on a prescription or sick note, or for younger patients.
- Patient confidence is decreasing due to a range of factors:
  1 Reduced access to primary care owing to appointment systems which were originally introduced to reduce waiting times;
  2 Less sympathetic treatment of minor problems due to the increasing number of serious illnesses dealt by GPs;
  3 More than one doctor dealing with each patient meaning there is less scope for developing a good doctor-patient relationship.
- Long consultations are essential to providing a good standard of care, as GPs have to deal with acute symptoms, health promotion, and manage chronic illnesses for each patient.

The authors conclude that the need for longer consultations is not in dispute. Research needs to determine how best to introduce these changes.

A concordance-based study of metaphoric expressions used by general practitioners and patients in consultation. Skelton, J.R., Wearn, A.M. and Hobb, F.D.R. Department of Primary Care and General Practice, University of Birmingham, Birmingham, UK.
Br. J. Gen. Pract., 52(475): 114-118, 1 February 2002.

This study analyses the metaphors used by doctors and patients in the consultation. Nearly 400 consultations were analyzed.

- Doctors tend to use metaphors relating to machines to describe how the body works e.g. system, waterworks, repair.
- Doctors view themselves as problem solvers and controllers of disease rather than curers of disease.
- Patients use vivid metaphors to describe their illness.
- Patients tend to view themselves (self) and their bodies as separate entities.

The use of depersonalised metaphors by the doctor may be a reassuring reinterpretation of the patients vivid descriptions. On the other hand it may be important for doctors to reflect upon their use of such metaphors.

OTHERS

EDITORIAL – Communications and emotions. Buckman, R. 55 Eglinton Avenue East, Suite 601, Toronto, Canada.
BMJ, 325(7366): 672, 28 September 2002.

Good communication skills are vital to being a good doctor, but such skills are not easy to acquire. Training in communication skills has been shown to improve the diagnosis and treatment of various conditions, and can be especially effective in palliative care and dealing with chronic illness.

Dealing with emotions both those of the doctor and of the patient is important for effective communication. The author breaks this down as identifying emotions and their sources, then communicating an acknowledgement of the connection between the two. The doctor does not, however, have to actually experience the emotion in order to empathise with the patient.

Various techniques are available for teaching communication skills, including the use of standardised patients, recording consultations for feedback using the video, and viewing pre-recorded sample consultations.

The author concludes that good communication skills make a good impression on patients, and are vital for meeting their expectations.

CLINICAL REVIEW SECTION – Key communication skills and how to acquire them.
Maguire, P. and Pitceathly, C. Cancer Research UK Psychological Medicine Group, Christie Hospital NHS Trust, Manchester, UK.
BMJ, **325**(7366): 697-700, 28 September 2002.

Effective communication greatly benefits doctors and patients alike, however many doctors are unskilled at this. The authors attribute this to lack of communication skills training, coupled with a lack of confidence in using such skills, owing to a perceived lack of support from colleagues. However, they acknowledge recent steps to improve these aspects of medical school teaching.

Key communication strategies doctors could use include:
- Establish eye contact, and encourage patients to explain their complaint chronologically. Summarise the information given, and enquire about psychosocial implications, empathising with the patient
- Ascertain patients understanding of their condition, and give information in a structured manner, confirming they have understood what has been said
- Include patients in decisions regarding their treatment.

Communication skills teaching should include:
- Information for participants, relating to existing communication deficiencies, their effect, and how they can be addressed, with evidence to support new techniques
- Videotaped consultations or simulated patients, supported by constructive feedback and suggestions as to how patient interaction can be improved

Doctors can most effectively learn good communication skills by attending relevant courses, and receiving ongoing feedback from real consultations. The authors suggest further research should compare the efficacy of learning in a multidisciplinary environment compared to within one discipline; and of residential courses compared to workshops.

Continuity of care in general practice: a survey of patients views. Schers, H., Webster, S. and van den Hoogen, H. *et al.* Department of General Practice, University Medical Centre, St. Radboud, Nijmegen, Netherlands.
Br. J. Gen. Pract., **52**(479): 459-462, 1 June 2002.

The main objectives of this study were to assess patients views on personal continuity of care and to determine the extent to which these views are related to patients characteristics. Postal questionnaires were completed by 644 patients across 35 different general practices throughout the Netherlands.

The authors highlight a number of points:

- Recent developments, including an increase in part-time working, GP specialisation, the enlargement of practices and more extensive out of hours services all serve to decrease personal doctor continuity of care

- Continuity of care in general practice is associated with a number of potential benefits, including increased levels of patient satisfaction, recovery and trust.

- Patients with family problems and serious medical conditions place considerable value on continuity of care.

- Patients rank an overall understanding of their medical condition, their personal and family background, together with feeling that it is easier to talk to their own GP, as being the main reasons for preferring personal continuity of care.

- Characteristics such as age, sex and frequency of visits to the GP have only a minor influence on patients views towards continuity of care.

Patient non-compliance with paper diaries. Stone, A.A., Shiffman, S. and Schwartz, J.E. *et al.* Department of Psychiatry and Behavioural Science, Stony Brook University, Stony Brook, New York, USA.
BMJ, **324**(7347): 1193-1194, 18 May 2002.

For some time doctors have asked patients to record health experiences, such as pain or fatigue, using diaries instead of recall. This leads to more accurate clinical data on which to base management decisions. In this study 80 adults with chronic pain were assigned to either a paper or electronic diary group, with 40 in each group. Patients were instructed to complete diary entries three times per day for 21 days. The author highlights several points:

- The patients in the paper diary group reported compliance of 90%, but actual compliance was found to be less than 20%.

- Three quarters of those completing paper diaries had at least one day when data was recorded retrospectively.

- With those in the electronic diary group, actual compliance was 94%.

Review: cognitive care and combined cognitive and emotional care interventions may influence patients health outcomes. Commentator, Paul Hadet, Houston Veterans Affairs Medical Center, Houston, Texas, USA.
Evidence-based Medicine, **6**(6): 181, Nov./Dec. 2001

Question: Do cognitive and emotional care interventions during patient-clinician interactions affect patients health outcomes?

The following article is briefly presented

Influence of context effects on health outcomes: a systematic review. Di Blasi, Z., Harkness, E. and Ernest, E. *et al.*
Lancet, **357**: 757–62, 10 March 2001

Twenty five randomized controlled trials met the inclusion criteria. A MA was not performed because of heterogeneity.

- Patients given a firm diagnosis and good prognosis did better than those given an uncertain diagnosis.
- Blood pressure was lower in patients told to expect a lower blood pressure at the next visit than patients told to expect a higher reading.
- A positive doctor-patient interaction decreased pain and increased recovery time more than neutral consultations.
- They conclude that doctor-patients interactions can affect health outcomes.

Commentary

Hadet concludes that clinical treatments must not be viewed in isolation but in the context of a doctor-patient relationship, which has the ability to modify therapeutic effectiveness.

Observational study of effect of patient centredness and positive approach on outcomes of general practice consultations. Little, P., Everitt, H. and Willamson, I. *et al.* Primary Care Group, Community Clinical Sciences Division, Faculty of Medicine, Health and Biological Sciences, Southampton University, Aldermoor Health Centre, Southampton, UK
BMJ, 323(7318): 908-911, 20 October 2001.

The aim of this questionnaire study was to examine which aspects of a patient centred approach are related to patient outcomes in primary care. Eight hundred and sixty five consecutive patients from three practices took part in the study, of which 76% completed questionnaires before and after their consultation.

Patient satisfaction was related to communication and partnership, which requires that the doctor takes an interest in the patient, and involves the patient in the decision making process.

Satisfaction was also related to a positive approach, which involves the doctor being clear about the nature of the problem and when it would resolve.

Patient enablement was related to the doctor being interested in the effect the condition would have on the patients life.

Patient enablement was also related to health promotion and a positive approach.

Referrals were reduced when the patient felt that they had a personal relationship with their doctor.

EDITORIAL – A key medical decision maker: the patient. Deyo, R.A. Professor of Medicine Center for Cost and Outcomes Research, Department of Medicine, University of Washington, Seattle, USA.
BMJ, **323**(7311): 466-467, 1 September 2001.

New types of decision support systems are being developed which will enable patients to take a more active role in the decision making process. The new tools tend to be interactive, use computer technology and best evidence (based on systematic reviews and Randomised trials).

Studies (see **further reading**) suggest that these tools reduce decisional conflict and are highly acceptable to doctors and patients. If these tools were web based, they would improve acceptability and reduce costs.

EDITORIAL – Engaging patients in medical decision making. Kravitz, R.L. and Melnikow, J. UC Davis Center for Health Services Research in Primary Care, Sacremento, CA, USA.
BMJ, **323**(7313): 584, 15 September 2001.

Ethicists have suggested that patient autonomy is more important than beneficence (doctor doing what he/she thinks is best). There is a growing belief that patients should be involved in decisions regarding their own care. Shared decision making is often a complex issue. The authors highlight a number of points.
- Decision making for the patient often depends on their attitude to risk.
- Family and health beliefs affect decision making. For example southeast Asian cultures belief that surgery will cause them to be physically incomplete in the next life. Some cultures belief that to talk about death is to hasten its onset.
- Patients generally want to be informed about the options available but they do not necessarily want to be involved in the decision making process.
- The authors suggest a first step might be to ask the patient about their understanding of their disease and how much they want to be involved in the decision making process.

Reasons for patient removals: results of a survey of 1005 GPs in Northern Ireland.
O'Reilly, D., Gilliland, A., Steele, K. and Kelly, C. Department of General Practice, The Queens University of Belfast, UK.
Br. J. Gen. Pract., **50**(469): 661-663, 1 August 2001.

This N. Ireland study was a survey of GPs reasons for removing patients from their lists. In 1999 they sent questionnaires to over 1000 GPs (response rate around 85%).

- Nearly 50% of those who responded had removed a patient in the previous 2 years.
- Nearly 50% of those removed were because of violent or threatening behaviour.
- One in six patients were removed for unrealistic demands e.g. inappropriate requests for home visits or inappropriate use of out-of-hours services.
- Incompatible doctor-patient expectations and breakdown of doctor-patient relationship, were also mentioned as reasons for removal.
- One of the recommendations by the Select Committee on Public Administration is that GPs should not be allowed to remove patients without a reason or without getting permission from the Health Authority. Most GPs (81%) agreed that GPs should not have to comply with such recommendations.

Practice size: impact on consultation length, workload and patient assessment of care. Campbell, J.L., Ramsay, J. and Green, J. Department of General Practice and Primary Care, Guys, Kings and St Thomass School of Medicine, London, UK.
Br. J. Gen. Pract., **50**(469): 644-650, 1 August 2001.

The aim of this study was to assess the impact of practice size on provision of care in general practice. Fifty-four practices from the London area took part in the study. They assessed practice workload over a 2-week period and issued a questionnaire to 2000 consecutive patients. They found that:

- practices with larger numbers of doctors providing care, had smaller average list sizes than practices with a smaller number of doctors;
- assessing the number of doctors providing care in a practice was more informative than using the number of GP principals in a practice;
- consultation length was longest in practices with a larger total practice size and shortest in those with a large number of patients per practice doctor;
- single-handed doctors had an average consultation length of 10.2 minutes. Group practice doctors had an average consultation length of 17.8 minutes;
- further analysis showed that the advantage gained by patients in larger practices (of longer consultations) was only true when the value for "patients cared for per doctor" was below 3000. This is lower than the 3500 patients allowed per doctor by the terms of service for UK GPs.

They conclude that "defining the optimum size of practice is a complex decision".

Deprivation, psychological distress and consultation length in general practice. Stirling, A.M., Wilson, P. and McConnachie, A. Department of General Practice, University of Glasgow, Glasgow, UK.
***Br. J. Gen. Pract.*, 51**(467): 456-460, June 2001.

This west of Scotland, cross-sectional survey, examines the relationship between deprivation, psychological distress (as measured by the general health questionnaire (GHQ)) and consultation length. Over 1000 consultations with 21 GPs from training practices were evaluated. The mean consultation length was 9 minutes. Consultation length was associated with:

- age of the patient. A 10 year increase in age was associated with a 3% increase in consultation length;
- the doctor rating of the patients psychological distress. A one point increase in the doctor's rating was associated with a 6% increase in the length of the consultation;
- patient self-reported psychological distress. A one point increase in the GHQ score was associated with a nearly 2% increase in consultation length;
- deprivation score. A one point increase in deprivation score was associated with around a 3% decrease in consultation length.

They point out that the most deprived patients have the shortest consultations. This is evidence that Tudor Harts inverse care law (*Lancet*, 1971) is still in operation i.e. those in need of the best care are the least likely to receive it.

FREQUENT ATTENDERS

Clinically inexplicable frequent attenders in general practice. Stewart, P. and O'Dowd, T. Department of General Practice, Trinity College, Dublin, UK.
***Br. J. Gen. Pract.*, 52**(12): 1000-1001, 1 December 2002.

Frequent attenders are a cause of much anguish and workload to family doctors. This study explored the issue further. This study defined a frequent attender as someone who attended their GP more than 12 times a year. A rural Irish practice of around 5000 patients was chosen. The records of frequent attenders were compared to a similar sample of practice patients matched for age and sex only. Frequent attenders were further divided into two groups based on whether the GPs felt their attendance level was necessary for their clinical condition or not.

- Around 100 (2%) patients were frequent attenders and had five times the attendance rate when compared to the other sample of practice patients.

- The GPs felt around half of these patients attended for clinically unexplainable reasons.
- Frequent attenders were more commonly female and had high psychiatric referral rates especially those in the clinically unexplainable group.

Defining frequent attendance: evidence for routine age and sex correction in studies from primary care settings. Howe, A., Parry, G., Pickvance, D. and Hockley, B. School of Medicine, Health Policy and Practice, University of East Anglia, Norwich, UK.
Br. J. Gen. Pract., **52**(480): 561-562, 1 July 2002.

This study aimed to modify cohort definition of frequent attenders so future investigators can identify patients whose consultation rate is elevated for their age and sex. The investigators utilised computerised routine attendance data from 10000 patients in two Sheffield General Practices. Consultation rates were investigated for patients aged 15–75, and those in the highest 2, 3 and 5 of attenders were analysed. The authors found:
- Women consistently consulted more than men up till age 65.
- Male consultation rates rose from age 65, while female rates remained constant.
- Without age-sex correction the top 3 of attenders was biased towards older women.

The authors conclude that male and females need to be considered separately when defining frequent attendance. The top 3 of male attenders in both the under and over 45 age group and the top 3 of female attenders can be considered "frequent attenders".

Psychosocial, lifestyle, and health status variables in predicting high attendance among adults. Little, P., Somerville, J. and Williamson, I. *et al.* Aldermoor Health Centre Practice, Southampton, UK.
Br. J. Gen. Pract., **51**(473): 987-994, 1 December 2001.

The aim of this cross-sectional survey is to assess the predictors of high attenders in general practice. Four thousand randomly chosen households were sent health questionnaires. They received around 2700 replies (response rate 74%). The following were predictors of high attendance:
- number of medical problems;
- poor physical health status;
- sociodemographic variables;
- multiple unexplained physical symptoms (MUPS);
- health anxiety;
- perceived health.

High attenders were:
- less likely to have negative attitudes towards doctors;
- have a low threshold for re-attending;
- less likely to have consulted the pharmacist first.

Family influences in a cross-sectional survey of higher child attendance. Little, P., Somerville, J. and Williamson, I. *et al.* Aldermoor Health Centre Practice, Southampton, UK. ***Br. J. Gen. Pract.,* 51**(473): 977-982, 1 December 2001.

This is a cross-sectional survey whose aim is to assess the relationship between parental factors and high childhood consultation rates in general practice. Four thousand randomly chosen households were sent health questionnaires. They received around 500 relevant replies. The following were associated with high consultation rates in the child:
- number of child medical problems;
- parents perceptions of severity of childs ill health;
- sociodemographic variables;
- parental perception of multiple unexplained physical symptoms (MUPS) in the child;
- parental willingness to tolerate somatic symptoms;
- parents own attendance rates;
- parental health anxiety was indirectly associated with high attendance, via the factors mentioned above.

They conclude that high attendance in a child can largely be explained by parental factors and parental anxiety/depression. Hence help may need to be directed at the parent.

Frequent attenders in general practice: a retrospective 20–year follow–up study. Carney, T.A., Guy, S. and Jeffrey, G. The Burn Brae Medical Group, Hencoates, Hexham, UK. ***Br. J. Gen. Pract.,* 51**(468): 567-569, July 2001.

This is a 20-year retrospective study of frequent attenders in one general practice in Northumbria. Records of 58 frequent attenders (>7 consultations per year) were compared with a similar number of controls over a 20 year period beginning in 1975.
- 1975 was the only year that a significant difference was found between the groups, in terms of attendance rates.
- The groups had similar consultation rates in 1990 and 1995.
- High attendance was associated with older age, being female, and having multiple physical illnesses.

The authors discuss the limitations of their study i.e. small numbers, retrospective and based in an 'atypical practice'. They conclude that frequent attendance is a function of chronic health problems. Doctors need to focus on adequate management of these problems when dealing with 'frequent attenders'.

FURTHER READING

Randomised controlled trial of an interactive multimedia decision aid on hormone replacement therapy in primary care. Department of Primary Care and Population Sciences, Royal Free and University College Medical School, University College, London.
BMJ, **323**(7311): 490-493, Jan. 2001.

Randomised controlled trial of an interactive multimedia decision aid on benign prostatic hypertrophy in primary care. Department of Primary Care and Population Sciences, Royal Free and University College Medical School, University College, London.
BMJ, **323**(7311): 493-496, Sept. 2001.

See 'Chronic disease' for

EDITORIAL - Patients as partners in managing chronic disease. Stanford University School of Medicine, Palo Alto, USA.
BMJ, **320**(7234): 526-572, 26 Feb. 2000.

DRUG MISUSERS

- Methadone can be prescribed safely in primary care.
- Analyzing the contents of amnesty bins at dance venues, may be a valuable method of keeping up to date with young peoples drug taking habits.
- The key to recognition of cardiovascular complications of recreational drugs is a high index of suspicion.
- Studies have repeatedly shown that GP care of problem drug users is feasible and can be effective

---

BACKGROUND

All indicators of illicit drug dependence have risen over the last 20 years. Although services in the UK are still very patchy, several studies have found methadone treatment programmes to be effective. Methadone is better than placebo in terms of illicit use of opioids, involvement in crime and mortality. Prescribing methadone results in lowered rates of HIV infection because of a reduction in risky injecting and decreased sharing behaviour. The government has tried to encourage GPs to be more involved in the care of problem drug users. Studies, however, have shown that more support services need to be made available to GPs. The additional workload may justify special payments. Community pharmacists may also need to play a key role in supervising the self-administration of methadone.

Methadone maintenance treatment can be provided in a primary care setting without increasing methadone-related mortality: the Sheffield experience 1997–2000. Keen, J., Oliver, P. and Mathers, N. Institute of General Practice and Primary Care, University of Sheffield, Sheffield, UK.
Br. J. Gen. Pract., 52: 387-389, 1 May 2002.

Methadone-maintenance treatment reduces mortality and morbidity among heroin users. However, there is concern that increasing the prescribing of methadone will lead to a rise in methadone-related deaths. This study examines methadone-related deaths in Sheffield during a 2-year period when 400 untreated patients were recruited to methadone treatment in primary care. Coroner records were searched and Prescription Pricing Authority records were used to calculate how much methadone was prescribed in Sheffield during this period.
- The amount of methadone prescribed rose more than twofold during the 2 years.
- The number of methadone deaths fell from six to two.

The authors conclude that methadone may be safely prescribed for large numbers of patients in a primary care setting without a rise in methadone deaths.

A method to monitor drugs at dance venues. Ramsey, J.D., Butcher, M.A. and Murphy, M.F. *et al.* St. Georges Hospital Medical School, London, UK.
***BMJ,* 323**(7313): 603, 15 September 2001.

In this brief study, the contents of 'amnesty bins' at dance venues were analyzed. The authors believe that this a valuable method of monitoring drug use at dance venues, which in turn gives an idea about what drugs young people are taking. This information could be used to inform health care providers about new drug formulations and also enable them to prepare appropriate preventative literature.

EDITORIAL – Cardiovascular complications of recreational drugs. Ghuran, A., van der Wicken, L.R. and Nolan, J. Department of Cardiological Sciences, St. Georges Hospital Medical School, London, UK.
***BMJ,* 323**(7311): 464-465, 1 September 2001.

The editorial details some of the cardiovascular complications of recreational drugs.

Cocaine, ecstasy and amphetamines have similar effects and activate the sympathetic nervous system. They can cause tachycardia, vasoconstriction and unpredictable blood pressure effects. There action on vessels may accelerate atherosclerosis and may cause aortic dissection. Cocaine and amphetamines may also cause non-cardiogenic pulmonary oedema and dilated cardiomyopathy.

Morphine and heroin increase parasympathetic activity and reduce sympathetic activity causing, bradycardia and hypotension. Arrhythmias, right sided bacterial endocarditis and non-cardiogenic pulmonary oedema can occur.

Volatile substances (e.g. butane gas from lighter refills) can cause arrhythmias and MIs have also been reported.

Cannabis alters sympathetic and parasympathetic activity. They can reduce the threshold for angina in predisposed individuals.They key to recognition of cardiovascular complications of recreational drugs is a high index of suspicion.

Difficult behaviour in drug-misusing and non-drug-misusing patients in general practice a comparison. Thompson, J. Principal in General Practice, Leeds, UK.
***Br. J. Gen. Pract.,* 51**(466): 391-393, 1 May 2001.

The aim of this study was to compare the incidence of difficult behaviour in drug misusers with non-drug misusers in a practice in Leeds. The staff reported difficult behaviour over a 3 month period (5200 appointments):

- drug misuers took up 12% of the total appointments;
- when offensive smell was excluded, drug misusers were twice as likely to exhibit difficult behaviour than non-drug misusers (1 per 316 appointments vs. 1 per 656 appointments). This difference did not reach significance.

Thompson concludes that drug misusers make a relatively small contribution to difficult behaviour in general practice.

ELDERLY

ALZHEIMER'S DISEASE
- A Finnish prospective study found that raised systolic (but not diastolic) blood pressure and serum cholesterol ⩾6.5 mmol/l was significantly associated with a high risk of Alzheimer's disease
- Guidelines for the management of people with Alzheimers disease may help to improve cognitive outcomes and independence.
- Patients well-being and prognosis are the main focus of treatment decisions for incompetent patients.
- Aromatherapy is beneficial for agitation and general quality of life, in patients with dementia. Bright light treatment is effective for seasonal affective disorder, restlessness, and sleep disturbances.

FALLS
- The national service framework for the care of elderly people was published in April 2001. They recommend the development of services to reduce the number of falls in the elderly
- A New Zealand study has found that a home based exercise programme delivered by a district nurse reduced falls in the elderly by 46%
- Urge incontinence may be one of the additional risk factors for falls
- Various measures can be taken to reduce the risk of falls in high-risk elderly people
- Exercise regimes for older people can prevent falls; other interventions have an additive effect
- Falls can be prevented in older people, if interventions are multifaceted and targeted

OTHERS
- It seems that a clinical iceberg exists in relation to the prevalence of urinary incontinence in the community with considerable unmet need
- An article by Gary Andrews argues that chronic disease and disability are not inevitable consequences of the ageing process
- Research is needed to address complications of diabetes specific to elderly people.
- Long-term care for older patients needs to be fully funded by the NHS to improve the quality of care
- A clinical review deals with strategies to maintain cognitive function during ageing
- Many trials assessing the efficacy of Parkinson's Disease treatment are too small or have methodological weakness
- Serious physical illness is associated with suicide in elderly people
- Home visiting with multidimensional assessment and multiple visits is effective in low risk elderly people.
- One study showed that outcomes for older people suffering from minor depression are not improved by follow-up mental health assessment
- Pharmacist review of repeat prescriptions can cut prescribing costs with no extra work for the doctor.
- Ageing well and dealing with the problems that will occur in most peoples lives as they get older presents challenges and opportunities for general practice.

- The majority of elderly patients without cancer would like to be told if they developed cancer
- The health and well being of older people should be a priority for PCGs and the primary health care team. Doctors should provide care for older people that is of the quality and responsiveness they would want for their own relatives.

ALZHEIMER'S DISEASE

EDITORIAL – Sensory stimulation in dementia. Burns, A., Byrne, J. and Ballard, C. *et al.* University of Manchester Department of Psychiatry, Education and Research Centre, Wythenshawe Hospital, Manchester, UK.
***BMJ,* 325**(7376): 1312-1313, 7 December 2002.

Many patients with dementia develop psychiatric symptoms or behavioural disturbances. Non-pharmacological approaches, such as behavioural management, are the recommended first line treatments for this. However drugs, such as neuroleptics and other sedatives, are often prescribed to control this situation, which is difficult for patients, carers and healthcare professionals. These drugs have modest short-term efficacies, but also carry hazardous side effects. Various alternative therapies have been tried, but reports are mainly qualitative and involve a small number of patients, with the exception of aromatherapy and bright light treatment.

- Three placebo-controlled trials for aromatherapy, each with almost 100% compliance, reported significant beneficial effects on agitation, coupled with marked improvement in patients quality of life. No extended periods of massage were used in these trials, so it is likely aromatherapy has a direct chemical effect, perhaps through terpines in essential oils.
- Bright light is an effective treatment for seasonal affective disorder. Three controlled trials in the past 3 years have shown benefits for restlessness, and significant benefits for sleep disturbances.

The authors conclude that while drugs are only moderately beneficial and carry significant hazardous side effects, aromatherapy and bright light seem safe and effective treatments for symptoms of dementia.

Review: pharmacological and non-pharmacological interventions improve outcomes in patients with dementia. Commentator, Mark Clarfield, Soroka Hospital Centre and Ben Gurion University of the Negev Beersheva, Israel.
***Evidence-based Medicine,* 6**(6): 183, Nov./Dec. 2001.

Question: Do pharmacotherapy, educational or other non-pharmacological interventions improve outcomes in patients with dementia or their caregivers?

The following article is briefly presented
Practice parameter: management of dementia (an evidence-based review). Report of the Quality Standards Subcommittee of the American Academy of Neurology. Doody, R.S., Stevens, J.C. and Beck, C. *et al.*
Neurology, **56:** 1154–1166, 8 May 2001.

Nearly 400 articles concerning the pharmacological and non-pharmacological management of Alzheimers disease (AD) were reviewed. The following guidelines emerged for the management of patients with AD
Pharmacological therapies
  • Cholinesterase inhibitors (tacrine, donepezil, tartrate, galantamine) improve cognitive outcomes in those with mild to moderate AD.
  • Antidepressants are useful in those with AD who are depressed.
  • Antipsychotic medication is useful for those with agitation or psychosis.
  • No benefit was seen for cholinesterase precursors (lecithin, xanomeline).
Non-pharmacological therapies
  • Education of caregivers delays time to institutionalization of the subject with AD.
  • Scheduled toileting reduced urinary incontinence.
  • Graded help and practicing skills together with positive reinforcement improved independence.

Midlife vascular risk factors and Alzheimer's disease in later life: longitudinal, population based study. Kivipelto, M., Helkala, E.-L. and Laakso, P. *et al.* Department of Neuroscience and Neurology, University of Kuopio, Finland.
BMJ, **322**(7300): 1447-1451, 16 June 2001.

This was a 21 year prospective follow up study, of random population based samples in Finland. The aim was to examine the relationship between blood pressure, cholesterol and later development of Alzheimer's disease. Around 1500 people participated in the study which began in 1972.
  • They found that raised systolic (but not diastolic) blood pressure and serum cholesterol $\geqslant 6.5$ mmol/l was significantly associated with a high risk of Alzheimer's disease.

FALLS

Review: Intrinsic and environmental risk factor modification reduces falls in elderly people. Hill, K. National Ageing Research Institute, Parkville, Victoria, Australia.
Evidence-based Medicine, **7**(4): 116, July/Aug. 2002.

Question: In community dwelling and institutionalised elderly people, how effective are programmes designed to reduce the incidence of falls?

The following article is briefly presented
Interventions for preventing falls in elderly people. Gillespie, J.D., Gillespie, W.J., Robertson, M.C. *et al.* University of Otago, Dunedin, New Zealand.
Cochrane Database Syst. Rev. **3**: CD000340 (latest version 19 May 2001)

Forty RCTs examining measures to minimise the incidence of or effects of falling were reviewed.
- Fourteen RCTs examined exercise or physiotherapy interventions. Exercise courses to improve muscle strength and balance, and also tai chi courses reduced fall rates
- Home safety interventions by occupational therapists resulted in a lower rate of falls amongst patients with previously recorded falls.
- Withdrawal from psychotropic medications decreased falls.
- Multidisciplinary, multifactorial, health, or intervention programmes decreased the rates of falls.

Commentary
Hill notes that most of the reviewed research took place in the community setting. He suggests that these results may not be generalisable to hospital or residential home settings, where further research is needed. In addition, Hill comments that multidisciplinary falls clinics, which use a comprehensive assessment and management programme for patients at high risk of falls, have not been evaluated in RCTs.
- Exercise regimes for older people can prevent falls; other interventions have an additive effect
- Falls can be prevented in older people, if interventions are multi-faceted and targeted

Randomised factorial trial of falls prevention among older people living in their own homes. Day, L., Fildes, B. and Gordon, I. *et al.* Accident Research Centre, Monash University, Clayton, Victoria, Australia.
BMJ, **325**(7356): 128-133, 20 July 2002.

This RCT tested the effectiveness of, and interactions between, three interventions to reduce falls among 1090 people over 70 years old and living in their own home. The interventions were group-based exercise, vision improvement and home hazard modification. Participants were randomly allocated to one of eight groups. Seven of these received at least one intervention, with the eighth group acting as a control.
- No interactive effect was found between interventions; rather they each had an additive effect.
- A supervised exercise programme for 15 weeks, coupled with home exercise for up to 12 months, was found to reduce falls, despite poor compliance with the home exercises. This was mainly due to improved balance, but possibly also due to behavioural change or social interaction, as awareness of these issues increased during the classes.

- Home hazard management had only a limited effect. This may have been due insufficiency of the intervention.
- Vision improvement also had a limited effect, perhaps because of the low number of subjects receiving treatment and the general lack of improved visual acuity.
- Participants were not blinded to which intervention group they were assigned, so may have under or over reported falls accordingly.

Further studies are needed to test the effectiveness of these interventions in populations with different characteristics, and to determine the cost effectiveness of exercise and other successful interventions, on the rate of falls in elderly populations.

Review: Falls can be prevented in older people, but interventions should be multifaceted and targeted. Commentator, Suzanne Fields, SUNY at Stony Brook, Stony Brook, New York, USA.
Evidence-based Medicine, **6**(3): 86, May/June 2001

Question: What is the evidence that risk factor modification and other interventions will reduce falls in people ⩾65 years of age?

The following article is briefly presented
Guidelines for the prevention of falls in people over 65. Feder, G., Cryer, C. and Donovan, S. *et al.*
BMJ, **321:** 1007–1011, 21 Oct. 2000.

- Eight RCTs looked at the effect of exercise intervention. Some showed a decreased risk of falling some showed an increased risk of falling.
- Five RCTs looked at the effect of multifaceted interventions. All of these showed a decreased risk of falls.
- Other findings were that hip protectors were useful in high risk individuals.
- Medical and occupational health follow up (after an emergency department attendance) reduced subsequent falls.
- Home-based interventions were not as effective as those based in residential settings.

Commentary
Patients at increased risk of falling should be identified and should have multidisciplinary assessment and intervention. Specific areas to be assessed would include:
- postural hypotension;
- vision;
- gait;
- balance;
- medication review;
- referral for occupational and physical therapy;
- home safety evaluation;
- hip protectors for the very frail.

EDUCATION AND DEBATE SECTION – Falls in late life and their consequences – implementing effective services. Cameron, Swift, Department of Health Care of the Elderly, Guy's, King's and St. Thomas's School of Medicine, London, UK.
BMJ, 322(7290): 855-857, 7 April 2001.

This article examines the reasons and implications for a 'falls service' as recommended by the national service framework for the care of older people. Each year 30% of people over the age of 65 have a fall. Half of these have at least two falls. Mortality from falls is high; for fractured femur over 30% die within the year. A multidisciplinary approach to reducing falls has the best results and falls can be reduced by between 30 and 50%. Important areas requiring attention include:

- **primary prevention** - including improved environmental safety, good diet and more physical activity;
- **identification of those at increased risk** - requires screening programmes or a means of opportunistic assessment;
- **'falls clinics'** - have been set up in some hospital outpatient departments, to deal with those at increased risk of falls;
- **management of those who fall** - requires collaboration between services.

Lessons learned from instigating adequate 'falls services' could be used to improve general care for the elderly population.

Weekly urge incontinence was associated with increased risk for falls and non-spiral fractures in older women. Commentator, Suzanne Fields, State University of New York at Stony Brook, Stony Brook, New York, USA.
Evidence–based Medicine, 6(2): 59, Mar./Apr. 2001.

Question: In community dwelling older white women, do urge and stress urinary incontinence increase risk for falls and non-spiral fracture?

The following article is briefly presented
Urinary incontinence: does it increase risk for falls and fractures? Brown, J.S., Vittinghoff, E. and Wyman, J.F. *et al.*
J. Am. Geriatr., **48:** 721–725, July 2000.

This USA study uses around 6000 women from the Study of Osteoporotic Fractures. Mean age 79 years.
- Urge incontinence was associated with falls and fractures ($P < 0.001$) whereas stress incontinence was not.

Commentary
This was a well-performed study. However the authors failed to make adjustments for patients with poor cognitive function. Poor cognitive function as found in dementia is often present alongside urge incontinence. Further studies will be required to validate this result.

Effectiveness and economic evaluation of a nurse delivered home exercise programme to prevent falls. 1: Randomised controlled trial. Robertson, M.C., Devlin, N., Gardner, M.M. and Campbell, A.J. *et al.* Department of Medical and Surgical Sciences, Otago Medical School, Dunedin, New Zealand.
BMJ, 322(7288): 696-701, 24 March 2001.

and

Effectiveness and economic evaluation of a nurse delivered home exercise programme to prevent falls. 2: Controlled trial in multiple centres. Robertson, M.C., Gardner, M.M. and Devlin, N. *et al.* Department of Medical and Surgical Sciences, Otago Medical School, Dunedin, New Zealand.
BMJ, 322(7288): 701-704, 24 March 2001.

These two New Zealand studies provide an evaluation (both clinical and economic) of a nurse delivered exercise programme to prevent falls in the elderly. The first study, involving 240 men and women aged 75 years and over, is an RCT looking at the effectiveness of a home based programme delivered by a trained district nurse. The second study involving 450 men and women aged 80 years and over, is a controlled trial using trained practice nurses to deliver exercise programmes from general practices. Both studies have a 1-year follow up period.

- In the home-based study, falls were reduced by 46%. In the practice-based study falls were reduced by 30%.
- The home-based study cost $NZ 432 per person to deliver compared with $NZ 418 for the practice-based study.
- For the practice-based study, hospital costs were not reduced. When reduced hospital costs were taken into consideration cost per fall prevented, in the home-based study was $NZ 155 compared with $NZ 1519 (£441) for the practice-based study.

The authors recommend a home-based exercise programme delivered by a district nurse. They report that such a programme is practical, feasible and may reduce health service costs.

OTHERS

EDITORIAL – Complications of diabetes in elderly people. Gregg, E.W., Engelgau, M.M. and Narayan, V. Division of Diabetes Translation, National Center for Chronic Disease Prevention and Health Promotion, Centers for Disease Control and Prevention, Atlanta, GA, USA.
BMJ, 325(7370): 916-917, 26 October 2002.

Diabetes is becoming increasingly common, with the most rapid rises in prevalence occurring in the elderly population. Understanding and prevention of the risk for traditional microvascular and macrovascular complications has been improving steadily over the years. However, the expanding population of elderly diabetics is bringing with it a number of less well recognised complications of diabetes, such as cognitive disorders, physical disability, falls and fractures. This editorial describes the challenges presented by such complications. The authors suggest that research programmes need to adapt to include the complications of diabetics specific to elderly individuals, which have a great impact on the quality of life and independence of these patients.

Review: Home visiting with multidimensional assessment and multiple visits is effective in low risk elderly people. Commentator, Hirsch C, University of California at Davis Sacremento, Sacremento, CA, USA.
Evidence-based Medicine, 7(5): 148, Sept./Oct. 2002

Question: In elderly people, what are the effects of preventative home visits on nursing home admission, functional status and mortality?

The following article is briefly presented:
Home visits to prevent nursing home admission and functional decline in elderly people. Systematic review and meta-regression analysis. Stuck, A.E., Egger, M., Hammer, A. *et al.*
JAMA **287:** 1022-1028 27 Feb. 2002
A Medline search isolated RCTs of effects of preventative in-home visits in elderly people living in the community. Data was excluded and analyzed:
- Over 50% of trials showed no difference in nursing home admissions between those receiving home visits and the control group.
- Four trials did show reduced nursing home admissions . In these trials more than nine follow up visits were carried out.
- If the home visit programme was multidisciplinary, patients functional decline was reduced.
- Home visiting had the most significant effect on those with the lowest mortality risk.
- Home visiting did not decrease mortality except in the youngest of the patients included.

Commentary
There is a general lack of data and a difficulty interpreting the data that exists regarding elderly evaluation and management.

At the centre of the uncertainty lies the question of where best to carry out the assessment process. Home visiting with intensive follow up now has evidence to support its effect in reducing admission to nursing homes, yet the benefit in functional status does not seem to be sustained.The implementation of eldery evaluation and management programmes and the selection of suitable patients is a task for care of the elderly physicians, not general practitioners.

EDUCATION AND DEBATE SECTION – Evaluating drug treatments for Parkinson's disease: How good are the trials? Wheatly, K., Stowe, R.L., Clarke, C.E. and Hills, R.K. *et al.*
BMJ, 324(7352): 1508-1511, 22 June 2002.

Parkinson's Disease is one of the commonest causes of disability in elderly individuals. The principle agents used to treat Parkinson's are levodopa, dopamine agonists, monamine oxidase type B inhibitors and catechol-O-methyltransferase inhibitors. Multiple RCT of these agents have been performed, but due to the inadequacies of these studies the efficacy of these treatments remains uncertain. The authors reviewed all randomised trials of treatment of Parkinson's Disease. The authors highlight the following problems with the published trials:

- The description of trial's methodology was often inadequate, hampering attempts to detect sources of bias.
- Most trials were too small to produce reliable results, 60 accrued less than 100 patients and so could not detect/refute small differences between treatments.
- The median length of patient follow up per trial was 2 years. As most patients with Parkinson's survive for 15 years current research does not give information on drug efficacy at all stages of disease.
- Most outcome measures related to standardised motor scores and not the treatment's impact on a patients' quality of life.

EDITORIAL – Long term care for older patients. Increasing pressure for change.
Heath, I. General Practitioner Caversham Group Practice, London, UK.
BMJ, 324(7353): 1534-1535, 29 June 2002.

Long-term care for older people is described as a 'political hot potato' fuelled by the perception of an unjust government policy and the increasing power of the older vote producing pressure for change. This has been intensified by the decision in Scotland to fund long-term care. In June 2000 the government ignored the main recommendation by a royal commission to divide long-term care into living costs, housing costs and personal care. Instead it is divided into health care (which the NHS covers) and social care (which is not covered). Social care is paid for by the patient.

Older people mainly require chronic care extending over months or years. However, as they enter into care homes their needs are no longer for health care but for social care. Ageism manifests itself in this division between health and social care. Social care forces older people to shift the emphasis away from their disease. It creates a barrier between themselves and healthcare professionals. It also implies families should be accountable for this care.

In addition the care that is provided is often delivered by 'unskilled', 'poorly trained' and 'poorly paid' care assistants. The standard of care for older people needs to be better and that full funding for long-term care is 'long overdue'.

CLINICAL REVIEW – What we need to know about age related memory loss. Small, G.W. UCLA Neuropsychiatric Institute, Los Angeles, CA, USA.
***BMJ, 324**(7352): 1502-1505, 22 June 2002.*

Age-related memory changes are common and cause much concern to patients. This review paper describes subtypes of memory loss and proposes measures to maintain cognitive health during ageing.
- Age-associated memory loss is defined as "self perception of memory loss" accompanied by a small decline in objective memory test scores.
- Mild cognitive impairment consists of more severe memory impairment combined with functional deficits.
- Dementia is irreversible impairment in several cognitive domains with severe loss of memory and functional disability.

The author suggests that the following factors should prompt formal memory assessment:
- Patient worrying about memory loss.
- Family history of dementia.
- Illness which increased risk of dementia.

To protect memory it is suggested:
- Cholinesterase inhibitors and vitamin E may slow the onset of dementia.
- Minimising stress may protect neuroanatomical structures involved in memory processing.
- Aerobic exercise reduces risk of Alzheimer's Disease in later life.
- Dietary changes: low fat, anti-oxidant rich fruit and vegetables (e.g. blueberries, broccoli), carbohydrates with low glycaemic index.
- Performing stimulating mental tasks.
- Avoidance of sports with a risk of head trauma.
- Not smoking.
- Light daily alcohol intake (2-4 drinks) protects against Alzheimer's Disease.

Burden of illness and suicide in elderly people: case-control study. Waern, M., Rubenowitz, E., Runeson, B., Skoog, I., Wilhelmson, K. and Allebeck, P. Section of Psychiatry, Institute of Clinical Neuroscience, Gothenburg University, Sahlgrenska University Hospital, Gothenburg, Sweden.
***BMJ, 324**(7350): 1355-1358, 8 June 2002.*

The aim of this case-control study was to examine the association between physical disorder and suicide in elderly people. This was determined from interviews with relatives of people who committed suicide and with control participants, and from medical records. Eighty-five study cases were included, and 153 controls participated. The main findings of the study were:
- Serious physical illness is independently associated with suicide (relative risk just 6.4). This was found to be a stronger predictor in men than in women.

- Impaired vision, neurological disorder and on-going malignant disease were all associated with an increased risk of suicide.

Evaluating a mental health assessment for older people with depressive symptoms in general practice: a randomised controlled trial. Arthur, A.J., Jagger, C., Lindesay, J. and Matthews, R.J. School of Nursing, Faculty of Medicine and Health Sciences, University of Nottingham, Queens Medical Centre, Nottingham, UK.
***Br. J. Gen. Pract.,* 52**(476): 202-207, 1 March 2002.

Minor depression is prevalent amongst older people. There remains, however, a lack of evidence describing the most effective method of its treatment. This randomised controlled trial, which was conducted in Leicester aimed to compare and evaluate the follow-up assessment of patients diagnosed with a depressive symptom at their over 75 health check. Nearly 100 patients were randomised between a community mental health team (CMHT) worker and their GP.

- A follow-up mental health assessment conducted 1 year to 8 months later did not improve the patients score on the Geriatric Depression Scale.

More research is required to determine the effect of CMHT involvement in the treatment of mildly depressed older patients. This study has shown the difficulty in evaluating health services provided jointly by different health bodies.

Randomised controlled trial of clinical medication review by a pharmacist of elderly patients receiving repeat prescriptions in general practice. Zermansky, A., Petty, D. and Raynor, D.K. *et al.* Division of academic Pharmacy Practice, School of Healthcare Studies, University of Leeds, Leeds, UK.
***BMJ,* 323**(7325): 1340-1343, 8 December 2001.

The aim of this RCT (involving around 1200 patients from four practices, and one pharmacist) is to assess whether a community pharmacist can review repeat prescriptions with elderly people. Elderly patients receiving repeat prescriptions were allocated to either intervention with the pharmacist, who performed consultations in the surgery or usual care.

- The pharmacist took around 20 minutes to review each patient.
- Pharmacist review resulted in more changes to drugs than the control group.
- Pharmacist care resulted in a cost saving even when the cost of the intervention was taken into consideration.
- Consultation rates were increased immediately after the review but there was no difference in consultation rates between the two groups at one year.

They discuss that the study may not be generalisable to other situations as it was a small study involving just one pharmacist.

Should elderly patients be told they have cancer? Questionnaire survey of older people. Ajaj, A., Singh, P. and Abdulla, J. Department of Elderly Care, Mid-Staffordshire General Hospitals, Stafford, UK.
BMJ, **323**(7322): 1160, 17 November 2001.

This questionnaire survey asked 315 patients aged between 65-94, (recruited from day hospitals, outpatients and the local senior citizens association), their views on how much they would want to know and whether they would want family informed should they be diagnosed with cancer. Mobility and living circumstances were also taken into account.

• Of the 270 who responded, nearly 90% wanted to be informed, 70% wanting relatives to be informed.
• Significantly more over-75s and those with poor mobility (requiring the aid of more than a stick) did not wish to be informed.

The authors comment that this study may help decision-making where relatives request elderly patients are not informed about a cancer diagnosis.

Urinary incontinence in older people in the community: a neglected problem? Stoddart, H., Donovan, J. and Whitley, E. *et al.* Division of Primary Health Care, Department of Clinical Medicine, University of Bristol, UK.
Br. J. Gen. Pract., **51**(468): 548-554, July 2001.

The aim of this cross sectional survey was to assess the prevalence of urinary incontinence in men and women aged over 65 in the community of a British city. Two thousand elderly men and women were sent questionnaires. The response rate was 79%.

• Prevalence of incontinence was just under 30% (higher in women than men).
• Over 60% of women and just over 50% of men reported their incontinence as moderate or severe.
• Women had more severe incontinence than men. One quarter of women reported wetting their outer clothing or urine running onto the floor compared with 16% of men.
• Less than half had accessed health service resources.

Simple measures such as bladder training could help a significant proportion of elderly in the community. It seems that a clinical iceberg exists in relation to the prevalence of urinary incontinence in the community with considerable unmet need.

EDUCATION AND DEBATE SECTION – Promoting health and function in an ageing population. Gary, Andrews, Centre for Ageing Studies, Flinders University, Science Park, Bedford Park, Australia.
BMJ, **322**(7288): 728-729, 24 March 2001.

This article asks whether chronic disease and disability are inevitable consequences of the ageing process. In 1995 the WHO launched an ageing and health programme. The programme encouraged a broader community approach to health promotion in the elderly. It also encouraged communities to consider social, mental, economic and environmental determinants of old age. Probably the most important factor responsible for maintaining health in older age is regular physical activity. Regular exercise is associated with reduced coronary heart disease, type 2 diabetes, colon cancer and osteoporosis. Studies have shown that lost fitness can be regained and most of the benefits can be achieved by taking moderate intensity exercise e.g. brisk walking. Dancing, bowling, and gardening should be encouraged as more standard types of exercise may alienate elderly exercisers. The social aspects of exercise should also be emphasized in a population where social isolation and loneliness is common.

Ageing Britain - challenges and opportunities for general practice. Drury, M. and Neuberger, J. University of Birmingham, UK.
Br. J. Gen. Pract., **51**(462): 5-6, 1 January 2001.

This editorial looks at important issues concerning primary cares role in dealing with elderly people. Discrimination in the NHS manifests itself in decisions such as Do Not Resuscitate, upper age limits for care, and the what do you expect at your age attitude. The authors advocate equal respect and consideration for the older person.

Elder abuse is largely unrecognised and hence reliable measures of its incidence or prevalence do not exist. It can be physical, psychological or financial exploitation. Vigilance is needed within the care team to ensure security for this vulnerable group.

Carers play an important role and the primary care team should be proactive in supporting this group.

Palliative care: General practices should have clear policies about their End of Life Issues such as patients refusal to accept treatment. Good quality information should also be provided for the patient.

Accessibility of services: At least a quarter of older people have some sort of mobility impairment and half do not have access to cars. Basic access requirements include good lighting, absence of stairs, an accessible toilet and good space. House calls may re-emerge as good practice for care in the community. Primary care teams need to explore the use of electronic technology for the better informed older person.

Medical care for older people in nursing and residential homes: Obtaining continuity of medical care, good medical supervision as well as emergency care for the older person can be difficult. These areas need to be within the Clinical Governance remit.

The health and well being of older people should be a priority for PCGs and the primary health care team. Doctors should provide care for older people that is of the quality and responsiveness they would want for their own relatives.

FURTHER READING

See 'Respiratory infections' for

Comparison of elderly people's technique in using two dry powder inhalers to deliver zanamivir: randomised controlled trial. Department of Elderly Care Medicine, Mayday Hospital, Croydon.
BMJ, 322 (7286): 577-579, 10 March 2001

Heat related mortality in warm and cold regions of Europe: Observational study. Keating, W.R., Donaldson, G.C., Cordioli, E. *et al.,* Medical Sciences Building, Queen Mary and Westfield College London.
BMJ, **321**(7286): 670-673, 16 Sept. 2000

EDUCATION AND DEBATE SECTION - Equity in the new NHS: hard lesson from implementing a local health care policy on donepezil. Doyle, Y., Merton, Sutton and Wandsworth Health Authority London.
BMJ, **323**(7306): 222-224, 28 July 2001

Ageing issue. This issue of the BMJ is devoted to issues concerning age and ageing.
BMJ, **315**(7115): 25 Oct. 1997

See 'Chronic disease' for

EDITORIAL - Building evidence on chronic disease in old age. Centre for Health Services Studies, University of Kent, Canterbury.
BMJ, **320**(7234): 528-529, 26 Feb. 2000

Inhibition of serotonin reuptake by antidepressants and upper gastrointestinal bleeding in elderly patients: retrospective cohort study. Clinical Epidemiology Unit, Ottawa Health Research Institute Ottawa Hospital - Civic Campus, Ottawa, Canada.
BMJ, **323**(7314): 655-658, 22 Sept. 2001

See 'Diet' for

EDUCATION AND DEBATE SECTION: Folic acid, ageing, depression and dementia. Institute of Epileptology, King's College, London.
Br. J. Gen. Pract., **324**(7352): 1512-1515, 22 June 2002

ETHNIC MINORITIES

- South Asians with asthma are at an increased risk of hospitalisation due to unique health beliefs, health behaviours and problems in accessing primary care.
- Self-reported health status is the most accurate predictor of the level of health service usage
- Children from south Asia have higher insulin, triglyceride, diastolic blood pressures and heart rates than white children.
- If patients consult in their own language, they are more able to cope with and understand their illness.
- Combined zinc and vitamin A has a beneficial effect on diarrhoea and dysentery but effects on lower respiratory disease are unsatisfactory.
- Lowering risk threshold for coronary heart disease would increase detection rates amongst certain ethnic groups and increase the potential for primary prevention.
- Contraceptive use in South Asian Women is below national levels.

BACKGROUND

'Triple jeopardy' describes a situation of ageism and racism combined with mental illness in people of ethnic minorities.

Application of Framingham risk estimates to ethnic minorities in United Kingdom and implications for primary prevention of heart disease in general practice: cross sectional population based study. Cappuccio, F.P., Oakeshott, P. and Strazzullo, P. *et al.* Department of General Practice and Primary Care, St Georges Hospital Medical School, London, UK. **BMJ, 325**(7375): 1271-1274, 30 November 2002.

This population based cross-sectional survey across nine general practices in London aimed to compare the 10 year risk of coronary heart disease, stroke and combined cardiovascular disease amongst patients from one population yet originating from a variety of ethnicities. Risk was assessed using the Framingham equation.

They found that:

- The risk thresholds that we currently use for coronary heart disease often underestimate the true risk of coronary heart disease in people of African or South Asian origin.

If risk thresholds were lowered in hypertensives of African and South Asian origin, there would be a higher probability of identifying and treating those with increased cardiovascular disease risk. Direct risk assessment of cardiovascular disease would be ideal.

Socioeconomic and ethnic group differences in self reported health status and use of health services by children and young people in England: cross sectional study. Saxen, S., Eliahoo, J. and Majeed, A. Research and Development Directorate, University College London Hospitals NHS Trust, London, UK.
***BMJ,* 325**(7363): 520-525, 7 September 2002.

This study examined whether there are inequalities in health status and use of services, between children and young adults of differing ethnicity and socio-economic status. Data was collected from the 1999 health survey for England, using firstly a general population sample, then adding a sample of only ethnic groups, and another of only Chinese people.

- The age and sex distribution was fairly even, however proportionally more Indian and Bangladeshi children were in lower socio-economic groups than the general population.
- The average number of consultations was 2.3 per person per year. Service usage did not vary according to socio-economic grouping, suggesting that some equality now exists in this respect.
- Indian and Pakistani children made greatest use of GP services, however Asian patients generally reported less ill health.
- Children from ethnic minorities were less likely to be referred to outpatient clinics.

The inequality in referrals for children from ethnic minorities needs further investigation. Usage of primary and secondary care services was best predicted by self-reported health status rather than by ethnicity or socio-economic grouping. The authors note that although actual health status does not reflect health service usage, this is often what is used to determine how resources are distributed.They comment too though, that high service usage is not necessarily inappropriate, as consultations may relate to preventative measures or routine health surveillance.

Contraceptive use among South Asian women attending general practices in southwest London. Saxena, S., Oakeshott, P. and Hilton, S. University College London Hospitals NHS Trust, Research And Development Office, London, UK.
***Br. J. Gen. Pract.,* 52**(478): 392-394, 1 May 2002.

In this cross-sectional survey a semi-structured questionnaire was used to investigate contraceptive use among 180 South Asian women, aged 16-50, seen at five different Wandsworth General Practices between 1999 and 2000. Ninety-five percent of the sampled group responded and 79% of the group was sexually active. The authors found:

- Sixty-three percent of women who were not trying for a baby used contraception.
- Use of contraception fell with age, with 71% of teenagers and 63% of women in their thirties using contraception.
- Unmarried women were more likely to use contraception (85%) than married women (60%).
- Oral contraception was the most commonly used form of contraception, none of the women's partners had a vasectomy.

The authors point out:
- South Asian women utilise contraception less frequently than white women.
- Despite cultural expectations single South Asian women are sexually active, and can, apparently, access contraception as required.

Early evidence of ethnic differences in cardiovascular risk: cross sectional comparison of British South Asian and white children. Whincup, P.H., Gilg, J.A., Papacosta, O. and Seymour, C. Department of Public Health Sciences, St Georges Hospital Medical School, London, UK.
BMJ, **324**(7338): 935-938, 16 March 2002.

The aim of this cross sectional study (the "ten towns health studies") was to compare cardiovascular risk factors in South Asian and British children. The children (73 South Asian and 1287 white) came from 10 British towns. They measured body build, BMI and took blood samples.
- South Asian children had higher diastolic blood pressures, heart rates, triglycerides, fibrinogen and insulin concentration than white children.
- Insulin levels were more sensitive to markers of adiposity in South Asian than white children.
- Serum total, LDL and HDL cholesterol concentrations were similar in the two groups.

This study shows that primary prevention of CHD in the South Asian population needs to start in childhood. They suggest concentrating on diet and physical activity.

Non-English speakers consulting with the GP in their own language: a cross-sectional survey. Freeman, G.K., Rai, H., Walker, J.J. and Howie, G.R. *et al.* Department of Community Health Sciences, General Practice, University of Edinburgh, UK.
Br. J. Gen. Pract., **52**(474): 36-38, 1 January 2002.

This study analyses patient enablement in a random sample of patients from 56 practices throughout the UK. Around 26 000 consultations were analyzed. Just over 2000 consultations came from patients who spoke non-English languages at home.
- People speaking non-English languages at home and speaking to the doctor in their own language had the highest patient enablement scores in the shortest consultation times. Hence, even though they had comparatively shorter consultations, consulting in their own language, facilitated understanding of their illness.

They conclude that if patients consult in their own language, they are more able to cope with and understand their illness.

Influences on hospital admission for asthma in south Asian and white adults: qualitative interview study. Griffiths, C., Kaur, G. and Gantley, M. *et al.* Department of General Practice and Primary Care, St Bartholomew and the Royal London School of Medicine and Dentistry, Queen Mary's School of Medicine and Dentistry, London, UK. *BMJ,* **323**(7319): 962-966, 27 October 2001.

A qualitative interview study based on a suburban London community (involving 58 south Asian and white patients, as well as 25 health care professionals) was conducted to determine the reasons for increased risk of hospital admission among south Asian populations with asthma. The authors of the study found that:

- Hospital admissions among south Asians are more common despite no consistent changes in asthma severity or prevalence, prescribed drugs, asthma education or interventions to reduce admission rates.
- Compared with white patients, south Asians coped differently with asthma. The latter are comparatively less confident in asthma control, are unfamiliar with preventative measures and have less confidence in their general practitioners.
- South Asians managed asthma exacerbation through family support, without systematic changes in prophylaxis or use of systemic corticosteroids.
- Patients unsatisfied with primary care access are often registered with practices without proper, integrated management strategies including policies for avoiding hospital admission.

To reduce hospital admissions involving south Asian patients, the authors highlighted the need for strategies to restore confidence in general practitioner, and to reinforce education on asthma control and prevention.

EVIDENCE–BASED MEDICINE

- RCTs are the most rigorous way of assessing a cause-effect relationship
- Implementing evidence based medicine is not a linear process, rather a complex fluid one involving both the doctor and the patient.
- The NHS Centre for Reviews and Dissemination recognises the role that qualitative studies play in providing evidence of effectiveness.

BACKGROUND

Evidence-based medicine is concerned with five key points:
(i)   clinical decisions should be based on the best available scientific data;
(ii) the clinical problem should determine the type of evidence sought;
(iii) identifying the best evidence means using epidemiological and biostatistical methods;
(iv) conclusions derived should be put into action in caring for patients;
(v)   performance should be evaluated regularly.

Research has shown that a physician's interpretation of clinical trial results depends on the way in which the results are presented. The same clinical trial results can be presented in four different ways:
- relative risk reduction;
- absolute risk reduction;
- proportion of event-free patients;
- number of patients who need to be treated to prevent an event (NNT).

Randomized trials usually present their results in one format only. This may affect the way results are interpreted. Health officials seem to be most familiar with relative risk reduction. This means that if the same results were presented in a different format, the results may be interpreted differently. This highlights the growing need for critical appraisal skills training amongst health professionals.

By convention $P > 0.05$ is taken to be 'not significant'. This is often inter-preted as meaning that there is no difference between two groups, or that a treatment or intervention is not effective. Often it simply represents the fact that there is insufficient evidence of a difference. One study found that only 30% (of 71 trials) were large enough to adequately detect whether the treatment was effective or not.

A meta-analysis is the mathematical combination of results from two or more primary studies that have dealt with the same hypothesis in the same way. They are usually represented in a standard format with an accompanying pictorial representation of the odds ratios called a 'forest plot'. The predictive value of small studies can be strengthened by combining the data in a meta-analysis. However, as far as possible, specific criteria should be met when formulating a meta-analysis.

Differences between trials, e.g.
- differences in types of patients studied;
- different dosage regimes;
- different outcomes measured;
- different length of follow-up;can result in 'clinical heterogeneity'. If marked, this may lead to skewed results and results that seem incompatible.

Communicating accuracy of tests to general practitioners: a controlled study.
Steurer, J., Fischer, J.E., Bachmann, L.M. and Koller, M. *et al.*, Horten-Sentrum für praxisorienterte Forschung and Wissenstranster, Universitätsspital, Zürich, Switzerland.
***BMJ,* 324**(7341): 824-826, 1 April 2002.

This study assesses the doctor's ability to interpret information concerning test accuracy. Two hundred and sixty three GPs were given questionnaires and clinical vignetttes which assessed their ability to evaluate sensitivity, specificity, predictive values and likelihood ratios. GPs were Swiss and attending conferences concerning evidence-based medicine.
- Most GPs were able to correctly identify definitions of sensitivity and predictive values.
- They were poor at interpreting numerical information concerning test accuracy.
- When test accuracy (as given by the likelihood ratio) was expressed in plain language many more GPs were able to interpret the results

They conclude that rather than GPs learning more about test accuracy, researchers need to explain the numerical values in plain language.

PRIMARY CARE – Obstacles to answering doctor's questions about patient care with evidence: qualitative study. Ely, J.W., Osheroff, J.A., Ebell, M.H. and Chambliss M.L. *et al.*, Department of Family Medicine, University of Iowa College of Medicine, Iowa City, USA.
***BMJ,* 324**(7339): 710-713, 23 March 2002.

Doctors are encouraged to seek evidence for answers to their questions about patient care but many remain unanswered. The main aim of this qualitative study was to ascertain the range of obstacles encountered when attempting to obtain evidence-based answers to real clinical questions. A total of 200 questions contributed by 103 family doctors were analyzed. In summary:
- Fifty-nine obstacles were found while attempting to provide evidence-based answers to questions and these were comprehensively organized.
- Six salient challenges were identified:
  1. Inadequate time to search for information;
  2. Difficulty modifying the original question, which was often vague and open to interpretation;

3. Difficulty selecting an optimal strategy to search for information;
4. Failure of resources to cover the topic;
5. Uncertainty about how to know when all the relevant evidence has been found so that the search can stop;
6. Inadequate synthesis of multiple bits of evidence into a clinically useful statement.

• Practising doctors often doubted the existence of useful information in available resources.

Why general practitioners do not implement evidence: qualitative study. Freeman, A.C. and Sweeney, K. Somerset and North and East Devon Primary Care Research Network, Institute of General Practice, School of Postgraduate Medicine and Health Sciences, Exeter, UK.
BMJ, 323(7321): 1100-1102, 10 November 2001.

This qualitative study uses focus groups of GPs (19 in total) to evaluate the reasons why GPs do not implement evidence-based medicine. They found that implementing evidence depended on:

• the doctors life experience and experience in hospital medicine;
• the doctor-patient relationship. The evidence was not ignored rather interpreted in the context of the patient. Patients could also simply refuse a particular treatment option;
• tension between primary and secondary care. Hospital consultants were seen to treat diseases whereas GPs were seen to treat patients. There was also difficulty with the concept of giving a well (asymptomatic) patient, medication which had side effects and which changed the quality of their lives;
• the logistical difficulties in starting new medication was highlighted. The patients personal circumstances need to be taken into consideration.

Implementing evidence-based medicine is not a linear process, rather a complex fluid one involving both the doctor and the patient.

Quality of Cochrane reviews: assessment of sample from 1998. Olsen, O., Middleton, P. and Ezzo J. *et al.*, Nordic Cochrane Centre, Copenhagen, Denmark.
BMJ, 323(7317): 829-832, 13 October 2001.

This study, coordinated from the Nordic Cochrane Centre, aimed to assess the quality of Cochrane reviews. Ten methodologists affiliated with the Cochrane Collaboration independently examined, in a semi-structured way, the quality of all 53 reviews first published in issue 4 of the Cochrane Library in 1998. The predominant types of problem were then categorized.

• No problems or only minor ones were found in most reviews.
• Major problems were identified in 15 reviews (29%); the evidence did not fully support the conclusion in nine reviews (17%), the conduct or reporting was unsatisfactory in 12 reviews (23%), and stylistic problems were identified in 12 reviews (23%).

Although a previous study found dubious or invalid statements in 76% of the conclusions or abstracts of drug trial reports, they occurred in only 17% of the Cochrane reviews. Since 1998, the Cochrane Collaboration has taken several additional steps to improve the quality of its reviews. However, readers should be particularly cautious of reviews with conclusions that favour experimental interventions when relatively little evidence is available for the review, as well as reviews with many typographical errors.

Qualitative research in systematic reviews. Dixon-Woods, M. and Fitzpatrick, R. *BMJ,* **323**(97316): 765-766, 6 October 2001.

The NHS Centre for Reviews and Dissemination have recently published its second edition concerning systematic reviews. It recognises the role that qualitative studies play in providing evidence of effectiveness. However, some difficulties are inherent in dealing with qualitative studies.
• There is no Cochrane-style register of qualitative studies, which means that searching for relevant studies may be difficult.
• Critically appraising qualitative studies requires alternative techniques to those required for quantitative studies.
• There is no consensus concerning how to assess the quality of qualitative studies.
• It may be difficult to combine studies in the same way as one would do for a meta-analysis.

EDITORIAL – Any casualties in the clash of randomised and observational evidence? Haidich, A.-B. and Lau, J. *BMJ,* **322**(7291): 879-880, 14 April 2001.

Observational studies are often thought of as the poor relation to RCT, the 'quick and dirty' method compared with the 'gold standard'. However, several analyses show that observational studies can produce the same results as RCTs. Indeed when several studies are compared with each other, the concordance between observational studies is higher than that between RCTs. However the variability amongst RCTs is produced because diverse and specific patient populations are being studied. Observational studies tend to group all sub-populations together which makes it harder to see which patient populations would benefit from a specific intervention. Haidich and Lau also point out that observational studies are only appropriate for certain clinical questions.

Treatment of acute otitis media: are children entered into clinical trials representative? Bain, J. Professor of General Practice, Tayside Centre for General Practice, University of Dundee, Dundee, UK.
Br. J. Gen. Pract., **51**(463): 132-133, February 2001.

This study asks whether children entered into clinical trials with otitis media are representative of the cases that we actually see in practice. Eight trials are analysed. He finds that when one considers the number of cases a typical GP would be expected to see, the recruitment of otitis media cases by doctors is low. Half of the exclusions in studies occur because the GP has judged that the child needs antibiotics. This would suggest that the children who are entered into trials are those with mild or moderate episodes of otitis media. This may account for the fact that meta-analyses show that antibiotics are not helpful in acute otitis media.

EDITORIAL – PubMed Central: creating an Aladdin's cave of ideas. Delamothe, T. and Smith, R.
BMJ, **322**(7277): 1-2, 6 January 2001.

PubMed central is a web based library run by the US National Institutes of Health. BMJ articles will be available in full text. It is hoped that PubMed Central will result in rapid and wider dissemination of research material.

HEART DISEASE

SECONDARY PREVENTION
• A study conducted for the ASSIST group concludes that the process of care can be improved by setting up a disease register with recall to a nurse-run service. However the outcome of care does not change

BOTH PRIMARY AND SECONDARY PREVENTION
• In terms of workload implications, it is more beneficial to concentrate on the over 65 year age group when targeting patients for assessment and treatment of cardiovascular risk factors
• Many patients currently eligible for drug therapy to combat CHD risk would be ineligible using the updated 4 year risk Framingham model
• The most appropriate primary prevention strategies are those that preselect patients who are at high risk of cardiovascular disease
• Focusing on informed choices by the patient may lower uptake of screening tests, but ultimately enhance the effectiveness of interventions
• Risk evaluation must improve if patients are to make genuinely informed choices to manage CHD risks
• Rehabilitation programmes, especially those containing exercise, are beneficial for the secondary prevention of CHD.
• The national service framework for primary care has marked workload implications for primary care.
• The British Womens Heart and Health study found that women still lag behind men in the secondary prevention of CHD.
• Some argue that screening for high risk individuals, as proposed by standard four of the NSF, will not be successful.

RISK FACTORS AND MORTALITY
• A new risk score (commissioned by the INDANA project steering committee) has been developed, which claims to be more generalizable than previous risk scores
• C reactive protein is a potential marker for future vascular disease
• The analysis of age related trends in coronary heart disease and breast cancer shows that the effect of oestrogen is small compared to environmental factors
• Many case notes do not contain the required information to allow doctors and nurses to accurately calculate risk of CHD.
• A study looking at a cohort of patients from the HOPE study has shown that the risk of cardiovascular events and all-cause mortality increased with increasing microalbuminuria.
• The Framingham scores should be recalibrated if used in non-black/white populations.
• More evidence showing that raised homocysteine levels are a cause of cardiovascular disease.

HEART FAILURE
• The CAPRICORN study showed that carvedilol reduced deaths after an MI, in patients with left ventricular dysfunction.

- Lack of open access to echocardiography and long waiting times to be seen, as well as fear of side effects and the hassle of dose titration with ACE inhibitors, were a significant barrier to effective management of heart failure in general practice.
- Carvedilol is beneficial in severe chronic heart failure as well as mild to moderate heart failure.
- Screening for heart failure should be confined to those with ischaemic heart disease.
- Specialist heart failure nurses might provide the necessary skills for appropriate palliative care of patients with heart failure.

OTHERS

- In the management of CHD, there is evidence that men are treated better than women
- Dothiepin (tricyclics antidepressant) has been shown to be associated with a 67% increased risk of ischaemic heart disease.
- A diet rich in potassium has a beneficial effect blood pressure, stroke, glucose tolerance, renal disease and cardiac arrhythmias.

BACKGROUND

It has been suggested that GPs are the most appropriate practitioners to offer effective care for patients with established CHD. Non-fatal and fatal outcomes can be reduced by lifestyle and pharmacological interventions.

- Observational studies show that those who stop smoking after an MI have a 50% lower mortality over 2 years than those who continue to smoke.
- A review of 22 RCTs involving around 4500 patients showed that cardiac rehabilitation reduced total mortality by 20% over 3 years of follow-up.
- The diet and reinfarction study involving 2000 men with a history of MI showed that those who add oily fish to their diets two or three times per week had a 29% reduction in all-cause mortality over 2 years.
- Eleven RCTs involving 20 000 patients with a history of MI have established that antiplatelet therapy prevents about 40 vascular events per 1000 patients in the first 2 years after an MI.
- Twenty-three randomized trials involving around 19 000 patients have shown that long-term treatment with β-blockers after an MI reduces mortality by 20%.
- In patients with left ventricular dysfunction after an MI, ACE inhibitors reduce all-cause mortality by nearly 20%.
- The Scandanavian simvastatin survival study of patients with angina or history of MI showed a 30% reduction in total mortality in patients with a total cholesterol of 5.5–8.0 mmol/l over a 5 year period.

SECONDARY PREVENTION

Secondary prevention in 24 431 patients with coronary heart disease: survey in primary care. Brady, A.J.B., Oliver, M.A. and Pittard, J.B. Department of Medical Cardiology, Glasgow Royal Infirmary University NHS Trust, Glasgow, UK.
***BMJ*, 322**(7300): 1463, 16 June 2001.

The Healthwise survey assessed the management of CHD (secondary prevention) in primary care. Over 24 000 patient records (around 500 GPs) were analysed from computerized practices throughout Britain.
- Between 20% and 26% of patients continued to smoke.
- Over 50% of diabetics were hypertensive.
- Up to 50% of patients did not have a recorded cholesterol level and few of those who did were taking statins.
- Less than a quarter of people post MI were taking β-blockers.
- Around 50% of heart failure patients were taking ACE inhibitors.

They conclude that there is still considerable room for improvement in the secondary prevention of CHD in primary care.

Cluster randomised controlled trial to compare three methods of promoting secondary prevention of coronary heart disease in primary care. Moher, M., Yudkin, P. and Wright, L. *et al.* for the Assessment of Implementation Strategies (ASSIST) Trial Collaborative Group.
***BMJ*, 322**(7298): 1338-1342, 2 June 2001.

This RCT conducted for the ASSIST group evaluates three health promotion strategies for secondary prevention of CHD in primary care. Twenty-one practices (around 1900 patients) from Warwickshire took part in the study. Practices were split into three groups: (1) had audit of their notes with feedback given at a practice meeting; (2) had help setting up a practice register and establishing a recall system to a GP; (3) had help setting up a practice register and establishing a recall system to a practice nurse. Follow up was after 18 months.
- Assessment of risk factors improved in all three groups.
- Assessment was better in the nurse group than the other two groups.
- Prescribing of antiplatelet drugs was highest in the nurse group.
- Blood pressure, cholesterol levels and cotinine levels did not differ between the groups after 18 months.

They conclude that although the process of care can be improved by setting up a disease register with recall to a nurse-run service. The outcome of care does not change.

BOTH PRIMARY AND SECONDARY PREVENTION

EDITORIAL – Primary prevention of coronary heart disease. Lawlor, D.A., Ebrahim, S. and Smith, G.D. Department of Social Medicine, University of Bristol, Bristol, UK.
***BMJ,* 325**(7359): 311-312, 10 August 2002.

The national service framework for CHD recommends asymptomatic patients at risk of CHD should be identified, and steps taken to minimise their risk.

There is little evidence that current screening programmes adequately meet Wilson-Junger criteria. Risk assessment should involve use of a clinical decision making aid based on a Framingham risk equation, though this tends to overestimate risk in populations with low CHD incidence.

Having estimated the patient's risk, dialogue must be opened between the clinician and patient to allow informed decisions to be made regarding minimising identified risk.

Patient motivation to change their lifestyle may be improved by facilitating their ability to make informed choices. The manner in which facts are presented influences patients; the national service framework advocated clinical decision aids present data only in absolute terms, and omit the risk reduction expected from interventions.

Analysis of predicted coronary heart disease risk in England based on Framingham study risk appraisal models published in 1991 and 2000. Nanchahal, K., Duncan, J.R. and Durrington, P.N. *et al.* Department of Public Health and Policy, London School of Hygeine and Tropical Medicine, London, UK.
***BMJ,* 325**(7357): 194-195, 27 July 2002.

This paper compares the predicted CHD risk calculated using Framingham coronary risk appraisal models of 1991 and the updated 2000 model, and makes an assessment of the implications for preventing CHD. The authors used data on 5518 patients from the 1998 health survey for England, to estimate the 4 and 10 year risk probabilities of developing CHD using the 1991 equation, and 4 year risk using the 2000 equation.

- The 1991 equation suggests 32% of men and 7% women in England aged 35–74 are at 15% risk of developing CHD in the next 10 years. The 2000 model gives 29% of men and 6% of women 5% risk of CHD in the next 4 years
- Only 1–2% of those currently ineligible for drug therapy would become eligible using the 2000 model, however 20% of men and 43% of women currently receiving drug treatment would become ineligible by assessing their 4 year risk with the 2000 model

Resource implications and health benefits of primary prevention strategies for cardiovascular disease in people aged 30 to 74: mathematical modelling study.
Marshall, T. and Rouse, A. Public Health and Epidemiology, University of Birmingham, Birmingham, UK.
***BMJ,* 325**(7357): 197-202, 27 July 2002.

The UK government policy framework for the prevention of coronary heart disease recommends that primary care teams should assess adult patients' risk of cardiovascular disease every 5 years and treat eligible patients. Such assessment of all adult patients is time-consuming and costly. In this study, such assessment policy was compared to alternative policies in which only certain patients (e.g. those with known cardiovascular risk factors) were invited for clinical assessment. Subjects were patients aged 30-74 selected from a population of 2000 General Practice patients. Outcome measures included the resource costs of assessing, treating, and following up eligible patients, and the number of cardiovascular events that this should prevent.

- It was found that strategies involving assessment of specific preselected patients prevented more cardiovascular disease, at lower cost, than those involving assessment of all adult patients.

The authors conclude that the most appropriate primary prevention strategies are those that preselect patients at high risk of cardiovascular disease and those that avoid the use of expensive drugs such as simvastatin and enalapril.

Screening for cardiovascular risk: public health imperative or matter for individual informed choice? Marteau, T.M. and Kinmonth, A.N. Psychology and Genetics Research Group, King's College London, London, UK.
***BMJ,* 325**(7355): 78-80, 13 July 2002.

This paper is a review of literature and examines the implications of offering primary preventative services for cardiovascular disease, with an emphasis on informed choice for patients.

Traditionally, invitations to participate in screening programmes have emphasised population benefits rather than potential risks of the procedure. National Screening Committee guidelines now state patients should be made aware of the risks and benefits, to make informed choices about whether to participate.

There is little evidence as to the effects of changing the emphasis of cardiovascular screening from population-based advice to individual informed choice. Labelling patients as being at high risk of cardiovascular disease may be harmful, as it prompts clinical monitoring and lifestyle changes the patient may find unacceptable in light of uncertain personal risk reductions.

The authors propose several implications of informed choices for screening programmes:

- Detailed invitations may promote fear and hence avoidance of the test, and may also exclude those with lower levels of literacy
- Lower uptake of screening procedures, however participants will have more realistic expectations of the procedures
- Participants may have more motivation to change following a positive result

The authors conclude that while informed choice may reduce uptake of screening procedures, interventions may improve in effectiveness.

Randomised trials of secondary prevention programmes in coronary heart disease: systematic review. McAlister, F.A., Lawson, F.M.E., Teo, K.K. and Armstrong, P.W. Division of General Internal Medicine, University of Alberta Hospital, Edmonton, Canada. **BMJ, 323**(7319): 957-962, 27 October 2001.

The aim of this systematic review was to assess the efficacy of rehabilitation programmes for the secondary prevention of CHD. Twelve trials met the inclusion criteria (longest period of follow up 48 months).

- People on rehabilitation programmes were more likely to be prescribed appropriate medication e.g. lipid lowering drugs and β blockers.
- Hospital admissions were reduced in those on rehabilitation programmes.
- Mortality was not significantly effected by the programmes. This study and other studies, particularly those that included exercise, showed that disease management programmes were beneficial for the secondary prevention of CHD. Longer studies will be needed to more accurately assess the effect of these programmes on survival.

Is population coronary heart disease risk screening justified? A discussion of the National Service Framework for coronary heart disease (standard 4). Rouse, A. and Adab, P. Department of Public Health and Epidemiology, Medical School, University of Birmingham, Edgbaston, Birmingham, UK. **Br. J. Gen. Pract., 51**(471): 834-837, 1 October 2001.

This discussion paper argues that standard 4 of the national service framework (NSF) for coronary heart disease will not be successful. Standard 4 states that all general practices should identify all those at increased risk of CHD and manage them accordingly.

Standard 4 does not mention screening, but this is effectively what it is asking GPs to do. Rouse and Adab highlight the likely problems with screening for CHD risk factors, based on established screening criteria.

- They argue that their needs to be adequate 'structure, co-ordination, management and appropriate resources', for the programme to be a success.
- The identification of high risk individuals is dependent upon which risk tables one uses.

- The social and ethical aspects of such screening programmes have not been evaluated.
- They point out that the British Family Heart Study and the Oxcheck study evaluated the management of high risk individuals in primary care and found that there were only minimal benefits.
- They site the cervical screening programme with all its quality control difficulties as an example of a poorly planned and run programme.
- Ideally an RCT should first be performed to determine if screening can actually reduce mortality.

Aspirin use for the prevention of cardiovascular disease: The British Womens Heart and Health Study. Lawlor, D.A., Bedford, C., Taylor, M. and Ebrahim, S. Department of Social Medicine, University of Bristol, Canynge Hall, Whiteladies Road, Bristol, UK. **Br. J. Gen. Pract., 51**(470): 743-745, 1 September 2001.

The British Womens Heart and Health Study comprises around 2100 women aged 60-79 registered with general practices in 13 towns in England, Wales and Scotland. Initial assessments took place in 1999 and 2000. This study presents aspirin use in this group of women.
- One in five women were taking aspirin; most of whom (~70%) were taking it for primary prevention.
- Of those requiring secondary prevention, around a third were taking aspirin.An update of the British Regional Heart Study found that 60% of men requiring secondary prevention were taking aspirin. The authors argue that an average GP will only need to identify 20 elderly women to comply with the national service framework

General practice workload implications of the national service framework for coronary heart disease: cross sectional survey. Hippisley-Cox, J. and Pringle, M. Division of General Practice, Nottingham University, Nottingham, UK. **BMJ, 323**(7307): 269-270, 4 August 2001.

The aim of this survey was to assess the workload implications of standards 1-4 of the national service framework for coronary heart disease. Sixty-five practices from the Trent region were surveyed and computer records were analyzed.
- They found a 14-fold variation in risk factor recording on the computer and a 4-fold variation in the need for disease intervention.
- For a practice with a list size of 10 000 patients, around 900 items would need to be recorded and around 2200 interventions would be needed.The national service framework for primary care has marked workload implications for primary care.

Meeting the National Service Framework for coronary heart disease: which patients have untreated high blood pressure? Marshall, T. and Rouse, A. Department of Public Health and Epidemiology, University of Birmingham, Edgbaston, Birmingham, UK. *Br. J. Gen. Pract.*, **51**(468): 571-574, July 2001.

Step 4 of the national service framework for coronary heart disease requires that patients with a 10 year risk of cardiovascular disease greater than 30% should be identified and offered treatment. This study used data from various sources, including the Health Survey for England and the general practice research database, to estimate workload implications if these targets are to be met. Data is calculated per primary care group (PCG) representing 100 000 patients.

- They estimate that each PCG would have around 6000 patients with high blood pressure plus a greater than 30%, 10 year risk of cardiovascular disease. The majority (80%) of these people would be aged over 65 years.
- If assessment were confined to people over the age of 65, 11 500 patients with high blood pressure would need to be assessed to identify the 6000 patients for treatment.
- Up to 600 cardiovascular events would be prevented every 5 years using this approach.
- Assessing people with high blood pressure under the age of 45 did not prevent any cardiovascular events. This was because almost no one in this group had a greater than 30%, 10 year risk of cardiovascular disease.

The authors recommend that PCGs concentrate on the over 65 age group for identification and treatment of cardiovascular risk factors.

EDITORIAL – The renaissance of C reactive protein. Pepys, M.B. and Berger, A. Department of Medicine, Royal Free and University College Medical School, London, UK. *BMJ*, **322**(7277): 4-5, 6 January 2001.

C reactive protein is a potential marker for future vascular disease. It seems that it may be valid in both primary and secondary prevention. Studies have shown a link between C reactive protein and coronary events in patients with angina and in patients who have had coronary angioplasty. In healthy individuals C reactive protein in the top third of normal range have twice the risk of a vascular disease (heart, stroke and peripheral disease) than those in the lower third.

RISK FACTORS AND MORTALITY

Homocysteine and cardiovascular disease: evidence on causality from a meta-analysis. Wald, D.S., Law, M. and Morris, J.K. Department of Cardiology, Southampton General Hospital, Southampton, UK.
***BMJ,* 325**(7374): 1202-1206, 23 November 2002.

The serum level of the amino acid homocysteine is positively associated with the risk of ischaemic heart disease, deep vein thrombosis and pulmonary embolism and stroke. Homocysteine levels can be reduced safely and easily by the B vitamin folic acid. Homocysteine levels are found to be raised in the rare autosomal recessive condition, homocystinuria, and in individuals carrying a mutation in the enzyme methylenetetrahydrofolate reducatase (MTHFR) which is involved in homocysteine metabolism. Previous analyses have had insufficient patient numbers to assess cardiovascular risk in individuals with and without the mutation. A search of the Cochrane Database resulted in 120 studies being included in the analysis. The main outcome measure was the odds ratio (OR) of the three diseases for a 5 mmol/l increase in serum homocysteine concentration.

- Homocysteine was shown to be significantly associated with the three diseases; IHD, DVT/PE and stroke.
- Both prospective and genetic studies showed a highly significant association

The authors concluded that their results provide strong evidence for the causal relationship between homocysteine and cardiovascular disease. Hence a reduction of 3 mmol/l in serum homocystiene concentration (achievable by daily intake of 0.8 mg folic acid) should reduce the risk of ischaemic heart disease by 16%, deep vein thrombosis by 25% and stroke by 24%.

Role of endogenous oestrogen in aetiology of coronary heart disease: analysis of age related trends in coronary heart disease and breast cancer in England and Wales and Japan. Lawlor, D.A., Ebrahim, S. and Smith, G.D. Department of Social Medicine, University of Bristol, Bristol, UK.
***BMJ,* 325**(7359): 311-312, 10 August 2002.

This study was an analysis of the effect of menopause on the age related trends in coronary heart disease and breast cancer in England and Wales and Japan. Specific mortality rates from coronary heart disease for men and women and from breast cancer in women were obtained in England and Wales and Japan. These were used to plot 5 year aggregate rates for each country. The results showed that:

- Coronary heart disease mortality in women increased with age and death rate decelerated in men at older ages in both countries.
- There was no affect on mortality from coronary heart disease around the age of menopause in either country.

• Breast cancer began to decelerate around the time of menopause. The author concludes that environmental factors are the most important determinants of coronary heart disease in women and men of the difference in coronary heart disease rates between them.

Comparison of estimates and calculations of risk of coronary heart disease by doctors and nurses using different calculation tools in general practice: cross sectional study. McManus, R.J., Mant, J. and Meulendijks, C.F.M. *et al.* on behalf of the Midlands Research Practice Consortium.
***BMJ,* 324**(7335): 459-464, 23 February 2002.

This study evaluates the ability of GPs and practice nurses to assess CHD risk levels in selected patients. Eighteen GPs and 18 practice nurses from practices forming part of the Midlands Research Practice Consortium, took part in the study. They were asked to subjectively assess risk in a selected group of patients and then calculate the risk using four risk tools: Sheffield tables, New Zealand tables, European recommendations, British recommendations (computer programme).
  • One fifth of the notes did not have HDL measurements, required by the New Zealand and British risk tools.
  • Sensitivity was highest for GPs and nurses using the British programme.
  • Many scores were calculated incorrectly or inappropriately e.g. in people with known CHD (these people automatically come under secondary prevention guidelines), or in patients who had missing HDL measurements (many assumed this level to be 1 mmol/l, when using the British and New Zealand risk tools).They state that with the exception of the British programme, subjective assessment is as good as using risk tools.

The Framingham scores overestimated the risk for coronary heart disease in Japanese, Hispanic and native American cohorts. Commentators, D. Kent and J. Griffiths New England Medical Center, Boston, MA, USA.
Evidence-based Medicine, 7(1): 31, Jan./Feb. 2002.

Question: Can the Framingham scores, originally developed in a white middle class population, predict the risk for coronary heart disease (CHD) in ethnically diverse populations?

The following article is briefly presented
Validation of the Framingham coronary heart disease prediction scores. Results of a multiple ethnic groups investigation. DArgostino, R.B. Sr, Grundy, S. and Sullivan, L.A. *et al.* for the CHD Risk Prediction Group. *JAMA,* **286**: 180–187, 11 July 2001.

The Framingham scores were validated against scores in studies looking at 6 ethnically diverse groups.

- The Framingham scores predicted risk over a 5-year period in white and black subjects.
- The Framingham scores overestimated risk in Japanese-American, Hispanic and native American women.

Commentary
The Framingham scores should be recalibrated if used in non-black/white populations.

Cardiovascular events were increased in patients with high cardiovascular risk who had albuminuria. Commentator, Donald Smith, Mount Sinai Medical Center New York, New York, USA.
Evidence-based Medicine, 7(1): 29, Jan./Feb. 2002

The following article is briefly presented
Albuminuria and risk of cardiovascular events, death and heart failure in diabetic and nondiabetic individuals. Gerstein, H.G., Mann, J.F. and Yi, Q. *et al.* for HOPE Study Investigators.
JAMA, **286:** 421–426, 25 July 2001.

This was a cohort of around 9000 patients enrolled in the Heart Outcomes Prevention Evaluation (HOPE) study. Patients came from practices in Europe, South and North America and had previous cardiovascular disease or diabetes plus one or more cardiovascular risk factors.
- Microalbuminuria was present in a third of those with diabetes and 15% of non-diabetic subjects.
- The risk of cardiovascular events and all-cause mortality increased with increasing microalbuminuria in both diabetic and non-diabetic individuals.
- Increased risk was present even at cut off levels below that for a diagnosis of microalbuminuria

Commentary
The HOPE study has already shown us that albuminuria is associated with an increased risk for MI, stroke, cardiovascular death, chronic heart failure and all-cause mortality. Further studies will be needed to ascertain whether albuminuria is a risk factor (that needs to be modified) or just a marker for cardiovascular disease.

A score for predicting risk of death from cardiovascular disease in adults with raised blood pressure, based on individual patient data from randomised controlled trials. Pocock, S.J., McCormack, V., Gueyffier, F. and Boutitie, F. *et al.* on behalf of the INDANA project steering committee. Department of Epidemiology and Population Health, London School of Hygeine and Tropical Medicine, London, UK.
***BMJ,* 323**(7304): 75-81, 14 July 2001.

This study involves the development of a new risk score for predicting risk of death from CVD. They analyse studies from the individual data analysis of antihypertensive intervention trials (INDANA) database.

- Eight RCTs of hypertensive treatment are identified.
- They use 11 risk factors, namely age, sex, systolic blood pressure, cholesterol, height, serum creatinine, smoking, diabetes, left ventricular hypertrophy and history of stroke or MI.
- Points are added for the presence of each risk factor. Men start with 12 more points than women, reflecting their increased risk. Smoking is more important in women than men. Antihypertensive therapy reduces the score.

The authors make reference to other risk scores e.g. Framingham, British regional heart study, Dundee, prospective cardiovascular Munster study. All of these use data from a single population. This present risk score uses data from subjects in North America and Europe, which improves the generalizability of the score. The authors state that the risk score complements the qualitative guidelines from the WHO and the International Society of Hypertension.

Cardiovascular risk factors and their effects on the decision to treat hypertension: evidence based review. Padwal, R., Straus, S.E. and McAlister, F.A. Division of General Internal Medicine, University of Alberta, Edmonton, Canada.
***BMJ,* 322**(7292): 977-980, 21 April 2001.

Blood pressure is related to risk of CVD in a graded fashion. International hypertension bodies differ in their chosen cut off points for the diagnosis of hypertension. Blood pressure is not the only risk factor for CVD and most risk tables take this into consideration when deciding upon a person's absolute risk of CVD. The *Framingham risk equation* is one of the most commonly used tables. *The cardiovascular disease life expectancy model* is in some aspects superior to the Framingham equations in that data is derived from people with and without CHD. The Framingham equations use only data from people who do not have CHD. Other risk tables include, *the Dundee coronary risk disk*, the *PROCAM risk function*, the *British regional heart study risk function.* The latter three have problems with generalizability to other populations. Modifiable risk factors include, cholesterol, smoking, diabetes, obesity, sedentary lifestyle and left ventricular hypertrophy. Alcohol in moderate amounts is associated with positive outcomes for CVD. Other risk factors have been studied but need further research. These include, triglycerides, lipoprotein a, microalbuminuria, uric acid, plasma renin A, fibrinogen, homocysteine, *chlamydia pneumonia,* inflammatory markers e.g. C-reactive protein.

HEART FAILURE

Primary Care: Prevalence of left ventricular systolic dysfunction and heart failure in high risk patients: community based epidemiological study. Davis, R.C., Hobbs, F.D.R. and Kenkre, J.E. *et al.* Department of Primary Care, University of Birmingham, Birmingham, UK.
***BMJ,* 325**(7373): 1156-1161, 16 November 2002.

This study conducted in Birmingham set out to see whether screening for heart failure and ventricular dysfunction improved disease pick-up and subsequent treatment rates. The commonest causes of ventricular dysfunction are MI, angina, hypertension and diabetes mellitus. The study also set out to see which of these risk factors are most important to enable cost-effective screening. Sixteen English GP practices were chosen at random and all patients with the above risk factors were identified. Of these around 1500 patients were chosen at random.

Each patient underwent a clinical history, ECG and echocardiogram. Overall around 65% of the patients attended for screening. Heart failure was defined as dyspnoea plus objective findings such as systolic dysfunction, atrial fibrillation or evidence of valvular disease.
- Heart failure was found in 16% of those with a previous MI; just over 8% of those with angina; nearly 3% of those with hypertension and nearly 8% of those with diabetes.
- Regression analysis showed that angina and diabetes were not independent risk factors for heart failure.

The authors conclude that previous MI is the best predictor of heart failure. They suggest that screening should be confined to patients with ischaemic heart disease.

The barriers to effective management of heart failure in general practice. Hickling, J.A., Nazareth, I. and Rogers, S. Department of Primary Care and Population Sciences, Royal Free and University College Medical School, University College London, UK.
***Br. J. Gen. Pract.,* 51**(469): 615-618, 1 August 2001.

The aim of this qualitative study is to explore the reasons for inadequate management of heart failure in general practice. They initially audit 10 practices from the Medical Research Council General Practice Research Framework. Thirty-nine principals and four registrars took part in group sessions designed to highlight barriers to effective management of heart failure. They found that:
- lack of open access to echocardiography and long waiting times to be seen were a significant barrier to referral for echocardiography;

- lack of perceived need for echocardiography was also stated, e.g. patient was already on ACE inhibitors or ACE inhibitors were not suitable;
- fear of side effects and lack of confidence in managing heart failure were reasons for not using ACE inhibitors;
- the "hassle" factor of dose titration, renal impairment and follow up were also sited as reasons for not using ACE inhibitors. They point out that these views may not be representative of general practice as a whole because these practices are part of the research framework. The views expressed are consistent with practitioners who are midway through a cycle of change.

Carvedilol reduced mortality and morbidity caused by myocardial infarction in patients with left ventricular dysfunction. Commentators, D. Jagasia and K. Shivkumar, University of Iowa Hospitals and Clinics, Iowa City, IA, USA.
Evidence-based Medicine, 7(1): 15, Jan./Feb. 2002.

Question: In patients with left ventricular dysfunction, does adding carvedilol to the management of myocardial infarction (MI) reduce mortality and non-fatal MI?

The following article is briefly presented
Effect of carvedilol on outcome after myocardial infarction in patients with left-ventricular dysfunction: the CAPRICORN randomised trial. The CAPRICORN Investigators.
Lancet, **357:** 1385–1390, 5 May 2001.

This was an RCT with 15 months follow up, involving around 1900 patients from 17 countries. All patients had had an MI between 3 days and 3 weeks prior to the study and also had left ventricular dysfunction. They received either carvedilol or placebo in addition to usual post MI management.
- The carvedilol group had lower all-cause and cardiovascular mortality rates compared with the placebo group.

Commentary
They highlight some of the limitations of the study. For example some of the studies were stopped early because of the perceived established benefits of β blockers post MI. They suggest that at the time of discharge after an MI, all eligible patients should receive:
- aspirin;
- a statin;
- ACE inhibitor.

Bucindolol reduced mortality and hospitalisation related to cardiovascular causes in advanced chronic heart failure. Commentator, Goutham Rao, University of Pittsburgh, Pittsburgh, PA, USA.
Evidence-based Medicine, **6**(6): 172, Nov./Dec. 2001

and

Carvedilol reduced mortality and hospitalisation in severe chronic heart failure. Commentator, Goutham Rao, University of Pittsburgh, Pittsburgh, PA, USA.
Evidence-based Medicine, **6**(6): 173, Nov./Dec. 2001

The following articles are briefly presented
A trial of the beta-blocker bucindolol in patients with advanced chronic heart failure. The Beta-blocker Evaluation of Survival Trial Investigators. [BEST].
N. Engl. J. Med., **344:** 1659–1667, 31 May 2001 **And**

Effect of carvedilol on survival in severe chronic heart failure. Packer, M., Coats, A.J. and Fowler, M.B. *et al.* for the Carvedilol Prospective Randomized Cumulative Survival Study Group. [COPERNICUS]
N. Engl. J. Med., **344:** 1651–1658, 31 May 2001.

The BEST study is an RCT involving just over 2700 patients from 90 centres in North America, with follow up of 2 years. Patients were assigned to either bucindolol or placebo.
 • All cause mortality was no different between the two groups at follow up.
 • Bucindolol patients had lower cardiovascular mortality and hospitalization rates than the placebo group.
The COPERNICUS study is an RCT involving around 2300 patients from 21 countries, with follow up of 10.4 months. Patients were given either carvedilol or placebo.
 • The carvedilol group had significantly lower death and hospitalization rates than the placebo group.

Combined commentary
Both trials were of good quality and both looked at patients with severe chronic heart failure. Carvedilol may have benefits over bucindolol which relate to its alpha-adrenergic, antioxidant and antiendothelial effects. Beta-blockers should be used routinely for mild to moderate heart failure. If the patient develops severe heart failure and is on a beta-blocker other than carvedilol, the patient should then be switched to carvedilolol. Studies directly comparing bucindolol and carvedilol may shed more light on this situation.

OTHERS

CLINICAL REVIEW SECTION: Beneficial effects of potassium. He, F.J. and MacGregor, G.A. Blood Pressure Unit, St. Georges Hospital Medical School, London, UK. *BMJ,* **323**(7311): 497-501, 1 September 2001.

This review analyses the beneficial effects of potassium. The easiest way to increase potassium in diet is to eat more fresh fruit and vegetables.

Blood pressure
The Intersalt study (*Am. J. Epidemiol.*, 1994) and other studies have shown that increased potassium intake either as supplements or in the diet, reduces blood pressure. Each 30-45 mmol increase in potassium is associated with a reduction in systolic blood pressure of 2-3 mmHg. It also seems that a reduction in sodium intake at the same time may have an additive effect.

Stroke
Studies also suggest that potassium may have a direct effect on stroke which is independent of its blood pressure effects. A 12 year prospective study (Khaw KT *NEJM* 1987) found a 10 mmol increase in potassium intake to be associated with a 40% reduction in death from stroke (independent of blood pressure). The Framingham study (20 year follow up study of around 800 middle aged men, JAMA 1995), showed that three daily helpings of fruit and vegetables was associated with a 22% decrease in risk of stroke (independent of blood pressure).

Renal damage and calcium balance
In rats increased potassium intake is associated with a reduced risk of renal disease. Increase potassium intake may be helpful in Black people who tend to have low potassium intakes and an increased prevalence of hypertensive renal disease.

Increased potassium intake is associated with reduced calcium excretion which may be beneficial for reducing the risk of kidney stones. A positive calcium balance would also help protect against osteoporosis.

Increased sodium intake has the opposite effect to potassium and hence, reducing sodium intake at the same time may have an additive effect.

Glucose intolerance
Hypokalaemia is associated with glucose intolerance. A 6-year prospective study in women found that high potassium intake is associated with reduced risk of type 2 diabetes.

Arrhythmias
Diuretics and heart failure predispose to hypokalaemia which is associated with cardiac arrhythmias. It is thought that one of the reasons that ACE inhibitors are so good in heart failure is because of their effect on potassium. The same is thought to be true of spironolactone. It has been

suggested that patients with heart failure should take a potassium supplement even if their initial potassium concentration was normal. Magnesium may need to be given as well as potassium as this is often low at the same time.

Adverse effects of high potassium intake.

The only real danger from high potassium comes when the individual has renal impairment or when it is given by intravenous injection.

Healthy levels of potassium intake are in excess of 200 mmol/day. Processed food has potassium removed. This together with the fact that our diets are poor in fruit and vegetables means that our usual intake is around 70 mmol/day.

Sex matters: secular and geographical trends in sex differences in coronary heart disease mortality. Lawlor, D.A., Ebrahim, S. and Davey Smith, G. Department of Social Medicine, University of Bristol, Bristol, UK.
BMJ, 323(7312): 541-5, 8 September 2001.

The aim of this study was to explore the relationship between sex and coronary heart disease. They use data from the UK and 50 other countries over a period spanning between 1921 and 1998. The study showed that:
- The increase in heart disease that occurred over the last century mainly affected men.
- Some countries show minimal sex differences for heart disease mortality.
- Fat intake in the diet correlates with mortality from coronary heart disease. Increasing fat intake is associated with increased mortality from coronary heart disease in men. The reverse is true in women.

They conclude that sex differences in heart disease mortality cannot be solely explained by oestrogen, but are also controlled by environmental factors.

Antidepressants as risk factor for ischaemic heart disease: case-control study in primary care. Hippisley-Cox, J., Pringle, M. and Hammersely, V. *et al.* Division of General Practice, University of Nottingham, Nottingham, UK.
BMJ, 323(7314): 666-669, 22 September 2001.

This case-control study involved around 930 cases (men and women with ischaemic heart disease) and around 5500 controls, from general practices in the Trent region. The aim of the study was to assess the relationship between antidepressants and heart disease.
- After controlling for confounding factors, tricyclic antidepressants were significantly associated with ischaemic heart disease.
- Dothiepin (dosulepin) alone seemed to account for this increased risk.
- Patients who had taken dothiepin had a 67% increased risk of ischaemic heart disease. This risk was regardless of how long ago the dothiepin was taken.

- The more prescriptions of dothiepin the greater the risk of ischaemic heart disease.The conclude that three out of five criteria for causality have been met concerning dothiepin and ischaemic heart disease. The five criteria are association, temporal relation, dose-response, specificity and biological explanation.Association and dose-response are clear from the results. A biological explanation can be given by the fact that tricyclics antidepressants:
- are class one antiarrhythmic drugs and can cause orthostatic hypotension, both of which are associated with MI;
- increase insulin resistance, which is associated with atheroma;
- there is also evidence that dothiepin is more toxic than other tricyclics antidepressants.

Sex inequalities in ischaemic heart disease in general practice: cross sectional survey. Hippisley-Cox, J., Pringle, M. and Crown, N. *et al.* Division of General Practice, Nottingham University, Nottingham, UK.
***BMJ,* 322**(7290): 832-834, 7 April 2001.

The aim of this study was to assess whether men and women with heart disease are managed differently in general practice. Data was extracted from the case notes of nearly 6000 men and women in the Trent region of the UK. There was evidence of bias towards men in that:
- women were more likely to have a raised cholesterol but were less likely to be taking lipid lowering drugs;
- risk factors were less likely to be recorded for women than men;
- men were more likely to be taking aspirin than women.

FURTHER READING

See 'Hypertension' for

CLINICAL REVIEW SECTION - Using cardiovascular risk profiles to individualise hypertensive treatment. Division of General Internal Medicine, University of North Carolina at Chapel Hill, Chapel Hill, NC, USA.
***BMJ,* 322**(7295): 1164-1166, 12 May 2001

See 'Lipids' for

Dietary fat intake and prevention of cardiovascular disease: systematic review. Manchester Dental and Education Centre (MANDEC). University Dental Hospital of Manchester, Manchester.
***BMJ,* 322**(7289): 757-763, 31 March 2001

Joint British recommendations on prevention of coronary heart disease in clinical practice: summary. British Cardiac Society, British Hyperlipidaemia Association, British Hypertension Society, British Diabetic Association.
***BMJ,* 320**(7236): 705, 11 March 2000

Updated New Zealand cardiovascular disease risk-benefit prediction guide. Jackson, R., Department of Community Health, University of Auckland, Auckland, New Zealand.
BMJ, **320**(7236): 709, 11 March 2000

Do patients with suspected heart failure and preserved left ventricular systolic function suffer from 'diastolic heart failure' or from misdiagnosis? A prospective descriptive study. Caruana, L., Petrie, M.C., Davie, A.P. and McMurray, J.J.V., Department of Cardiology, Western Infirmary, Glasgow.
BMJ, **321**(7255): 215-219, 22 July 2000.

Individualised multifactorial lifestyle intervention trial for high-risk cardiovascular patients in primary care. Ketola, E. and Mäkelä, M., Klockars National Research and Development Centre for Welfare and Health Helsinki.
Br. J. Gen. Pract., **51**(465): 291-294, April 2001.

Cardiovascular risk factors and disease in general practice; results of the Nijmegen Cohort Study. Bakx, J.C., Van den Hoogen, H.J.M., Van den Bosch, W.J.H.M. *et al.,* University of Nijmegen, The Netherlands.
Br. J. Gen. Pract., **52**(475): 135-137, Feb. 2002.

See 'Antiplatelet therapy' for

Aspirin but not vitamin E prevented cardiovascular events in patients at risk. Providence-St Vincent Medical Center, Portland, OR, USA.
Evidence-based Medicine, **6**(4): 112, July 2001.

See 'Ethnic minorities' for

Early evidence of ethnic differences in cardiovascular risk: cross sectional comparison of British South Asian and white children. Department of Public Health Sciences, St Georges Hospital Medical School, London.
BMJ, **324**(7338): 935-938, 16 March 2002.

HELICOBACTER PYLORI

- Young, healthy people with ulcer-like dyspepsia who are HP positive should be treated empirically rather than being referred for endoscopy
- A meta-analysis has shown that HP eradication therapy may be useful for non-ulcer dyspepsia
- Antibiotic susceptibility testing of *H. pylori* is likely to become a prerequisite for successful eradication of *H. pylori* from individual patients
- A study published in the *Lancet* has found that a test-and-treat strategy for the management of dyspeptic symptoms is as effective as prompt endoscopy.
- The authors of a Dutch study have concluded that choosing empirical treatment based on symptom subgroups is a reasonable approach.

BACKGROUND

EPIDEMIOLOGY

H. pylori (HP) is part of a large and enormously diverse family of bacteria that are likely to have been around for thousands of years. They can be regarded as normal flora which are acquired during childhood, probably from a family member, via the faeco-oral route. Colonization rates of HP seem to be decreasing which may reflect environmental circumstances e.g. better living conditions. Indeed those from low socio-economic backgrounds and those living in overcrowded conditions have the highest prevalence rates. Vaccination against HP may soon be available.

Carriers of HP are known to be at a 3-10 fold increased risk of the following:

- peptic ulcer;
- adenocarcinoma of the antrum and body of the stomach;
- non-Hodgkin's (MALTomas) of the stomach.

Ulcer disease and adenocarcinoma have been decreasing alongside the decline in HP colonization rates. However, it is thought that some strains of HP offer a protective effect against oesophageal reflux and adenocarcinoma of the distal oesophagus. So that, whilst colonization rates have been decreasing the rates of these conditions have been increasing. Some have therefore suggested that asymptomatic individuals should be left untreated unless they have a first degree relative with adenocarcinoma of the stomach.

NON-INVASIVE DIAGNOSIS OF INFECTION

Breath tests

The patient swallows a fixed amount of urea, labelled with a carbon isotope (13C or 14C) as a test meal after a 4 hour fast. If HP is present, the urea is rapidly broken down to 13C or 14C carbon dioxide which is measured in a breath sample taken 30 minutes later. As yet, no urea breath test is licensed in the UK, so it is only available on a named patient basis. Urea breath tests are the only non-invasive tests that are specific for active infection. They have a sensitivity of 90-95%. They require careful supervision and cost more than serological assays. In order to be sure that HP eradication therapy has succeeded and not just simply suppressed the infection, the test must be done at least 28 days after completing treatment and 14 days after stopping any antibiotic or proton pump inhibitor.

Serological tests

The immune response to HP infection is complex. Two percent of people fail to mount a response despite proven infection. Serological tests will remain positive for at least 6 months after eradication of the bacteria, so their use to confirm cure is not practical. Laboratory based serological assays have a wide range of sensitivities and specificities and tests should be validated locally amongst the relevant population. GP based tests (near-patient) that can be used without laboratory support are also available. Some tests use finger capillary blood and can produce a result within minutes. The Medical Devices Agency has published a report of the poor specificity of these kits compared to breath testing, histology or culture.

COST-EFFECTIVENESS

A decision analysis model has found that the cost savings associated with eradication therapy and a reduction in H_2 antagonists, may take many years to materialize (*BMJ*, May 1996). A further decision analysis model (*BMJ*, May 1998) found that the most cost-effective regimen for eradication of HP was omeprazole, chlarithromycin and metronidazole.

MANAGEMENT

> **TESTING: Randomised trial of endoscopy with testing for Helicobacter pylori compared with non-invasive H. pylori testing alone in the management of dyspepsia.** McColl, K.E.L., Murray, S. and Gillen, D. *et al.* University Department of Medicine and Therapeutics, Western Infirmary, Glasgow, UK.
> **BMJ, 324**(7344): 999-1002, 27 April 2002.

The aim of this RCT was to compare non-invasive *H. pylori* testing (C-urea breath testing) with endoscopy plus *H. pylori* testing. Nearly 590 patients from gastroenterology clinics in Glasgow were followed up for 12 months. They found that:
- Outcomes were similar between the two groups in terms of change in dyspepsia scores and satisfaction.
- No serious pathology was missed in the non-invasive group.

TREATMENT PRIMARY CARE: Treating Helicobacter pylori infection in primary care patients with uninvestigated dyspepsia: the Canadian adult dyspepsia empiric treatment – Helicobacter pylori positive (CADET-Hp) randomised controlled trial. Chiab, N., van Zanten, S.J.O.V. and Sinclair, P. *et al.*, Division of Gastroenterology, McMaster University, Hamilton, Canada.
BMJ, 324(7344): 1012-1016, 27 April 2002.

This was an RCT involving around 290 patients from 36 family practices in Canada. The aim of the study was to assess whether a "test and treat" strategy for *H. pylori* associated dyspepsia without prior endoscopic investigation, confers any symptomatic relief after 1 year. All patients were *H. pylori* positive on C-urea breath testing. Patients were randomised to receive either triple therapy (omeprazole, metronidazole and clarithromycin) twice a day for 7 days or the same therapy as placebo. They found that:

- Triple therapy was better than placebo (NNT 7).
- Eighty percent of the triple therapy group were cured.
- Eradication therapy was cheaper after 1 year than placebo.

Testing for Helicobacter pylori in dyspeptic patients suspected of peptic ulcer disease in primary care: cross sectional study. Weignen, C.F., Numans, M.E. and de Wit, N.J. *et al.*, Julius Centre for General Practice and Patient Orientated Research, University Medical Centre Utrecht, Location Stratenum, Universiteitsweg, Utrecht, Netherlands.
BMJ, 323(7304): 71-75, 14 July 2001.

The aim of this study was to develop a scoring method to help diagnose peptic ulcers in dyspeptic patients in primary care. This was achieved by investigating whether *H. pylori* testing adds any value to history taking. This was a cross-sectional study performed in the Netherlands, involving 565 patients who consulted a GP about dyspeptic symptoms.

- Three simple questions; history of peptic ulcer, pain on an empty stomach, and smoking can distinguish between 'low' and 'high' risk patients of peptic ulcer disease. The odds ratio for the three questions respectively were 5.5 (95 confidence interval 2.6 to 11.8), 2.8 (1.0 to 4.0) and 2.0 (1.4 to 6.0).
- Applying *H. pylori* testing in all patients with dyspepsia in primary care added no value to history taking in the diagnosis of peptic ulcer. But *H. pylori* testing only in 'high' risk patients improved the predictive value of history taking from 16 to 26.

H. pylori testing is only of value in high-risk patients. For low-risk patients, history taking alone is sufficient.

MANAGEMENT : TESTING FOR *H. PYLORI*

EDITORIAL – Causes of failure of eradication of Helicobacter pylori. Antibiotic resistance is the major cause, and susceptibility testing may help. Jenks, P. Institute of Infections and Immunity, University Hospital, Nottingham, UK.
***BMJ*, 325**(7354): 3-4, 6 July 2002.

In the management of peptic ulcer disease, the eradication of *II. pylori* from infected patients is the most important goal. At present basing therapy on susceptibility data obtained from the laboratory before treatment is rarely performed because of cost implications and because of "methodological problems". The author predicts that susceptibility testing will be of growing importance based on the following main points:
* The current refinement of protocols will "improve reproducibility of tests and allow surveillance of antibiotic resistance". This will enable the prevalence of resistant strains to be monitored and guide empirical treatment on the basis of local resistance.
* Antibiotic resistance is the major cause of treatment failure and the rising proportion of patients colonized with resistant strains will mean that the savings made by "avoiding follow up of patients and costs for repeated treatment will outweigh the expense of acquiring the specimens by endoscopy".

The author stresses the need for "future interpretative criteria" to be based on "trials where the *in vitro* susceptibility of a population of isolates is correlated with the clinical efficacy of the regimen".

Helicobacter pylori testing and endoscopy were less cost-effective than usual management for patients with dyspepsia. Commentator, Nicholas Talley, University of Sydney, Penrith, Australia.
***Evidence-based Medicine*, 6**(6): 189, Nov./Dec. 2001

Question: In patients who had had dyspepsia for > 4 weeks, are testing and endoscopy as cost-effective as usual management for dyspepsia?

The following article is briefly presented
Randomised controlled trial Helicobacter pylori testing and endoscopy for dyspepsia in primary care. Delaney, B.C, Wilson, S. and Roalfe, A. *et al.*
***BMJ*, 322:** 898–901, 14 April 2001

This was an RCT involving around 470 patients from 31 primary care centres in the UK, with 18 months follow up. Patients with dyspepsia either had an *H. pylori* (Helisal) test followed by endoscopy (in those who were positive) or usual general practitioner care.
* At follow up they found no difference between the two groups for outcomes.
* Testing and endoscopy cost on average £368, whereas usual care cost £253.

Commentary

The British Society of Gastroenterology recommends testing followed by endoscopy in those who are positive. The study by Delaney suggests that this strategy is not as cost-effective as usual care. Usual care resulted in less than half the number of endoscopies compared with the test and endoscopy group. The results in this study may have been hampered by the use of the Helisal test which is not very accurate.

'Test and treat' seems to be more cost-effective than 'test and endoscope'. However, in younger patents (for whom there is a lower prevalence of *H.pylori*, peptic ulcer disease and more serious pathology) the most cost-effective strategy may be a short trial of proton pump inhibitor.

EDITORIAL – Dyspepsia in primary care to prescribe or to investigate. Ghosh, S. and Kinnear, M. Gastrointestinal Unit, Department of Medical Sciences, University of Edinburgh, Western General Hospital, UK.
***Br. J. Gen. Pract.*, 51**(469): 612-613, 1 August 2001.

There is still much debate concerning the management of dyspepsia in primary care.

Early endoscopy
Referral for early endoscopy is indicated particularly if there are alarm symptoms, e.g. weight loss, vomiting, early satiety and anaemia. Using age alone as an indication for referral is unlikely to be helpful.

Investigation of uncomplicated dyspepsia
There is little evidence to support prompt referral for endoscopy in uncomplicated dyspepsia. A Danish study (*Lancet*, 1994) and a Swiss survey (*Eur. J. Gastroenterol. Hepatol.* 1997) both found no benefit from prompt endoscopy.

Test and treat vs. early endoscopy for H. pylori
Two randomized trials (*Gastroenterology*, 1998; *Gut*, 1999) looking at this issue were subject to bias (patients aged over 45 were excluded).

H. pylori eradication therapy in non-ulcer dyspepsia
Five large and good quality studies have addressed this issue. Four out of five found no evidence of a benefit from eradication therapy. None of these trials had sufficient power to be conclusive about these results.

Prokinetic therapies in dyspepsia
A MA showed a 10% RRR for patients with dyspepsia. The problem here is that cisapride has fallen from grace and other prokinetics e.g. domperidone and metaclopramide are still being evaluated.

Reflux symptoms

A Cochrane MA found prokinetc agents and H2 antagonists useful in this situation. Updated dyspepsia criteria will not include reflux-like symptoms (Rome criteria: *Gut* 1999)

> **A randomised controlled trial of four management strategies for dyspepsia: relationships between symptom subgroup and strategy outcome.** Lewin-van den Broek, N., Numans, M.E. and Buskens, E. *et al.* Jullius Centre for General Practice and Patient Oriented Research, University Medical Center, Utrecht, The Netherlands.
> **Br. J. Gen. Pract., 51**(469): 619-624, 1 August 2001.

This Dutch study was a randomized controlled trial comparing four treatment strategies for the management of dyspepsia in primary care. Just over 300 patients were randomized into either:

1. symptom based therapy i.e. patients with reflux-like and ulcer-like symptoms were given acid suppressants. Patients with non-specific symptoms were given prokinetic agents (cisapride). All for 8 weeks;
2. empirical treatment with omeprazole for 8 weeks;
3. empirical treatment with cisapride for 8 weeks;
4. prompt endoscopy.

Follow up was at regular intervals up to 1 year.

- Outcomes (proportion of patients with strategy failure) were not significantly different between the groups.

They found some non-significant trends e.g.

- Patients with reflux-like symptoms benefited most from treatment with omeprazole, cisapride or endoscopy.
- Patients with ulcer-like symptoms benefited most from treatment with omeprazole.
- Patients with non-specific symptoms benefited most from cisapride.
- The non-specific group had poorer outcomes overall.
- The presence of *H. pylori* did not influence outcome.

Whilst noting that the overall power of the study is low, they conclude with the following recommendations.

- Choosing empirical treatment based on symptom subgroups is a reasonable approach.
- Acid suppression drugs should be reserved for those whose symptoms clearly indicate an acid problem.
- Omeprazole rather than an H2 antagonists is preferred when pain is the main symptom.
- Give prokinetic drugs to those with non-specific symptoms

Helicobacter pylori testing plus eradication was as effective and safe as prompt endoscopy for dyspepsia. Commentator, J.O. Sander, Velduyzen van Zanten, Queen Elizabeth II Health Sciences Center, Halifax, Nova Scotia, Canada.
Evidence-based Medicine, 6(2): 48, March/April 2001

The following paper is briefly presented

Helicobacter pylori **test-and-eradication versus prompt endoscopy for management of dyspeptic patients: a randomised trial**. Lassen, A.T., Pedersen, F.M. and Bytzer, P. *et al.*
Lancet, **356:** 455–460, 5 Aug. 2000.

This randomised controlled trial, involved 500 Danish patients with at least a 2 week history of dyspeptic symptoms. Half of the patients were in the test-and-treat group and half were in the prompt endoscopy group. Those found to be positive in the test-and-treat group received a 2 week course of lansoprazole, metronidazole and amoxicillin.

- At 1 year follow up, there was no difference between the two groups for days off work, days without symptoms or quality of life.
- Patients in the prompt endoscopy group were more satisfied with care than the test-and-treat group.

Commentary

The commentator describes this as a well performed study. They note that patients with alarm symptoms were excluded from this study, but otherwise there was no upper age limit for entry into the study. Other guidelines recommend endoscopy for anyone aged between 50 and 55 years.

HORMONE REPLACEMENT THERAPY

> • A postal survey of post-menopausal women found that increasing rates of use of HRT is attributable to a desire for relief of menopausal symptoms and to a lesser extent for disease prevention.
>
> • A cochrane meta-analysis, ultrasonography and a recent paper all agree with the case-controlled studies in showing that continuous combined hormone replacement therapy reduces the incidence of endometrial cancer.
>
> • A 5 year follow up study found that long term continuous combined HRT does not increase the risk of endometrial cancer.

EDITORIAL – Continuous combined hormone replacement therapy and endometrial hyperplasia. Risk of developing cancer is very low. Archer, D.F. Director, Clinical Research Centre and Professor of Obstetrics and Gynaecology, The Jones Institute for Reproductive Medicine, Colley Avenue, Norfolk, UK.
***BMJ,* 325**(7358): 231-232, 3 August 2002.

The possible benefits of combined hormone replacement therapy, consisting of an oestrogen and a progestogen, include prevention of endometrial hyperplasia and reduction of endometrial bleeding. Exposure to oestrogen and progestin continuously maybe more important than using oestrogen intermittently. Endometrial cancer is a major concern for women using cyclic hormone replacement. However, continuous combined hormone replacement therapy as well as not increasing the incidence of endometrial cancer, could even be protective. Endometrial hyperplasia is used as the end point in clinical trials.

- All clinical trials of unopposed oestrogen at moderate and high doses have shown an increase in the incidence of endometrial hyperplasia, related to dose and duration.
- A Cochrane meta-analysis has shown no difference in the rate of endometrial hyperplasia between continuous combined hormone replacement and placebo.
- Ultrasonography has failed to document any malignant cause for endometrial bleeding in postmenopausal bleeding women taking continuous combined hormone replacement therapy.
- A paper has found no evidence of endometrial hyperplasia after 5 years of continuous combined hormone replacement.

These data agree with the case-controlled studies showing a reduction in the incidence of endometrial cancer in women taking continuous combined hormone replacement therapy.

Effect of long term treatment with continuous combined oestrogen-progesterone replacement therapy: follow-up study. Wells, M., Sturdee, D.W. and Barlow, D.H. *et al.* Academic Unit of Pathology, Section of Oncology and Pathology, Division of Genomic Medicine, University of Sheffield Medical School, Sheffield, UK.
***BMJ*, 325**(7358): 239-242, 3 August 2002.

The aim of this follow up study in post-menopausal women was to determine the effect on endometrial histology of 5 years of continuous combined oestrogen-progesterone replacement therapy. A total of 534 women, from 31 menopause clinics in the UK, all with an intact uterus, and who had all undergone a 9 month course of combined 2 mg 17-oestradiol and 1 mg norethisterone acetate were followed up for 5 years (including the original 9 month trial). Endometrial aspiration biopsies were taken before the continuous combined hormone replacement (HRT) was commenced, at 9 months, between 24 and 36 months, and at the end of treatment (or withdrawal from the study).

- No cases of endometrial hyperplasia or malignancy were detected by a single independent pathologist assessing the samples.
- Prior to the study, 21 women were found to have complex hyperplasia, which reverted to normal after 9 months of continuous combined HRT.

Previous studies have demonstrated that while long term use of sequential oestrogen-progesterone HRT increases the risk of endometrial cancer, continuous combined HRT does not. This study supports the latter finding in a long term follow-up and provides reassurance that this therapy does not increase the risk of endometrial cancer.

Women's use of hormone replacement therapy for disease prevention; results of a community survey. Ballard, K. Department of General Practice and Primary Care, Guys, Kings and St. Thomas' School of Medicine, London, UK.
***Br. J. Gen. Pract.*, 483**(52): 835-838, 1 October 2002.

Use of Hormone Replacement Therapy (HRT) by menopausal women in the UK has risen from 19% having tried HRT in 1990 to 45% of women age 50 in 2000. There is also data suggesting that duration of use of HRT by women over 50 is increasing. It has been suggested that this increased use of HRT may be attributable to either a desire for palliation of menopausal symptoms or the potential benefits from disease prevention (e.g. prevention of osteoporosis). The authors utilised a postal questionnaire, sent to 650 randomly selected women (from West Surrey), to evaluate the reasons for women aged 51–57 to take HRT. The authors found:

- Of the 66% (413) of women who responded, 60% had tried HRT and 42% were currently using HRT.
- The median length of time women used HRT for was 4.0 years.
- The commonest reason for taking HRT was relief of hot flushes (70%).

- Fifty eight percent stated that they took HRT for osteoporosis prevention, while only 20% took it for prevention of coronary heart disease.

They conclude that both the prevalence and duration of HRT use continue to increase, and, that the principle reason for using HRT is relief of menopausal symptoms.

HYPERTENSION

- Short acting calcium channel blockers have been shown to increase the incidence of CHD by 12% and possibly of heart failure by 12%
- GPs management of hypertension in a Dutch study was inadequate. Sixty three percent of patients analysed had a diastolic blood pressure over 90 mmHg
- White coat hypertension is responsible for unnecessary treatment initiation and alteration
- The ideal method of blood pressure monitoring needs to be acceptable to patients and be medically accurate. Ambulatory monitoring does not meet these requirements
- Antihypertensive treatment of older patients with isolated systolic hypertension is beneficial regardless of cardiovascular risk status
- One study found that reducing sodium intake by 40 mmol/l per day lowered blood pressure by 4.3/2 mmHg.

BACKGROUND

Internationally there are currently at least five different sets of guidelines regarding the treatment of hypertension; arising from New Zealand, Canada, Britain, USA and the WHO. All are said to be evidence-based and yet they all differ in content and emphasis. Nevertheless, what is clear is that lowering blood pressure in hypertensives, results in decreased coronary events and strokes. A decrease in diastolic blood pressure of 5–6 mmHg and of systolic blood pressure of 10 mmHg has been shown to decrease strokes by one third and coronary events by one sixth.

Non-pharmacological methods have been shown to decrease blood pressure by 10 systolic and 8 diastolic. Subjects are advised to:
- stop smoking;
- avoid excess alcohol;
- increase exercise;
- decrease energy intake to achieve ideal body weight;
- decrease salt intake;
- decrease intake of saturated fats.

The risk of smoking and the benefit in those who stop outweigh the benefit of treating mild hypertension.

SALT

Replacing common salt with mineral salt can lower diastolic and systolic blood pressure. However, much of the battle with salt needs to be fought at the food processing level.

Salt intake in the UK and USA (9–12 g/day) is much higher than the recommended daily requirements (500 mg/day). Little (15%) of our salt intake comes from salt added during cooking/mealtimes and only 10% comes from the natural salt content of food. A staggering 75% comes from salt added during food processing procedures.

ELDERLY HYPERTENSIVES

There had previously been some debate about whether or not to treat elderly hypertensives. Most of the evidence suggests that those over the age of 60 years should be treated and treatment reduces coronary events and strokes. Some of the questions concerning treating elderly hypertensives may have arisen because some studies suggested that elderly people with lower blood pressures have a higher mortality than those with higher blood pressures. This finding may arise because low blood pressures are associated with cancers and heart failure and those with higher blood pressures are more likely to be identified and treated.

DRUG THERAPIES

The HOT trial (*Lancet* 1998: RCT, 19 000 patients, 4 year follow-up) found that low dose aspirin significantly reduces cardiovascular events in people with hypertension. Lowering diastolic blood pressure to between 85 and 90 mmHg should be our aim (80 mmHg in diabetics).
   A meta-analysis of 12 studies (*JAMA*, 1998) suggests that diuretics should be used as first line in elderly hypertensives. The study found that:
* diuretics reduced cerebrovascular events, coronary heart disease, strokes, cardiovascular mortality and all-cause mortality;
* β-blockers only reduced cerebrovascular events.

DRUG THERAPIES

CLINICAL REVIEW SECTION – What are the elements of good treatment for hypertension? Mulrow, C.D. and Pignone, M. Division of General Internal Medicine, University of Texas, San Antonio, USA.
BMJ, 322(7294): 1107-1109, 5 May 2001.

This forms one of a series of 5 articles published between April and May 2001 under the title 'Evidence based management of hypertension'. Information is taken from a book entitled 'Evidence-based Hypertension' by Michael Pignone and Cynthia Mulrow. This article assesses the benefits and harms of drug management of hypertension. Drug treatments reduce the risk of stroke, cardiac events and death. Those with the highest initial risk e.g. elderly and those with other risk factors, gain the most from treatment. It is not clear whether the benefits come from a direct antihypertensive effect or from other indirect actions.

Thiazides
High and low doses reduce strokes and death rates. Low doses only, reduce coronary artery disease (CAD).

β-blockers
Data suggests (but is not conclusive) that β-blockers reduce strokes but not CAD or death.

ACE inhibitors
One study (*NEJM*, 2000) found that ramipril reduced cardiovascular events (CVEs) by 22% and death by 16% in high risk subjects. A review of 4 RCTs (*Lancet*, 2000) showed that ACE inhibitors reduced strokes by 30% and CHD by 20%.

Calcium channel blockers
One study (*Lancet*, 1997) showed that a long acting calcium channel blocker reduced CVEs by 31%.

Comparisons between different antihypertensive agents
- The new antihypertensives have not been shown to be more effective than diuretics and β-blockers in reducing cardiovascular morbidity and mortality.
- Thiazides seem to reduce CVEs more than β-blockers (12% difference). Both are equally effective at lowering blood pressure.
- In type 2 diabetes, UKPDS 39 (*BMJ*, 1998) found no difference in blood pressure or CVEs between β-blockers and ACE inhibitors.
- Studies comparing long acting calcium channel blockers with diuretics and β-blockers have found no difference in CVEs.

Serious adverse events
- Short acting calcium channel blockers have been shown to increase the incidence of CHD by 12% and possibly of heart failure by 12% (whilst reducing strokes by 13%).
- A study showed that doxazosin (α agonist) increases the risk of CVEs, especially heart failure, compared with a thiazide diuretic.
- Long term use of diuretics doubles the (already low) risk of renal carcinoma.

Long acting nifedipine was as effective as hydrochlorothiazide plus amiloride for reducing mortality and morbidity in hypertension. Commentator, Cynthia Mulrow, Audie L. Murphy Memorial Veterans Hospital, San Antonio, Texas, USA.
***Evidence–based Medicine, 6**(1): 10–11, Jan./Feb. 2001.*

Question: In patients with hypertension who are at high risk for cardiovascular (CV) events, is long acting nifedipine, a calcium channel blocker, as effective as co-amilozide (hyrdochlorothiazide and amiloride) for preventing CV and cerebrovascular mortality and morbidity?

and

Question: In middle aged patients with hypertension, is diltiazem a non-dihydropyridine calcium antagonist, as effective as diuretics, β-blockers, or both at preventing cardiovascular (CV) events?

The following article is briefly presented
Morbidity and mortality in patients randomized to double–blind treatment with a long–acting calcium–channel blocker or diuretic in the International Nifedipine GITS study: Intervention as a Goal in Hypertension Treatment (INSIGHT). Brown, M.J., Palmer, C.R. and Castaigne, A. *et al. Lancet,* **356:** 366–372, 29 July 2000.

Diltiazem was as effective as diuretics or β–blockers or both at preventing cardiovascular mortality and morbidity. Commentator, Cynthia Mulrow, Audie L. Murphy Memorial Veterans Hospital, San Antonio, Texas, USA.
Evidence–based Medicine, **6**(1): 10–11, Jan./Feb. 2001.

The following article is briefly presented
Randomised trial of effects of calcium antagonists compared with diuretics and β–blockers on cardiovascular morbidity and mortality in hypertension: Nordic Diltiazem (NORDIL) study. Hansson, L., Hedner, T. and Lund–Johansen, P. *et al. Lancet,* **356:** 359–365, 29 July 2000.

Both studies look at the effect of calcium antagonists on cardiovascular morbidity and mortality in the treatment of hypertension. The INSIGHT study compares calcium antagonists with a diuretic. The NORDIL study compares calcium antagonists with a diuretic, β-blocker or both.
The INSIGHT trial is an RCT involving around 7000 patients from eight countries, with a 3 years or greater follow up.
  • Both the calcium antagonist group and the diuretic group were equally effective at reducing cardiovascular morbidity and mortality.
  • Adverse events and non-fatal heart failure were more common in the nifedipine group.
In the NORDIL study, patients (over 10 000 of them) were randomized to either calcium antagonist, or β-blocker or diuretic or both. Follow up was for greater than 4 years.
  • There was no difference between the groups for combined cardio-vascular end points.

Commentary
Mulrow comments that these two trials 'add to the acronymic litany of recent trials'. There are now 10 trials which compare calcium antagonists with other hypertensives. The trials tend to be too small and the findings are variable and difficult to interpret. Adverse effects are more frequent in the current second line antihypertensive agents e.g. 30% have cough with ACE inhibitors, 25% have peripheral oedema with calcium antagonists. Calcium antagonists are more expensive than current first line treatments.

ELDERLY HYPERTENSIVES

Treating isolated systolic hypertension prevented major cardiovascular events across strata of risk in older patients. Gray, J. Queen Elizabeth II Health Sciences Centre, Halifax, Nova Scotia, Canada.
Evidence-based Medicine, 7(4): 109, July/Aug. 2002.

Question: In older patients with isolated systolic hypertension (ISH), is blood pressure (BP) lowering treatment more effective than placebo for preventing major cardiovascular disease (CVD) events in those at high risk than in those at low risk?

The following article is briefly presented

Treatment of isolated systolic hypertension is most effective in older patients with high-risk profile. Ferrucci, L., Furberg, C.D., Penninx, B.W. *et al.* INRCA Geriatric Department, Florence, Italy.
Circulation **104:** 1923-1926, 16 Oct. 2001

This study was a subgroup analysis of the SHEP (Systolic ypertension in the Elderly Program) trial, and involved just under 4200, 60 year old patients from five centres in the US. All had isolated systolic hypertension. Follow up was for 4.5 years. Patients were allocated to treatment (stepped programme involving chlorthalidone, followed by atenolol or reserpine) or placebo groups. The main outcome measure was the first occurring major cardiovascular disease event (stroke, MI or congestive cardiac failure).

The rates of major cardiovascular events were lower in the treatment vs placebo group.

Commentary

Gray notes that the results of Ferrucci et al. suggest that even though patients of all levels of risk benefit from antihypertensive treatment, the extent of this benefit is greater for those patients in the higher risk groups.

The Swedish Trial in Old Patients with Hypertension-2 (*Lancet* 1999) looked at the effect of ACE inhibitors and calcium channel blockers and showed similar beneficial effects to SHEP (which originally started in 1984). Further trials also need to consider the effect of reduced fat and reduced sodium diets.

CLINICAL REVIEW SECTION – What to do when blood pressure is difficult to control. O'Rorke, J.E. and Richardson, W.S. Division of General Internal Medicine, University of Texas at San Antonio, San Antonio, USA.
BMJ, **322**(7296): 1229-1232, 19 May 2001.

This forms one of a series of five articles published between April and May 2001 under the title 'Evidence based management of hypertension'. Information is taken from a book entitled 'Evidence-based Hypertension' by Michael Pignone and Cynthia Mulrow. This article discusses what to do when blood pressure is poorly controlled. The following reasons should be considered:

- **Inaccurate measurement.** Ensure that correct measurement technique is used;
- **White coat hypertension.** Use different measuring strategies e.g. home, self-monitoring, ambulatory, practice nurse;
- **Disease progression.** Exclude other causes before concluding that the disease has progressed;
- **Suboptimal treatment.** In one hypertension trial, more than 70% of patients needed more than one drug to control blood pressure. Also reassess diet and exercise;
- **Non-compliance.** Direct and non-judgmental questioning may illicit non-compliance;
- **Antagonizing substances.** For example, steroids, alcohol, caffeine, cocaine, amphetamines, contraceptive pill, NSAIDs.
- **Co-existing conditions.** Conditions such as anxiety, obesity, pain, smoking, sleep apnoea can raise blood pressure;
- **Secondary hypertension.** This is an uncommon reason, but if it is suspected, the patient will require specialist investigations.

CLINICAL REVIEW SECTION – Using cardiovascular risk profiles to individualise hypertensive treatment. Pignone, M. and Mulrow, C. Division of General Internal Medicine, University of North Carolina at Chapel Hill, Chapel Hill, NC, USA.
***BMJ*, 322**(7295): 1164-1166, 12 May 2001.

This forms one of a series of articles published between April and May 2001 under the title 'Evidence based management of hypertension'. Information is taken from a book entitled 'Evidence-based Hypertension' by Michael Pignone and Cynthia Mulrow. This article discusses the difficulties of treating patients who are at increased risk of CVD. They also look at strategies (including decision tools) for managing patients who also have other serious conditions, that might impact upon the decision or importance of treating hypertension. They give factors that need to be considered when prioritizing treatments, which include:

- benefits and harm of treatments;
- cost and availability of treatments;
- likelihood of compliance;
- risks associated with other conditions and whether or not these conditions will negate the need for antihypertensive treatment e.g. patient with end stage dementia and high blood pressure;
- interactions between treatments;
- patient and provider preferences.

Blood pressure control in treated hypertensive patients: clinical performance of general practitioners. Frijling, B.D., Spies, T.H. and Lobo, C.M. *et al.* Centre for Quality of Care Research, University of Nijmegen, The Netherlands.
Br. J. Gen. Pract., **51**(462): 9-14, Jan. 2001.

This Dutch study examines general practitioner's performance in the management of hypertension. Nearly 200 GPs agreed to complete self report forms immediately after their consultation with a hypertensive patient. The study took place between 1996 and 1997.

- They found that 63% of patients had a diastolic blood pressure over 90 mmHg.
- The median performance rate of GPs (compared with the Dutch hypertension guidelines) was 51%.
- GPs seemed to act more when the diastolic blood pressure was over 100 mmHg.
- Intensity of management varied considerably between individual GPs.
- Patient and GP factors did not have a large effect on the performance of GPs.
- GPs seemed to look at blood pressure in isolation rather than taking other cardiovascular risk factors into consideration.

They conclude that more aggressive treatment of hypertension in general practice may reduce cardiovascular morbidity and mortality.

OTHERS

Comparison of agreement between different measures of blood pressure in primary care and daytime ambulatory blood pressure. Little, P., Barnett, J. and Barnsley, L. *et al.* Community Clinical Sciences Division (Primary Medical Care Group), Faculty of Medicine, Health and Biological Sciences, Southampton University, Aldermoor Health Centre, Southampton, UK.
BMJ, **325**(7358): 254, 3 August 2002.

The White coat hypertension resulting from patients having their blood pressure monitored by a doctor is thought to be at the root of much unnecessary treatment and alterations of treatments. In order to eliminate this, a suitable alternative method of monitoring needs to be found. Ambulatory blood pressure monitoring has been proven as a more accurate predictor of hypertensive target organ damage and the resultant adverse effects than blood pressure monitoring within a clinic environment. Two hundred newly diagnosed or poorly controlled hypertensive patients from three GP practices in England, were monitored by each of the above methods over a period of time. They found the following

- Readings made by doctors had consistently higher systolic values as compared to ambulatory monitoring
- The white coat effect was equally applicable to patients who were established long-term hypertensives with poor control and was not an artefact of research

- Ambulatory monitoring was again proven to be reliable
- Nurse readings provide better reliability than doctors readings
- Self-measurement by patients in clinic provided results comparable with ambulatory monitoring

They make the following conclusions

- Measurement by a nurse and ambulatory monitoring are effective but carry a huge financial burden.
- Home measurement also incurs significant staff and equipment costs.
- Self-measurement by patients in clinic is more financially viable.
- Most importantly, white coat hypertension is not a research artefact and action must be taken in order to reduce the number of treatment decisions based on blood pressure readings influenced by this well documented effect.

Comparison of acceptability of and preferences for different methods of measuring blood pressure in primary care. Little, P., Barnett, J. and Barnsley, L. *et al.* Community Clinical Sciences Division (Primary Medical Care Group), Faculty of Medicine, Health and Biological Sciences, Southampton University, Aldermoor Health Centre, Southampton, UK. *BMJ,* **325**(7358): 258-259, 3 August 2002.

Ambulatory monitoring has recently been proposed as an effective method of diagnosing and monitoring hypertensive patients but its acceptability must be explored.

Two hundred newly diagnosed or poorly controlled patients from a wide range of ages and cultures from three practices in England, were selected and their blood pressure monitored by

- Nurses
- Doctors
- Home monitoring
- Ambulatory monitoring
- Seventy patients also measured their own blood pressure.

Patients then used their experiences to compare the methods of measurement available.Conclusions reached included:

- All methods were acceptable if they provided accurate results.
- Ambulatory monitoring was least acceptable because of sleep disturbance, discomfort and disruption of everyday living.
- Home measurement was most favoured.
- Few patients felt that recordings made by a doctor were the most acceptable.

Further research is required to establish methods that are acceptable to patients and practitioners, in addition to providing a high degree of medical accuracy.

Home monitoring service was more effective than usual care in patients with essential hypertension. Commentator, Richard Davidson, University of Florida College of Medicine, Gainesville, FL, USA.
Evidence-based Medicine, 7(1): 18, Jan./Feb. 2002

Question: In patients with essential hypertension, does a home monitoring service (HMS) improve mean arterial pressure more than usual care?

The following article is briefly presented

Home monitoring service improves mean arterial pressure with essential hypertension. A randomised, controlled trial. Rogers, M.A., Small, D. and Buchan, D.A. *et al.*
Ann. Intern. Med., **134:** 1024–1032, 5 June 2001.

This was an RCT with 11 weeks follow up, involving 121 patients with essential hypertension, from outpatient clinics in the USA. Patients either had usual care or had automatic blood pressure readings that were transmitted to the physician via telephone. Advice about medication changes were then relayed to the patient at outpatient visit or by phone.

• Those who received the HMS had lower blood pressure readings that those undergoing usual care.

Commentary

Arguably those receiving HMS had more intense treatment than those undergoing usual care. Hence, further studies would need to look at the mechanism of blood pressure lowering together with the cost of HMS.

Reduced sodium intake lowered blood pressure and need for antihypertensive medication. Commentator, Bruce Arroll, University of Auckland, Auckland, New Zealand.
Evidence-based Medicine, 6(5): 151, Sept./Oct. 2001

Question: In older adults with hypertension, is a reduced dietary sodium (RS) intervention more effective than usual lifestyle (UL) in controlling blood pressure and preventing cardiovascular events?

The following article is briefly presented

Effects of reduced sodium intake on hypertension control in older individuals. Results from the Trial of Nonpharmacologic Internvetion in the Elderly (TONE). Appel, L.J., Espeland, M.A. and Easter, L. *et al.*
Arch. Intern. Med., **161:** 685–693, 12 March 2001.

This was an RCT involving around 680 elderly patients (aged 60-80 years) from four centres in the US. They were allocated to either a reduced salt intervention, (group and individual sessions with a dietician), or usual lifestyle, (similar sessions to reduced salt, but without reference to hypertension and cardiovascular disease). At 30 months follow up they found:

- blood pressure was lower in the reduced salt group compared with the usual lifestyle group;
- more people in the reduced salt group remained off medication than in the control group;
- reducing sodium intake by 40 mmol/l per day lowered blood pressure by 4.3/2 mmHg.

Commentary

This magnitude of blood pressure reduction may not seem like much, but it may translate into decreased mortality. However, reducing salt in the diet is difficult because most of our salt comes from processed foods. He recommends starting with other non-pharmacological interventions before prescribing salt reduction, unless the person is motivated enough to prepare their own low salt foods.

FURTHER READING

Meeting the National Service Framework for coronary heart disease: which patients have untreated high blood pressure? Department of Public Health and Epidemiology, University of Birmingham, Edgbaston, Birmingham.
***Br. J. Gen. Pract., 51**(468): 571-574, July 2001.*

See 'Diabetes mellitus' for

Review: intensive blood pressure control and drugs reduce morbidity and mortality in hypertension and diabetes mellitus. Mayo Clinic, Rochester, MN, USA.
***Evidence-based Medicine, 6**(2): 44, April 2001.*

Measurement of blood pressure: an evidence based review. McAlister, F.A. and Straus, S.E., Division of General Internal Medicine, University of Alberta Edmonton, Canada.
***BMJ, 322**(7291): 908-911, 14 April 2001.*

Blood pressure measuring devices: recommendations of the European Society of Hypertension. O'Brien, E., Waeber, B., Parati, G. *et al.* on behalf of the European Society of Hypertension Working Group on Blood Pressure Monitoring.
***BMJ, 322**(7285): 531-536, 3 March 2001.*

IMMUNIZATION

INFLUENZA

- Combining home health checks with influenza vaccination boosts vaccination uptake in older patients
- Offering influenza immunisation appointments by telephone can boost uptake rates by around 6%
- Influenza immunisation for both high risk and non-high risk groups is central to decreasing mortality and morbidity

MMR

- Several studies have concluded that there is no link between the MMR vaccine and autism.
- For some mothers, the media made a lasting impression about possible side effects of the MMR vaccine.
- One study has found wide variations amongst health professionals in their knowledge and attitude towards the MMR vaccine.
- Tom Heller wonders whether, the financial inducements that go along with immunizations targets have influenced the direction of the MMR debate.

OTHERS

- Surveillance of pertussis shows a re-emergence in countries with high vaccination coverage and a low mortality rate
- The varicella zoster vaccine has been shown to be effective.
- Immunization is not a cause of SIDS and may offer some protection against it.
- Carefully instigated educational outreach practices can significantly increase uptake of valuable healthcare interventions in high-risk patients.

INFLUENZA

Improving uptake of influenza vaccination among older people: a randomised controlled trial. Arthur, A.J., Matthews, R.J. and Jagger, C. *et al.* School of Nursing, Faculty of Health and Medical Sciences, University of Nottingham, Queens Medical Centre, Nottingham, UK. *Br. J. Gen. Pract.*, **52**(482): 717-722, 1 September 2002.

In older patients, contact with a doctor or nurse has been associated with increased uptake of the influenza vaccination. In this study, different approaches to improve uptake of vaccination in patients over 75 years were examined.

Just over 2000 patients from a single rural GP practice in Leicestershire were randomised to one of two groups. One group were offered influenza vaccination as part of an over-75 health check performed at the patients home by a practice nurse. The second group were sent a letter inviting them to attend an influenza vaccination clinic. Uptakes of vaccine for the two groups were determined.

- Of those patients in the health check group, 74.3% underwent vaccination
- Of the letter of invitation group, 67.9% underwent vaccination

The authors conclude that combined over-75 checks and influenza vaccination at home can improve immunization rates. However, given that the increase in immunization rates was small, targeting only those patients who do not routinely attend immunization clinics for the combined health check and vaccination regime might be a cost-effective way to boost immunization uptake.

Boosting uptake of influenza immunization: a randomised controlled trial of telephone appointing in general practice. Hull, S., Hagdrup, N. and Hart, B. *et al.* Department of General Practice and Primary Care, Medical Sciences Building, Queen Mary College, London, UK.
Br. J. Gen. Pract., **52**(482): 712-716, 1 September 2002.

This study examined whether a simple telephone appointment system increased the uptake of inflenza immunization. Just under 2000, low-risk East London GP patients aged over 65 years were randomised to control or intervention groups. The intervention involved a telephone call made by the practice reception, offering a nurse apppointment for immunization. The numbers of patients of each group receiving immunization, and the practice costs of the telephone-appointment intervention were calculated.

- Fifty per cent of telephone appointment group patients were immunized, compared to 44% of the control group.
- In the control group, £11.35 income was generated per immunization
- In the intervention group £5.20 income was generated for each additional immunization achieved, taking into account the costs of the telephoning system

The authors conclude that a simple telephone appointment system can result in a 6% increase in influenza immunization uptake in older patients of inner city general practices. They suggest that the current item-of-service system of payments to practices for immunizations must be retained if this intervention is to be cost effective.

EDITORIAL – Boosting influenza immunisation for the over-65s. Kassianos, G. The Birch Hill Medical Centre, Leppington, Bracknell, Berks, UK.
Br. J. Gen. Pract., **52**(482): 710-711, 1 September 2002.

Influenza carries a significant annual burden in terms of cost and bed space.

Immunization against influenza has been reduced the cases of hospitalization, pneumonia and death by 50%. This effect is increased significantly by regular annual immunization.

In the USA, implementation of vaccination programmes in non-high-risk groups such as those 50-64 years, has lead to a significant decrease in absenteeism, medical visits and prescribing. The UK programme does not currently incorporate those who are non-high-risk. However, by following the USA and targeting the general population, those carrying the virus and transmitting it to high-risk patients would be prevented from doing so.

In order to achieve this, GP practices must reassess their methods of boosting immunization by addressing the barriers to uptake currently in place such as:

- The belief influenza is mild
- The hope of not catching it
- Fear of vaccine efficacy and side effects
- Lack of awareness/ general apathy
- Inability to attend the surgery due to lack of time or being housebound.

No single change will be effective in increasing immunization rates. Implementation of measures to encourage uptake will need to be tailored to the particular needs of the practice population and will involve many members of the multidisciplinary team.

MMR

Measles, mumps and rubella vaccination and bowel problems or developmental regression in children with autism: population study. Taylor, B., Miller, E. and Lingam, *et al.* Centre for Community Child Health, Royal Free and University College Medical School, University College, London, UK.
BMJ, 324(7334): 393-396, 16 February 2002.

The existence of a 'new variant' autism has been postulated. This involves developmental regression after MMR vaccination and bowel symptoms. This population survey involving nearly 500 autistic children from 1979, investigates the existence of this condition.

- During the 20 years from 1979, they found no significant trends in the incidence of the proposed "new variant" autism, including after 1988 (when the MMR vaccine was introduced)
- Neither bowel symptoms nor regression were associated with the MMR vaccine. However, bowel problems were more frequently reported with regression (than without regression). There is no evidence to support the idea of a "new variant" autism

Parents perspectives on the MMR immunization: a focus group. Evans, M., Stoddart, H. and Condon, L. Division of Primary Health Care, University of Bristol, Bristol, UK.
Br. J. Gen. Pract., 51(472): 904-910, 1 November 2001.

The aim of this qualitative study was to evaluate parents perspectives on the MMR vaccine. Six focus groups involving 48 parents were conducted in Avon and Gloucestershire. Focus groups contained parents who had both immunized and not immunized their child. Some of the themes that emerged were.

- Beliefs about the risks and benefits of the MMR vaccine. Even those who immunized their child felt anxious about the decision they had made. Those who had not immunized their child felt that they could reduce complications (if their child got the disease) by maintaining good general health.
- Many had been affected by media reports and were sceptical about government reassurances, particularly after the BSE crisis.
- Many found it difficult to have honest conversations with health professionals and were afraid to be labelled as a 'nuisance'.
- Many expressed concerns about the financial incentives offered to GPs for reaching immunization targets. Some also resented having to subject their child to an intervention just because it was better for the whole population.
- Many were prepared to give their child one or all of the single vaccines.

Vaccination against mumps, measles and rubella: is there a case for deepening the debate? Commentators, Tom Heller, Dick Heller and Stephen Pattison. **BMJ, 323**(7317): 838-840, 13 October 2001.

This is a summary of three opinions concerning the mumps, measles and rubella (MMR) vaccine. Tom Heller is a GP, Dick Heller is an epidemiologist and Stephen Pattison is an ethicist. Tom Heller states that he has become increasingly uncomfortable about offering the MMR vaccine and wonders whether he would give it to his own children if they were the appropriate age. We are encouraged to allow patients to take part in the decision making process and yet with MMR choice seems to be restricted. He wonders whether, the financial inducements that go along with immunizations targets have influenced the direction of the debate.

Dick Heller states that the evidence for a link between MMR and autism is anecdotal and that the risks and complications associated with getting these infections (as a result of non-vaccination) far outweigh the risk, if any, of developing autism after the MMR vaccine.

Pattison comments that Tom Hellers thoughts reflect his moral judgment of the situation. Simply ignoring these moral judgments will not make them go away. He also questions, whether, the doctor, in striving for the financial rewards associated with immunization targets, is acting in the best interests of the patient. He points out that although the government determines the protocol, it is the GP and parents who have to live with the consequences of such strategies.

Tom Heller concludes that "informed refusal must remain an acceptable choice."

Do children who become autistic consult more often after MMR vaccination?
DeWilde, S., Carey, I.M., Richards, N., Hilton, S.R. and Cook, D.G. Department of Public Health Sciences, St. Georges Hospital Medical School, London, UK.
Br. J. Gen. Pract., **51**(464): 226-227, 1 March 2001.

This study analyzes GP attendance rates 2 and 6 months before and after the MMR vaccination in a cohort of children who become autistic and compare this with controls. They use data from the Doctors Independent Network (DIN) database. Data from around 70 cases are compared with four times as many controls.

- They found no difference in the consultation rates between cases and controls pre and post the MMR vaccination.
- For those diagnosed with autism, attendance rates were significantly higher than controls for the 5 months prior to diagnosis.
- The mean time between MMR vaccine and diagnosis of autism was around 1000 days. The authors conclude that there is no link between MMR vaccination and autism. The results of previous studies suggesting a link probably arose due to recall or selection bias.

Mumps, measles and rubella vaccine and the incidence of autism recorded by general practitioners. A time trend analysis. Kaye, J.A., del Mar Melero-Montes, M. and Jick, H. Boston Collaborative Drug Surveillance Program, Boston University School of Medicine, Lexington, MA, USA.
BMJ, **322**(7284): 460-463, 24 February 2001.

The authors use the UK general practice research database (GPRD) to evaluate the relationship between the MMR vaccine and the incidence of autism. They analyze data for just over 300 children aged 12 or younger and around 100 boys (born between 1980 and 1993) with a first recorded diagnosis of autism during 1988 to 1999 .

- The estimated yearly incidence of diagnosed autism increased sevenfold, from 0.3 (per 10 000 persons) in 1988 to 2.1 in 1999.
- The median age at first recorded diagnosis of autism was 4.6 years.
- They found that whilst the incidence of autism increased four times between 1988 and 1993, the vaccination rate remained constant at around 97%.
- No time correlation was found between the prevalence of MMR vaccine and the incidence of autism.They conclude that exposure to the MMR vaccine cannot be the explanation for the increase in autism. The increase could be due to:
- raised awareness of the condition by parents, carers and GPs;
- changing diagnostic criteria and
- unidentified environmental factors.

Second dose of measles, mumps, and rubella vaccine: questionnaire survey of health professionals. Petrovic, M., Roberts, R. and Ramsay, M. Department of Public Health, North Wales Authority, Preswylfa, Mold, Flintshire, UK.
BMJ, 322(7278): 82-85, 13 January 2001.

The authors describe this as the first published questionnaire survey of the knowledge, attitudes and practices of health professionals regarding the second dose of the MMR vaccine, in the UK. The study was carried out in a North Wales Health Authority in 1998 and involved health visitors, practice nurses and general practitioners. Self-administered postal questionnaire were used (response rate 80% of GPs and 88% of Health Visitors).The main findings were:

Knowledge: Nearly 50% of GPs, and three quarters of the practice nurses and health visitors would like more information and training in the MMR vaccine and the rationale behind the introduction of the second MMR dose. Knowledge about the adverse effects was variable.

Attitude: Many GPs (40%), health visitors (49%), and practice nurses (54%) had reservations about the policy of the second dose.

Practice: Health visitors are the first point of advice and are more confident in explaining the rationale behind the MMR second dose. Confidence in explaining to an informed parent was strongly associated with agreeing with the policy.

OTHERS

PAPERS: Cluster randomised controlled trial of an educational outreach visit to improve influenza and pneumococcal immunisation rates in primary care.
Siriwardena, A.N., Rashid, A. and Johnson, R.D. *et al*. North Dene, Langworth Road, Scothern, Lincoln, UK.
Br. J. Gen. Pract., 52(482): 735-740, 1 September 2002.

Influenza and pneumococcal vaccinations in high-risk patients provide well-documented protection from potentially life-threatening infections. However, knowledge and uptake of these interventions amongst high-risk groups is poor.

A cluster randomised control trial was carried out across 30 practices in Central England to establish the effect of an educational outreach programme on uptake of the vaccinations within primary care.

- The educational outreach programme was shown to increase uptake in some subgroups of the population considered at high risk (e.g. coronary and diabetic patients), but not in others (e.g. splenectomy patients)
- The effect of this practice based education works best when applied within the context of the multidisciplinary team.

High costs and questions surrounding the sustained effect of educational outreach over time need to be addressed to further increase efficacy.

Ultimately, the effect of educational outreach depends on the willingness of the particular practice to involve themselves completely in the process.

EDITORIAL – Whooping cough – a continuing problem. Crowcroft, N.S. and Britto, J. Immunisation Division, Public Health Laboratory Service, Communicable Diseases Surveillance Centre, London, UK.
BMJ, **324**(7373): 1537-1538, 29 June 2002.

Pertussis is one of the top causes of vaccine-preventable death, of which infants are at greatest risk of death or severe complications. It has recently been reported that there has been a global resurgence of whooping cough in countries with low mortality and high vaccination coverage, possibly as a result of:
- A vaccine-driven evolution of circulating strains resulting in a fall in vaccine efficacy.
- Underdiagnosis: methods such as ELISA and PMR have increased diagnostic sensitivity and have only recently been available in some countries.
- The vaccine may be more effective at preventing disease than infection.

Participants of a recent WHO conference on pertussis concluded that it has been neglected as a disease, and that research and basic laboratory surveillance and control measures need strengthening globally.

Review: varicella vaccination is effective in children. Skull, A.S. and Wang, E.E. Commentator, Matt Uhari University of Oulu, Oulu, Finland.
Evidence-based Medicine, **7**(1): 9, Jan./Feb. 2002

Question: What are the benefits and harms of varicella vaccination in children?

The following article is briefly presented
Varicella vaccination a critical review of the evidence. Skull, A.S. and Wang, E.E.
Arch. Dis. Child., **85**: 83–90, Aug. 2001.

Eight RCTs were reviewed.
- The NNT for vaccination to prevent one additional case of varicella was 6–12.
- Injection site reactions occurred in 7–30% of subjects.

Commentary
Herd immunity is difficult because those vaccinated may still get zoster from the wild virus. However, Uhari notes that the vaccine is effective and the time has come to consider routine vaccination in children.

The UK accelerated immunisation programme and sudden unexpected death in infancy: case control study. Fleming, P.J., Blair, P.S., Platt, M.W., Tripp, J., Smith, I.J. and Golding, J. and the CESDI SUDI research group. Institute of Child Health, Royal Hospital for Children, Bedford, UK.
Br. J. Gen. Pract., **322**(7290): 822-825, 7 April 2001.

Previous studies have suggested a link between Sudden Infant Death Syndrome (SIDS) and immunization. This study analyses the relationship between the UK accelerated immunization programme and SIDS. It is a population based case control study conducted over 3 years and involving five regions in England with a total study population of 17.7 million people. Data was collected using questionnaires, medical records (child health records) and post mortem records and interviews. They control for possible confounding factors e.g. moving house, social class, low birthweight.

- Fewer SIDs cases had completed or begun the immunization programme compared with controls
- There was no correlation between recent immunization, signs or symptoms of illness and death.They conclude that SIDS is not associated with the accelerated immunization programme. The immunization programme may even have a protective effect.

LIPIDS

- An analysis of data from the EPIC-Norfolk study has shown that eating six times a day is associated with reduced total and LDL cholesterol levels.
- Gemfibrozil reduces non-fatal strokes in men with low HDL levels.
- A Durham study showed that laboratory based interventions can improve requests for lipid tests in general practice
- The evidence for the effects of modification of dietary fat on cardiovascular morbidity and mortality is still inconclusive
- Forty percent of people with familial hypercholesterolaemia have a normal life expectancy. Further research needs to identify which people with hypercholesterolaemia are at high risk of death
- Kasterlein states that the screening criteria as developed by Wilson and Jungner in 1968 can be applied to testing for familial hypercholesterolaemia
- A Netherlands study found that there is room for improvement in the care of patients identified as having familial hypercholesterolaemia.
- Cost-effective primary prevention of familial hypercholesterolamia can be achieved by population screening.
- Bezafibrate reduces the incidence of non-fatal vascular incidents, but has no significant effect on fatal incidents, possibly due to it increasing homocysteine concentrations.

BACKGROUND

Primary prevention

The West of Scotland coronary prevention (WOSCOP) study (*N. Engl. J. Med.*, 1995) showed that pravastatin (40 mg/day for 5 years) was useful for the primary prevention of cardiovascular disease in men (around 6500 aged 45-64) with hypercholesterolaemia (mean cholesterol 7.0 mmol/l).

Secondary prevention

The Scandinavian Simvastatin Survival Study (4S: *Lancet*, 1994) involving more than 4000 patients, found that after an MI, a 35% reduction in LDL resulted in 30% fewer deaths and 42% fewer coronary events. There was no increase in non-coronary events.

The results of the 4S and CARE (*N. Engl. J. Med.*, 1996) (cholesterol and recurrent events) studies suggest that aggressive lipid lowering treatment is indicated for both men and women with proven ischaemic heart disease across a wide range of LDL cholesterol concentrations.

Also, the CARE study shows that pravastatin is effective in both men and women with 'normal range' LDL concentrations.

In August 1997 a statement was issued to health authorities and GPs from the Standing Medical Advisory Committee (SMAC) on the use of lipid-lowering drugs. The statement recommends treatment for three groups:

- those with a history of previous MI with LDL ⩾3.2 mmol/l;
- those with a history of angina or other atherosclerotic disease with LDL ⩾3.7 mmol/l;
- those at high risk of developing coronary heart disease according to the revised Sheffield tables (the Sheffield tables are derived from epidemiological data from the Framingham population).

DIET

Dietary fat intake and prevention of cardiovascular disease: systematic review. Hooper, L., Summerbell, C.D. and Higgins, J.P.T. *et al.* Manchester Dental and Education Centre (MANDEC). University Dental Hospital of Manchester, Manchester, UK. ***BMJ, 322***(7289): 757-763, 31 March 2001.

This was a systematic review, looking at the effects of modification of dietary fat on cardiovascular disease morbidity and mortality. Interventions included, the reduction in total fat, dietary cholesterol or saturated fat or a change from saturated to unsaturated fat. Twenty-seven RCTs met the inclusion criteria, representing around 31 000 person years of observation.
- Modification of dietary fat had no or little effect on total mortality.
- Cardiovascular mortality was reduced by 9% (confidence intervals for the rate ratio passed through one).
- Cardiovascular events were reduced by around 16% (confidence intervals for the rate ratio came close to one)
- Meta-regression showed that greater reduction in cholesterol was associated with greater reduction in cardiovascular events and cardiovascular mortality. However, this association was very weak.

They conclude that in spite of the many trials, the evidence for the effects of modification of dietary fat on cardiovascular morbidity and mortality is still inconclusive.

DRUG THERAPIES

Bezafibrate in men with lower extremity arterial disease: randomised controlled trial. Meade, T., Zuhrie, R. and Cook, C. *et al.* Department of Epidemiology and Population Health, London School of Hygeine and Tropical Medicine, London, UK. ***BMJ, 325***(7373): 1139-1143, 16 November 2002.

This placebo controlled RCT examined the effect of bezafibrate, on lower extremity arterial disease events in 1568 men (from 85 general practices in the UK) with lower extremity artery disease. Subjects took either bezafibrate or placebo tablets identical in appearance, with dosage depending on plasma creatinine concentration. The dosage was adjusted as creatinine concentration varied during the trial. Most placebo group withdrawals were due to starting a drug incompatible with bezafibrate; most intervention group withdrawals were due to raised creatinine concentrations. Similar overall proportions of each group withdrew. Total cholesterol and LDL cholesterol decreased by 7.6% and 8.1%, respectively; HDL cholesterol increased by 8.0% and triglyceride and fibrinogen concentrations decreased by 23.3% and 13%, respectively.

- Bezafibrate had no significant effect on combined CHD and stroke incidence (odds ratio 0.96%).
- Intervention group had 19% fewer CHD incidents.
- Non-fatal coronary events reduced by 62% in men aged <65 years, taking bezafibrate.
- Intervention group showed significantly better improvement in severity of claudication at 1, 2 and 3 years, though not thereafter.

The authors suggest the low incidence of non-fatal events, may be due to participants taking platelet anti-aggregating agents.They conclude there was no significant difference in all-cause death rates between placebo and intervention group, with a greater effect being seen on non-fatal events. This agrees with other studies. Bezafibrate may also improve claudication for a year or two. Bezafibrate increases homocysteine concentrations, a risk factor for vascular disease. Future trials should investigate whether concurrent folic acid supplementation significantly reduces the incidence of strokes and heart attacks.

FAMILIAL HYPERCHOLESTEROLAEMIA

Follow up after a family based genetic screening programme for familial hypercholesterolaemia: is screening alone enough? Van Maarle, M.C., Stouthard, M.E.A. and Marang-van de Mheen, P.J. *et al.* Department of Social Medicine, Academic Medical Centre, University of Amsterdam, Amsterdam, Netherlands.
BMJ, 324(7350): 1367-1368, 8 June 2002.

In 1994, a family based genetic screening programme for familial hypercholesterolaemia was established in the Netherlands. This study examines the short-term outcome of this screening programme, in terms of preventive care and early clinical outcome of patients testing positive at screening.

Information from all 215 patients who tested positive at screening was analysed. Questionnaires were completed by subjects at screening, at 7 months and at 18 months after receiving the screening test result.

Outcome measures were: Quality of treatment (according to Dutch hypercholesterolaemia guidelines); cholesterol level; body mass index; and smoking status.

- Quality of treatment and clinical outcome improved significantly over time. However, quality of treatment was still insufficient in 20, and clinical outcome was still unsatisfactory in 45.

The authors suggest that closer adherence to guidelines, physician education, and improved links between diagnosis and follow up care are needed.

Cost effectiveness analysis of different approaches of screening for familial hypercholesterolamia. Marks, D., Wonderling, D., Thorogood, M. and Lambert, H. London School of Hygiene and Tropical Medicine, London, UK.
***BMJ*, 324**(7349): 1303-1306, 1 June 2002.

This paper summarises the findings from a cost effectiveness analysis of a number of screening initiatives for familial hypercholesterolamia (FH). About 110,000 people in the UK are affected by hypercholesterolamia with at least 75 undiagnosed currently.

The screening strategies examined were:

1. Identification and treatment of patients with F.H. by universal population screening.
2. Opportunistic screening at primary care consultations.
3. Opportunistic screening in acute setting of patients with premature myocardial infarction.
4. Systematic screening of family members of affected individuals.

They found:

- An increase in life expectancy was noted when treatment was given early (16-24 years) with the highest gain in life years found in women. This effect decreases linearly with increasing age.
- The number needed to screen ranged from 2202 in the general population to three in first degree relatives of index cases.
- Targeted strategies were more clinically effective though they were more expensive per individual screened, but cheaper per case detected.
- The earlier the diagnosis, the more cost effective the screening strategy. There was a 10-fold increase in the cost per life year gained between the oldest and the youngest age group using the screening of relative's strategy.
- For all age groups, identification and screening of the relatives of patients is the most cost effective strategy.

Mortality over two centuries in large pedigree with familial hypercholesterolae- mia: family tree mortality study. Sijbrands, E.J.G., Westendorp, R.G.J. and Defesche, J.C. *et al.* Department of Vascular Medicine and General Internal Medicine, Academic Medical Centre, Amsterdam, The Netherlands.
***BMJ*, 322**(7293): 1019-1023, 28 April 2001.

This Dutch study is a family tree mortality study of familial hypercholesterolaemia. They trace three probands back through 2 centuries to a single pair of ancestors. This involved the identification of around 400 descendants in eight generations.

- They found that before 1915, mortality was lower than that in the general population.

- After 1915 the mortality rate rose to a peak in the 1950s before decreasing.
- Within the years of increased mortality there was a large variation in death rates with some people having a normal life expectancy.

They suggest that hypercholesterolaemia may have conferred a protective effect on the subject during the 19th century. Alternatively, lifestyle factors may have a significant role to play alongside genetic make-up. Forty percent of people with familial hypercholesterolaemia have a normal life expectancy. Further research needs to identify which people with hypercholesterolaemia are at high risk of death.

OTHERS

Frequency of eating and concentrations of serum cholesterol in the Norfolk population of the European prospective investigation into cancer (EPIC-Norfolk): cross sectional study. Titan, S.M.O., Bingham, S. and Welch, A. *et al.* Institute of Public Health, University of Cambridge, UK.
BMJ, **323**(7324): 1286-1288, 1 December 2001.

Using data from the EPIC-Norfolk study (ongoing prospective study of 25 000 Norfolk residents aged 45–75), they analyze the relationship between frequency of eating and serum cholesterol.
- Frequency of eating was significantly associated with total and LDL cholesterol levels. After adjustment for confounders, the difference in total cholesterol between those eating six times a day and those eating once or twice was 0.15 mmol/l.
- Those eating more frequently had higher daily energy, fat, carbohydrate and protein intakes
- Women eating more frequently had lower waist-hip ratios than those eating less frequently. These findings are consistent with other studies performed on metabolic ward patients. On a population level, a reduction in total cholesterol of 0.15 mmol/l represents 10-20% reduction in CHD. This advice may be especially important for the elderly who have a higher absolute risk of CHD.

Gemfibrozil reduced the risk for stroke in men with coronary heart disease and low concentrations of high-density lipoprotein cholesterol. Commentator, Geoffrey Donnan, National Stroke Research Institute, Melbourne, Victoria, Australia.
Evidence-based Medicine, **6**(6): 175, Nov./Dec. 2001

Question: In men with coronary artery disease and low concentrations of high-density lipoprotein (HDL) cholesterol, is gemfibrozil effective for preventing stroke?

The following article is briefly presented

Reduction in stroke with gemfibrozil in men with coronary heart disease and low HDL. The Veterans affairs HDL Intervention Trial (VA-HIT). Rubins, H.B., Davenport, J. and Babikian, V. *et al.*
Circulation, **103:** 2828–2833, 12 June 2001

The study was an RCT involving around 2500 men from 20 Veterans Affairs centres in America. All had an HDL less than 1.03 mmol/l, LDL less than 3.6 mmol/l and triglycerides of less than 3.39 mmol/l.
- The gemfibrozil group had fewer strokes than the placebo group.
- There was no difference between the groups for fatal strokes.
- The greatest benefit from gemfibrozil was seen for athero-thrombotic strokes.

Commentary
The VA-HIT study reports similar findings to the LIPID (Long-Term Intervention with Pravastatin in Ischaemic Disease, NEJM 2000) study which involved statins. The difference between the two studies is that the VA-HIT study looked at men with a low HDL level, whereas the LIPID study included a wide range of cholesterol concentrations.

A laboratory based intervention to improve appropriateness of lipid tests and audit cholesterol lowering in primary care. Smellie, W.S.A., Lowrie, R. and Wilkinson, E. Clinical Laboratory General Hospital, Bishop Auckland, County Durham, UK.
BMJ, **323**(7323): 1224-1227, 24 November 2001.

This paper describes a laboratory based intervention aimed at improving requests for lipid tests in general practice. It involved 22 practices in the Durham area of northern England. An intervention was introduced which involved altering the request form so that GPs could select one of four options relating to primary or secondary prevention testing strategies. The GP could also opt not to use the initiative. Two practices opted out of the initiative.
- The intervention had no effect on the number of requests for total cholesterol and triglycerides.
- There was a 44% reduction in requests for HDL tests.
- The marked interpractice difference seen before the introduction of the intervention was reduced.They conclude that laboratory based interventions can help in the management of CHD in primary care.

Cholesterol reduction and non–illness mortality: meta–analysis of randomised clinical trials. Muldoon, M.F., Manuck, S.B., Mendelsohn, A.B. and Kaplan, J.R. *et al.* Center for Clinical Pharmacology, University of Pittsburg, School of Medicine, Pittsburgh, USA.
BMJ, **322**(7277): 11-15, 6 January 2001.

This study was a meta-analysis whose aim was to analyse the effect of cholesterol lowering interventions on non-illness causes of death e.g. accidents, suicides. Nineteen studies were analysed.

- In both primary and secondary prevention trials, statins had no effect on non-illness causes of death.
- There is a suggestion that dietary intervention and non-statins drugs are associated with a slight increase in non-illness mortality (odds ratio 1.32, $P = 0.06$).

They discuss the limitations of this study. The numbers dying from non-illness causes were small. Those susceptible to non-illness causes of death e.g. the mentally ill are less likely to enrol in clinical trials and hence this may have resulted in selection bias.

FURTHER READING

What is the optimal age for starting lipid lowering treatment? A mathematical model. Ulrich, S., Hinhorani, A.D., Martin, J. and Vallance, P., Centre for Clinical Pharmacology and Therapeutics, University College London. **BMJ, 320**(7242): 1134-1140, 22 April 2000.

MEDICALISATION

- Eventually, doctors will suffer from the practice of medicalisation.
- Medical authority has gradually replaced religion in influencing society's sexual behaviour.
- Is the evolution of the speciality of palliative care medicalising death?
- The problems of elderly people should be medicalised
- Genetic tests need thorough evaluation of predictive capability before their introduction
- Spending on preventative treatments that help a few may be unaffordable
- Pharmaceutical companies are actively sponsoring the defining of diseases and promoting them to prescribers and consumers.
- Targeting beliefs about birth, implementation of evidence based practice and team working can prevent the 'medicalisation' of childbirth.

EDITORIAL – Medicalisation: peering from inside medicine. Leibovici, L. and Lievre, M. Department of Medicine, Beilinson Campus, Rabin Medical Center, 49100 Petah-Tiqva, Israel. **BMJ, 324**(7342): 866, 13 April 2002.

The medicalisation of life events is believed to have benefited the medical practitioners through the gain of power and control over patients. Conversely, this practice can be detrimental to the doctor-patient relationship. The authors noted the following in the practice of medicalisation of old age, death, pain and handicap in society:
- Physicians may feel frustrated, angry and eventually harm the patient.
- Physicians may have to live up to the patient's unreasonable expectations.
- Physicians have to balance the competing interests of patients against that of their relatives.
- Consequently physicians may be coerced into making decisions for patients against their will.

To overcome these conflicts, the authors argued for a greater and improved patient-doctor partnership.

EDUCATION AND DEBATE – Sexual behaviour and its medicalisation: in sickness and in health. Gart, G. and Wellings, K. MRC Social and Public Health Science Unit, University of Glasgow, Glasgow, UK. **BMJ, 324**(7342): 896-900, 13 April 2002.

Historically, the medicalisation of sexual behaviour had been widespread with varying consequences. Medical authority has gradually replaced religion in influencing society's sexual behaviour.
- Medical authority over sexual behaviour began in the 19th century with doctors describing sexually deviant behaviours.
- In the following century, the medicalisation of sexual behaviour was dominated by views of non-medically qualified doctors.

- Since the mid-20th century, psychiatry offered the option of "treatable" sexual behaviours, in contrast to previous behaviours that were deemed morally unacceptable.
- Later, there was a tendency to associate women with the source of unhealthy sexual behaviour.
- The latter half of 20th century saw the expansion of the role of sex from procreation to being a form of healthy human relationship and pleasure. The latter had become an acceptable foci for doctors when dealing with sexual health and behaviour of their clients.
- Therapeutic advances had enabled this change of attitude to take place with minimal adverse effects. However, the medicalisation of sexual health had created demands for the use of drugs and surgery to enhance sexual pleasure.
- Mass surveillance, regulation, and control of sexual behaviour by the medical professionals can trigger feelings of insecurity within the society.
- Overmedicalisation of sex has adverse consequences in that social and interpersonal dynamics may be ignored.

EDUCATION AND DEBATE – Between hope and acceptance: The medicalisation of dying. Clark, D. Academic Palliative Medicine Unit, University Of Sheffield, Trent Palliative Care Centre, Sykes House, Sheffield, UK.
BMJ, **324**(7342): 905-907, 13 April 2002.

The specialty of Palliative care developed during the late 1960s and 1970s as a result of growing concern within the medical profession regarding the medicalisation of death and the process of dying. At the heart of palliative care lies an attempt to preserve dignity and identity during the processes of dying, and recognition of the interdependence of mental and physical distress. The author summarises the current challenges to the specialty:
- Recent technical advances have increased the pressure on physicians to attempt to intervene in the process of dying, resulting in high levels of invasive treatment (e.g. enteral feeding tubes) amongst the terminally ill.
- Despite technological advances, interventions which prolong life/ support vital functions still isolate patients and impede "dignified dying".
- Current attempts to integrate palliative care with earlier, pre-terminal, phases of patient management may shift the focus of the specialty away from the process of dying, leading to sub-optimal terminal care.
- The "modernisation" of palliative care, by adopting evidence-based medicine and focussing on symptom relief, may, by shifting emphasis away from psycho-social and spiritual issues, paradoxically, lead to further medicalisation of the process of dying.
- Achieving a balance between medical intervention and holistic and humanistic patient care is the central challenge in the field of palliative care.

EDITORIAL – The medicalisation of old age. Ebrahim, S. Professor of Epidemiology of ageing. Department of Social Medicine, University of Bristol, Canynge Hall, Bristol, UK. *BMJ,* **320**(7342): 861-863, 13 April 2002.

Over the last ten years, problems that accompany ageing have been "de-medicalised", with decreased medical care in hospitals and increased social care in nursing homes. This editorial discusses this issue, and argues that the problems of elderly people should be medicalised.

- Although ageing is a natural process, diseases associated with ageing should not be considered to be natural.
- Studies examining antihypertensive and cholesterol-lowering medications have demonstrated that elderly people gain greater absolute benefits from these treatments than younger people, because of their higher levels of risk.
- Given the wide range of physical needs of elderly people, arguments promoting the rationing of medical treatment for elderly patients because they have "had a good innings" are flawed.

EDITORIAL – Genetics and medicalisation. Melzer, D., Zimmern, R. and Melzer, David. The Department of Public Health and Primary Care, University of Cambridge, Cambridge, UK. *BMJ,* **324**(7342): 863-864, 13 April 2002.

The public image of genetic testing is one of high penetrance, single gene disorders such as Huntington's disease for which a positive test result implies inevitable future disease. However, the genes implicated in most disorders are not such definite determiners of disease. This editorial argues that the predictive value of genetic tests must be thoroughly evaluated before such tests are offered to patients. A number of points are made.

- Other than in the high penetrance, single gene disorders, most genetic tests can only offer statistics of risk. Their predictive value is often low.
- "Medicalisation" of abnormal genes can be unhelpful. For example, it may be inappropriate to treat an individual who is predisposed to but not definitely destined to develop a certain disease.
- Increased availability of genetic tests would risk unfair treatment of people carrying polymorphisms, for example by employers and insurers.
- Genetic tests should be subject to the same rigorous evaluation as other medical tests and interventions.

EDITORIAL – Medicalisation, limits to medicine, or never enough money to go around. Freemantle, N. and Hill, S. Department of Primary Care and General Practice, University of Birmingham, Birmingham, UK.
***BMJ, 324**(7342): 864-865, 13 April 2002.*

Developed world countries are now investing greatly in developing and prescribing preventative therapies which benefit only a minority of patients. The best example is the use of statins, whose use is scarcely affordable in the developing world. The benefits of statin use have been shown in very large studies, hence amplifying the reported efficacy data. The WOSCOP (West of Scotland Coronary Prevention Study) showed that in 10,000 patients treated with statins, 9755 would receive no benefit.

Although the use of statins may be best clinical practice, the cost of providing so few with benefit may not be affordable. Other cases of cost vs. benefit include the availability of interferon beta on the NHS. Health economics data may indicate feasibility, but most economic conclusions are based on strong assumptions and hypothetical benefits not shown by trials. Health spending on such evidence may be affordable in the UK, but may not be feasible for other health systems.

The overall implications of the increasing use of pharmaceuticals are unclear. The OECD (Organisation for Economic Co-operation and Development) has reported that health spending in the UK has increased on average 1.5 more than GDP growth. Therefore, all countries face difficult decisions regarding which treatments to provide in the future.

EDUCATION AND DEBATE – Selling Sickness: the pharmaceutical industry and disease mongering. Moynihan, R, Heath, I and Henry, D Caversham Group, London, UK.
***BMJ, 324**(7342): 886-891, 13 April 2002.*

Pharmaceutical companies are actively sponsoring the defining of diseases and promoting them to prescribers and consumers. They arrange alliances to facilitate this including manufacturers, doctors, and patient support groups. The end result may be orchestrated campaigns which can result in inappropriate medicalisation of disease. This carries the danger of unnecessary labelling, poor treatment decisions and economic waste.

The authors in this article used Australian cases to draw attention to fields where such 'disease mongering' was occurring;

- Baldness: an ordinary process that has been promoted as a medical problem with medical solutions.
- Irritable Bowel Syndrome: a mild, functional disorder promoted as a serious disease in order to promote a drug treatment.
- Social Phobia: exaggeration of prevalence figures to encourage medicalisation and hence treatment of a personal or social problem.
- Osteoporosis: a risk associated with age that has been conceptualised as a disease through sponsored meetings and research.

• Erectile Dysfunction: the use of undefined figures to maximise the size of the problem.

These observations were selective and aimed to promote debate. The authors proposed recommendations which may 'de-medicalise' normal conditions. They felt that information should be corporately funded, and as the Cochrane Database independently assesses therapies, illness should also be independently assessed with an aim to prevent corporate disease mongering.

EDUCATION AND DEBATE – Has the medicalisation of childbirth gone too far?
Johnson, R, Newburn, M and Macfarlane A, A. National Childbirth Trust, Alexandra House, Oldham Terrace, London, UK.
BMJ, **324**(7342): 892-895, 13 April 2002.

Maternal mortality fell dramatically in the 20th century due to the growing influence of medical care and improved standards of living. Obstetric care today is becoming more medicalised with obstetricians taking over responsibility for normal births. There are many possible reasons for this:

• Private practice.
• Medicolegal issues - public expectations change with introductions of sophisticated care, with people believing that all deaths are preventable, perhaps reflected in a doubling in the NHS medicolegal bill since 1997.
• Midwives role: many midwives have felt a blame culture which has contributed to a mechanistic and medicalised understanding of childbirth.

The authors reported on a Canadian study and proposed that birth can be demedicalised by taking pride in a low caesarean rate, developing a culture of birth as a normal physiological process, and having a commitment to one-to-one supportive care during active labour. Furthermore, community based care results in the highest proportions of normal births, and all the above, coupled with an end to the 'blame and claim' culture should reverse the growing trend of medicalisation.

MENTAL ILLNESS

- Routinely administering psychiatric questionnaires prior to consultation does not increase the detection, management or outcome of patients suffering with anxiety or depression
- Exercise may be beneficial for the management of depression but better quality studies need to confirm this
- Web based information concerning depression is generally of poor quality
- Health professionals need to be more aware of the physical needs of people with mental illness and attention to physical needs should be part of routine care
- Reattribution can help patients with MUPS to deal with their symptoms
- Basic training for GP's in Cognitive Behavioural Therapy for Depression does not improve patient outcome.
- A WHO study found that depression is still being poorly managed.
- Self-help audio cassette is useful in treating depression, and especially valuable for patients unwilling to take antidepressant medications.
- A longitudinal study of patients in primary care concludes that approximately 50% of those attending have depression or anxiety. Roughly 40% of these are diagnosed at the initial consultation and a further 25% are diagnosed over the next 3 years. Of the remaining 35% half resolve without a general practitioners diagnosis and half remain undiagnosed, suffering from clinically severe symptoms.
- A retrospective analysis found that the Hampshire Depression Project did not significantly improve management of depression in primary care.
- Patients with schizophrenia using olanzapine are at an increased risk of diabetes.
- Social stigma experienced by patients is a core issue which must be dealt with before optimal care can be achieved for those suffering with long term mental ill health.
- Equally successful outcome following psychological disorders can be achieved irrespective of whether a patient presents with somatic or emotional symptoms.
- Patients who received a psychological assessment after self-poisoning were half as likely to poison themselves compared with those who did not receive an assessment.
- A practice based, multifaceted disease management plan for depression can reduce morbidity but success necessitates a committed practice with financial backing, serving a relatively affluent population.
- Managing depression as a chronic condition can increase remission rates at 2 years.
- The prevalence of DSH in adolescents calls for promotion of mental health in schools
- History of parasuicide remains a strong predictor of suicide two decades after the parasuicidal incident
- Further evidence supports a link between psychotic illness, certain antipsychotics and an increased risk of sudden death due to cardiac arrythmias.
- Consultation techniques of doctors may cause problems in terms of facilitating good patient interaction and compliance
- Seratoninergics generally have less fatal toxicity than other anti-depressants, however, venlafaxine has greater rates of fatal toxicity than other seratoninergic drugs.
- There is an increased incidence of cardiac arrest and sudden death in schizophrenic patients taking antipsychotics as compared to the general population. These effects differ with the particular antipsychotic and are dose specific.

- Sertraline maintenance treatment reduced relapse and dropouts in post-traumatic stress disorder.
- Mental health interventions offer effective treatments for somatic symptoms of unexplainable cause.

BACKGROUND

DEPRESSION

We miss 50% of depression and we are said to prescribe lower doses than psychiatrists. A study in the *BJGP* (1998) compared outcomes in those with recognized and unrecognized depression and those taking anti-depressants with those not taking antidepressants. Outcomes at 12 months were similar in all groups. So the fact that we miss half of the cases may not be so bad after all. It may be that those who are unrecognized and those not prescribed antidepressants are less severe and would have got better anyway. A Dutch study of 200 patients with a 10 year follow up found that 60% of patients only have one episode of depression and the mean duration of these episodes are 100 days ($\sim$3 months). If depression is reasonably self-limiting, missing less severe cases may be more acceptable. The Dutch study also found that 12% of subjects had more than three episodes of depression. Trying to identify this group may be more important than identifying every single case. Especially as there is still a negative public perception of depression and antidepressants. There is still a widely held view that antidepressants are addictive.

DRUG THERAPIES

Several RCTs and meta-analyses have been published since 1998 confirming that SSRIs are as effective as older antidepressants and are better tolerated. *Evidence-based Medicine* in 1998 reported that SSRIs were less cost- effective than the older group. We must also be alert to the serotonin syndrome which can be potentially fatal.

HYPERICUM

An MA of 23 RCTs has found hypericum to be more effective than placebo for the management of mild to moderate depression. Compared with imipramine, hypericum has similar efficacy with fewer adverse effects. Hypericum costs more than imipramine and there is also a potential problem with drug interactions. Hypericum stimulates the cytochrome P450 system and hence may interfere with a number of drugs including the contraceptive pill.

DEPRESSION

The Defeat Depression Campaign (DDC) was instigated in 1992 by the RCGP and the Royal College of Psychiatrists. It sought to heighten the profession's awareness of depression in the community. It is reported that GPs miss 50% of cases of depression. Patients are more likely to have their depression diagnosed if they mention their symptoms early on in the consultation.

Antidepressant prescribing is as topical as ever. As part of the DDC, we are encouraged to prescribe adequate doses of antidepressants (125–150 mg of amitriptyline or equivalent) for a continuation period of 4-6 months. GPs have been criticized for prescribing suboptimal doses of antidepressants. This largely applies to tricyclic antidepressants (TCAs), which seem to be less well tolerated than the newer selective serotonin reuptake inhibitors (SSRIs).

A meta-analysis of 23 RCTs found that the plant extract *Hypericum perforatum* (or St John's wort) was better than placebo and as effective as standard antidepressants in the treatment of depression. There were fewer side effects and dropouts in the St John's wort group than in the standard antidepressants group. St John's wort may become an important tool in the treatment of depression, especially considering that in one survey of 2000 patients, nearly 80% felt that antidepressants were addictive.

SUICIDE AND DELIBERATE SELF-HARM

In 1974, Barraclough *et al.* reported that two-thirds of suicide victims consulted their GP within a month of death and 40% within a week of death. However, Matthews *et al.* (*BMJ*, 1994) looking at 1100 deaths in Scotland, found the figures to be lower than this. Sixteen per cent had seen their GP in the week before death and 40% in the month before death (these figures rise to 25 and 50%, respectively, for those with a previous psychiatric history).

Fourteen per cent of suicides are wholly or partly due to anti-depressant overdose. Suicide by this method is more likely if tricyclic antidepressants are prescribed. However, if alternative anti-depressants are given, suicide occurs by some other means.

A study (*BMJ*, 1997) looking at the GP attendance rates of suicide patients, found that, in the 10 year period before death, suicide patients are more likely to have attended their GP, have a diagnosis of mental illness, receive a prescription for psychotropic drugs and be referred to a psychiatrist.

DETECTING DEPRESSION

PRIMARY CARE SECTION. Detection of depression and anxiety in primary care: follow up study. Kessler, D., Bennewith, O. and Lewis, G. *et al.* Division of Primary Health Care, University of Bristol, Bristol, UK.
***BMJ, 325**(7371): 1016-1017, 2 November 2002.*

A number of studies have indicated that general practitioners fail to diagnose as many as 50% of patients presenting with clinical depression or anxiety.

The majority of these studies have been cross-sectional and do not take into account the diagnosis being made at subsequent consultations.

In this longitudinal study conducted at a general practice in Bristol, around 180 consecutive patients were screened using questionnaires to determine the number suffering from clinical depression or anxiety.

Roughly half of these patients were shown to be suffering from depression or anxiety. These patients were then followed up over a 3 year period, with the intention of determining whether depression or anxiety not diagnosed during their initial consultation is either diagnosed during subsequent visits or is self limiting and of no clinical importance.

The authors highlight a number of points:

- At least 1 in 6 patients presenting to their general practitioner with severe symptoms of depression or anxiety remain undiagnosed 3 years after their initial presentation.
- Only 40% of patients presenting with clinical depression or anxiety are diagnosed on the first consultation. A further 25% are diagnosed over the next 3 years at subsequent consultations.
- 75% of patients diagnosed with depression or anxiety in primary care receive antidepressants.

General practitioners have felt unfairly criticised for missing up to half of the patients with depression that present to them. This study supports their view and indicates that undiagnosed depression may not be as great a problem as previously thought.

The outcome for patients with undetected depression needs to be reviewed, as these patients usually have severe symptoms and would benefit from treatment.

Routinely administered questionnaires for depression and anxiety: systematic review. Gilbody, S.M., House, A.O. and Sheldon, T.A. NHS Centre for Reviews and Dissemination, University of York, York, UK.
***BMJ, 322**(7283): 406-409, 17 February 2001.*

It is thought that the routine use of psychiatric questionnaires may aid in the detection, management and outcome of anxiety and depression. The aim of this systematic review was to evaluate the effect of routinely giving psychiatric questionnaires to non-psychiatric patients consulting GPs and hospital outpatients. Nine randomized trials were analyzed. Six were performed in general practice.

- Routine administration of questionnaires did not increase the rate of recognition of anxiety and depression by clinicians.
- When only severe cases were highlighted, detection did increase, although detection of these cases did not alter the management.
- Patient outcome was not altered by routinely administering questionnaires.

ANTIDEPRESSANTS

Fatal toxicity of serotoninergic and other antidepressant drugs: analysis of United Kingdom mortality data. Buckley, N.A. and McManus, P.R. Department of Clinical Pharmacology and Toxicology, Canberra Hospital, Canberra, ACT, Australia. *BMJ,* **325**(7376): 1332-1333, 7 December 2002.

This study aimed to determine the relative frequency of fatal poisoning with serotoninergic anti-depressants, particularly venlafaxine, and other new anti-depressants. The authors calculated a fatal toxicity index for each drug, expressed as the number of deaths per million prescriptions (excluding hospital prescriptions).

- Seratoninergic drugs had a lower overall index than monoamine oxidase inhibitors or tricyclic antidepressants. However, the venlafaxine index was greater than the individual and combined values for all other seratoninergic drugs, and similar to that of less toxic tricyclic anti-depressants.

The authors suggest overdose toxicity be considered when choosing an anti-depressant, but decisions should be based on individual drug information, rather than generalized data for drug classes or drug effects. Suicide from anti-depressant poisoning accounts for large numbers of suicide among those prescribed such drugs; doctors should thus consider factors relating to risk in each patient, when prescribing venlafaxine.

Antidepressants and generic counselling for treatment of major depression in primary care: randomised trial with patient preference arms. Chilvers, C., Dewey, D. and Fielding, K. *et al.* for the Counselling versus Antidepressants in Primary Care Study Group. *BMJ,* **322**(7289): 772-775, 31 March 2001.

The aim of this study was to compare counselling with antidepressants for the treatment of mild to moderate depression. Patients came from general practices in the Trent region of England. They were offered the choice of either:

- randomization to antidepressant or counselling; or
- choosing for themselves either antidepressants or counselling.

Around 100 patients took part in the randomized part of the trial and 220 in the patient preference arm of the study.

- Patients choosing counselling were less severely depressed than the randomized group, or those choosing antidepressants.
- With both groups combined, at 12 months, there was no difference in outcome between antidepressants and counselling.
- People who chose counselling tended to do better than those in the randomized group.
- The antidepressant group got better faster than the counselling group.

They discuss a number of issues. The counsellors in this study were very experienced. They had difficulty recruiting people to the randomized part of the study. They suggest that for patients who do not express a preference, antidepressants should be used. Counselling is a scarce resource and should be reserved for those who express a preference.

MANAGEMENT OF DEPRESSION

EDUCATION AND DEBATE: Quality improvement report Effect of a multifaceted approach to detecting and managing depression in primary care. Scott, J., Thorne, A. and Horn, P. Division of Psychological Medicine, Institute of Psychiatry, London, UK. *BMJ*, **325**(7370): 951-954, 26 October 2002.

This paper describes attempts to introduce a multifaceted management model for depression. The use a chronic disease management approach to identify and manage cases in an attempt to establish an integrated care pathway.

The two practices in the north of England taking part in the study each represented either end of a spectrum in terms of resource availability and socio-economic status of the patient population. The numbers of cases of depression diagnosed, the number of cases on the depression register and the adherence to the practices clinical management guidelines were documented.

The practice with six partners serving a relatively affluent population found that:
- Detection of depression increased by 23%
- Prescriptions for subtheraputic doses of antidepressants was decreased by 36%
- Adherence to preferred management regimes increased.

The practice with three partners across two surgeries in a deprived inner city area found that:
- An increase in sensitivity for detecting depression but decreased specificity.
- The practice was not able to sustain the management model. An agreement regarding guidelines was not reached.

A practice based, multifaceted disease management plan for depression can reduce morbidity but success necessitates a committed practice with financial backing, serving a relatively affluent population.

PRIMARY CARE: Managing depression as a chronic disease: a randomised trial of ongoing treatment in primary care. Rost, K., Nutting, P. and Smith, J.L. *et al.* Center for Studies in Family Medicine, University of Colorado Health Sciences Center, Aurora, CO, USA. **BMJ, 325**(7370): 934, 26 October 2002.

Adopting the increasing view of depression as a chronic condition, this RCT, involving 211 patient, across 12 primary care practices in the United States aimed to ascertain whether adopting principles of chronic disease management and applying them to depression could lead to significant symptom reduction and remission over a 2 year period.

Interventions included a structured care plan involving both doctors and nurses. Patient contact (telephone calls and visits) and patient education were emphasised and increased with hopes of patients becoming more actively involved in management.

They found that:

- Antidepressant tablets were used for a longer time period.
- Mental health counselling rates increased in the first 12 months of major depressive illness.
- The interventions improved symptoms and patient functioning so that by 24 months, 74% of patients met with remission criteria.

Time and cost limit widespread implementation of such increased interventions.

PRIMARY CARE: Effectiveness of teaching general practitioners skills in brief cognitive behavioural therapy to treat with depression: randomised controlled trial. King, M., Davidson, O. and Taylor, F. *et al.* Department of Psychiatry and Behavioural Sciences, Royal Free and University College Medical School, UK. **BMJ, 324:** 947-950, 20 April 2002.

In this RCT the authors attempted to assess the effectiveness of teaching GP's brief cognitive behavioural therapy (CBT) techniques as applied to the treatment of depression. They wished to discover if gaining skills in brief CBT improved their attitudes to the management if depression and the outcomes of their patients. Eighty four GP's and 272 patients were recruited to the study. Training was given as a package of 4 half days.

- Their results showed that doctor's knowledge of depression and attitudes towards its treatment was not altered by receiving training.
- Trained doctors referred more patients, suggesting that the training made them feel unable to deal with more complex cases.
- Patients of trained GP's had no difference in outcome to the control group.

The authors concluded that GP's may require more extensive training to acquire skills in brief CBT that will result in positive impact on patient outcomes.

Hampshire Depression Project: changes in the process of care and cost consequences. Kendrick, T., Stevens, L. and Bryant, A. *et al.* Aldmoor Health Centre, Aldmoor Close. Department of Primary Care, University of Southampton, Southampton, UK.
Br. J. Gen. Pract., 51(472): 911-913, 1 November 2001.

The Hampton Depression project aimed to improve recognition and management of depression in primary care by utilising educational seminars. This current paper examined the effect of this intervention on the process of care for depression in General Practice. The records of 205 patients from practices receiving the intervention, and 412 patients from control practices were analysed for recognition of depression and prescription of antidepressants. The authors found:

- There was no significant difference in the recognition of depressed patients by GPs in the intervention and control groups.
- There was no significant difference in the rate of prescription of antidepressants, dose administered or duration of treatment between control and intervention groups.
- Only 15% of patients with possible major depression received a therapeutic dose of antidepressants, the figure for probable major depression was 26%.
- The intervention did not result in significant reduction of cost of care.

The authors conclude that significant changes in the management of depression in primary care are unlikely to be achieved by educational interventions alone.

Coping with depression: a pilot study to assess the efficacy of a self-help audio cassette. Blenkiron, P. Academic Unit of Psychiatry and Behavioural Sciences, University of Leeds School of Medicine, Leeds, UK.
Br. J. Gen. Pract., 51(466): 366-370, 1 May 2001.

Little assessment has been made of self-help resources for patients with depressive disorders. This study intended to preliminarily evaluate the use of an audio cassette that suggests coping strategies to patients. Seventy-one patients diagnosed as having depressive disorders were given a copy of the tape. A questionnaire was completed in their GP's surgery before listening to the tape, and another completed after listening to the tape at home (70 response rate). GPs were interviewed to gather their opinions on use of the tapes.

- Generally, patients had a positive response to the tape, and were enthusiastic about trying some of the strategies it suggested.
- The biggest improvement was in patients not taking antidepressant medication.
- Despite relatively little of the tape being dedicated to antidepressant drugs, the most significant finding was that it made such patient less cautious of antidepressants. Blenkiron suggests the tape may therefore

be useful in helping patients not taking medication, to reconsider this option.

The limitations of the study were emphasised - it was not a RCT and there was no control group; the outcomes were qualitative, and factors other than the tapes may have caused the reported improvements; the 30 who failed to return the second questionnaire may have had a negative experience that would significantly influence the results. Blenkiron concludes that more RCTs are needed to assess the use of self-help in Primary Care.

The effectiveness of exercise as an intervention in the management of depression: systematic review and meta–regression analysis of randomised controlled trials.
Lawlor, D.A. and Hopker, S.W. Department of Social Medicine, University of Bristol, Bristol, UK.
BMJ, 322(7289): 763-767, 31 March 2001.

The aim of this systematic review was to determine the effectiveness of exercise for the treatment of depression. Fourteen studies were analysed. All studies were poorly designed, using non-clinical subjects and with short follow up periods.

• All types of exercise seemed to be beneficial.
• The effects did not seem to last beyond the intervention period.

They conclude that more rigorously designed studies will have to be done to adequately address this topic.

DEPRESSION : OUTCOME

EDITORIAL – Improving outcomes in depression. Von Korff, M. and Goldberg, D.
BMJ, 323(7319): 948-949, 27 October 2001.

Numerous studies have suggested that patients suffering from depression are not receiving adequate care, which is affecting the outcome of their condition. The World Health Organisation carried out a study looking into the treatment of depression in 14 countries and found that patients were being treated as frequently with sedatives as with antidepressants, despite the fact that treatment with antidepressants has a more favourable outcome. The authors make the following suggestions for care of depressed patients:

• A case manager (e.g. a practice nurse) should take responsibility for the follow up of these patients.
• Patient compliance to treatment and outcomes of treatment should be monitored.
• Treatment plans should be flexible and change if the patient is not benefiting from current treatment.
• The case manager and primary care physician should foster good working relationships with psychiatric services to be able to refer patients if necessary.

MEDICALLY UNEXPLAINED PHYSICAL SYMPTOMS (MUPS)

Systematic review of mental health interventions for patients with common somatic symptoms: can research evidence from secondary care be extrapolated to primary care? Raine, R., Haines, A. and Sensky, T. *et al.* Department of Public Health and Policy, London School of Hygiene and Tropical Medicine, London, UK.
BMJ, 325(7372): 1082-1085, 9 November 2002.

Evidence has shown that in patients with somatic symptoms for which no specific cause can be found, mental health interventions can be effective. However, in general practice, such treatments are rarely implemented, partly because of questions over the strength of the evidence showing effectiveness. This systematic review addresses this question. Sixty-one RCTs examining mental health interventions for chronic fatigue syndrome, irritable bowel syndrome and chronic back pain were reviewed.

- Results of meta-analyses and of RCTs suggest that behavioural therapies are effective for chronic back pain and chronic fatigue syndrome, and that antidepressant therapies are effective for irritable bowel syndrome.
- The interventions described above were all effective in primary care as well as specialised settings, although they were more effective in specialised settings.

The authors suggested that further large trials are needed with adequately trained staff in primary care settings, to determine whether such treatments might be as effective in primary care as in specialised settings.

What to do about medical unexplained symptoms.
Drug and Therapeutics Bulletin, 39(1): 5–8, 1 January 2001.

Patients with medically unexplained physical symptoms (MUPS) represent 20% of new consultations in primary care. Most symptoms resolve spontaneously, but 30% will be persistent. Other terms used to describe MUPS are psychosomatic illness and somatization. These descriptions can be unhelpful because they assume that physical symptoms have a psychological origin and that symptoms are 'all in the mind'.

Explanation of symptoms
Some people may attribute normal bodily reactions as evidence of serious disease. Studies have shown that people who, during their childhood, have witnessed illness amongst close relatives are more likely to experience MUPS later on. MUPS can also be associated with social and psychological issues and psychiatric illness.

Management
Patients with MUPS generally have thick case notes. It may be necessary to give the patient a long appointment so that a thorough and in depth

history and examination can be performed. Ideally, the consultation will allow the patient to discuss social and psychological issues. Explaining 'why?' can be helpful for the patient. A study has shown that the following types of explanation can be helpful.

- Giving a good explanation for the cause or mechanism of symptoms.
- Explaining that the symptoms are due to something that the patient cannot be blamed for.
- Encouraging self-help strategies.

Doctor and patient should plan a 'problem list' and set realistic goals. The aim is to help the patient cope with the problems rather than to try to find a cure. Follow up consultations should be arranged and the patient should be discouraged from visiting multiple doctors and being re-examined for the same symptoms. Antidepressants have been shown to be helpful for both sleep and pain, regardless of whether or not the patient is depressed. Patients should be told that they are being given the treatment for symptoms and not because they are depressed. Treatment usually starts working within 1-7 days.

Reattribution

This is a technique whereby the doctor demonstrates that he/she understands the patients concerns. It involves taking a thorough and adequate history in a listening and supportive manner. The doctor needs to show interest in the patient and an acceptance of their problems. The doctor also needs to make the link between physical and psychological symptoms e.g. overbreathing and anxiety, lowered pain threshold and depression.

Referral

Referral to secondary care may be necessary and this should be tailored to the individual patient. Cognitive behavioural therapy has been shown to help people with MUPS. Self-help techniques are encouraged.

SUICIDE AND DELIBERATE SELF HARM

Deliberate self harm in adolescents: self report survey in schools in England.
Hawton, K., Rodham, K. and Evans, E. Department of Psychiatry, Warneford Hospital, Oxford, UK.
BMJ, 325(7374): 1207-1211, 23 November 2002.

This questionnaire study conducted in the Midlands area of England set out to determine the prevalence of deliberate self harm (DSH) in adolescents in English schools and the factors associated with it. Various schools in the area were chosen to gain a representative sample. Around 6000 pupils were recruited overall.

- Overall around 800 pupils reported a history of DSH with around 400 of these (7%) having carried out an act of DSH in the previous year. The main methods used were cutting and poisoning.

- DSH was more common in females (11%) than males (3%). Also DSH was less common in Asian females compared to white females.
- Other factors such as cigarettes, alcohol and drugs increase the risk of DSH.

DSH is more common than indicated by presentation to hospital as this is usually only for cutting injuries. The authors suggest the development of school based programmes for the promotion of mental health.

EDITORIAL – Suicide after parasuicide. Runeson, Bo S. Karolinska Institute, Department of Clinical Neuroscience, Section for Psychiatry, St Gorans Hospital, Stockholm, Sweden. **BMJ, 325**(7373): 1125-1126, 16 November 2002.

Patients with a history of parasuicide have a suicide risk 40 times greater than that of the general population. Parasuicide thus confers a greater suicide risk than other mental health disorders. This effect of parasuicide on suicide risk does not decline for two decades, however it seems most prominent immediately following psychiatric care.

The interval between first suicidal behaviour and suicide depends on the patients sex and mental disorder, with women having higher parasuicide rates than men.

Previous thinking that parasuicide and suicide involves different populations has been shown to be untrue. Higher risk is indicated by planned, repeated or severe parasuicide, or psychiatric comorbidity. The circumstances of parasuicide also influence the risk of future suicide.

The author concludes that a history of parasuicide is the best predictor of future suicide, and that the risk does not decline for several decades after the parasuicidal incident.

Suicide rate 22 years after parasuicide: cohort study. Jenkins, G., Hale, R. and Crawford, M. *et al.* Department of Psychiatry, East Ham Hospital, London, UK. **BMJ, 325**(7373): 1155, 16 November 2002.

Suicide rates for people with an episode of parasuicide are 100 times higher in the year following the incident than the general population. The long-term risk of suicide in these patients in the UK is uncertain. This study looked at a sample of patients 22 years after they presented to a London hospital with parasuicide.

The patients used presented to psychiatric services over a 3 year period in the late 1970s. Attempts were made to trace them at the current time. Any patients who died because of suicide or probable suicide were recorded.

- Around two-thirds of the patients interviewed in the 1970s were traced and of these 18% had died in the time period up to June 2000. Half of these deaths were attributed to suicides.
- The overall rate of suicide was 4.3 per 1000 per year. The rate did not decline with time.

Even if deliberate self-harm occurred many years ago it still remains an important risk factor for subsequent suicide.

Effect of general hospital management on repeat episodes of deliberate self poisoning: cohort study. Kapur, N., House, A. and Dodgson, K. *et al.* Department of Psychiatry, Manchester Royal Infirmary, Manchester, UK.
***BMJ*, 325**(7369): 866-867, 19 October 2002.

Patients who deliberately self-poison tend to receive variable treatment in the United Kingdom in terms of psychiatric assessment and referral. The authors here looked at whether aspects of management had any effect on repeat episodes of poisoning. Patients were prospectively identified over 8 weeks for self-poisoning at six hospitals in north west England. Care was taken to ensure no patients were missed and clinical data was collected regarding each patient including whether they received a psychosocial assessment as recommended. Patients were followed up for 12 weeks after their first episode.

- Overall around 600 people poisoned themselves of whom 15% did so again within 12 weeks.
- Ten percent of the patients who had received an assessment poisoned again compared to 18% of patients that did not.
- After adjustment for other risk factors for repetition patients who had not received a psychosocial assessment were still twice as more likely to poison themselves again.

Assessments have a number of elements and research is needed to refine the components that reduce the risk of repeated self-poisoning.

MENTAL ILLNESS: OTHERS

EDITORIAL – Arrythmias and sudden death in patients taking antipsychotic drugs. Herxheimer, A. Emeritus Fellow, UK Cochrane Centre and Healy, D. University of Wales College of Medicine, Bangor, UK.
***Br. J. Gen. Pract.*, 325**(7375): 1253-1254, 30 November 2002.

It seems that drugs have a contributory role in causing cardiac arrythmias in addition to a predisposition conferred by the psychotic illness itself.

Mortality due to all causes is increased in schizophrenia when compared with other conditions such as glaucoma or psoriasis which both necessitate long term medications.

Risk of sudden death due to cardiac arrythmias is increased with specific antipsychotics (thioridazine) and at specific doses.

The true risk remains unclear but it is wise to avoid use of such medications in conjunction with other drugs which may increase QT interval (e.g. erythromycin) and to avoid use in patients with pre-existing cardiac disease. There is a place for ECG monitoring in psychotic patients.

EDITORIAL – Improving the management of acute myocardial infarction. Savage, W.M. and Channer, K.S. Royal Hallamshire Hospital, Sheffield, UK.
***BMJ*, 325**(7374): 1185, 23 November 2002.

The benefits of thrombolysis for acute myocardial infarction are well established, however it is currently under utilised within NHS hospitals. Confusion amongst physicians regarding indications and contraindications for thrombolysis contribute to this. The authors review these:

- Many clinicians are unsure whether to give thrombolysis to patients presenting 12 hours after onset of chest pain; however, evidence suggests that such patients may still benefit from treatment.

- Given the high risk of death after myocardial infarction in the over 75 age group, the authors conclude age should not be a barrier to treatment.

- The authors point out that diabetic retinopathy and cardiopulmonary resuscitation after arrest are not contrary to popular opinion-contraindications to thrombolysis.

- To deliver thrombolysis effectively clinicians must be aware that myocardial infarction frequently presents atypically.

Engagement of psychosis in the consultation: conversation analytic study. McCabe, R., Heath, C. and Burns, T. *et al.* Unit of Community Psychiatry, Barts and the London School of Medicine, London, UK.
***BMJ*, 325**(7373): 1148-1151, 16 November 2002.

New NHS funding has been earmarked for mental health. One initiative is that patients with severe psychotic symptoms are involved with the mental health teams as a matter of urgency. This study conducted in London analyzed how psychiatrists and psychotic patients interacted with each other in routine consultations.

Patients were chosen from psychiatric outpatient clinics that met criteria for diagnosis of schizophrenia. The consultations were videotaped and analyzed for things like speech delivery and body language.

- On analysis the average consultation involved the psychiatrist reviewing the patients psychiatric history and then asking questions regarding symptoms. Overall the patients role in the consultation was to answer the psychiatrists questions and inform him/her of any changes since the last consultation.

- Patients with psychotic illness attempted to talk about their symptoms and content. However on hearing their symptoms doctors tended to hesitate, avoided answering patients questions and even responded with a question. Some even laughed or smiled and this indicated a reluctance on the doctors part to engage in the patients concerns.

Addressing patients concerns about psychotic symptoms may lead to patients accessing mental health service more readily.

Cardiac arrest and ventricular arrhythmia in patients taking antipsychotic drugs: cohort study using administrative data. Hennessy, S., Bilker, W.B. and Knauss, J.S. *et al.* Center for Clinical Epidemiology and Biostatistics, University of Pensylvania, School of Medicine, Philadelphia, PA, USA.
BMJ, 325(7375): 1070-1072, 9 November 2002.

A link between certain antipsychotics and sudden death due to cardiac arrythmias has been implicated for over 4 decades now. This study looked at data from three Medicaid programmes across the USA and compared rates of cardiac arrest and ventricular arrhythmia in schizophrenic patients taking antipsychotics and non-schizophrenic controls on long term medication treatments for glaucoma and psoriasis.

- Patients taking antipsychoticcs had an increased rate of cardiac arrest and sudden death as compared to patient from either the psoriasis or glaucoma groups.
- Risperidone was the antipsychotic that had the highest rates of cardiac arrest and sudden death.
- The risk associated with each antipsychotic varied with dose.
- For risperidone, the highest risk occurred with the lowest dose. (However, it must be remembered that risperidone is used primarily in weak, frail elderly patients, and it is used at lowest doses within this group.)
- The true effect of thioridazine as compared to haloperidol in terms of cardiotoxicity remains unclear.

These results may be confounded by several factors such as lack of information regarding the indications for commencing these drugs in patients, and that fact that all the cases studies were based on oral therapy not parenteral.

Review: Sertraline maintenance treatment reduced relapse and dropouts in post-traumatic stress disorder. Commentator, Bisson, Jonathon I. University Hospital of Wales, Cardiff, UK.
Evidence-based Medicine, 7(5): 149, Sept./Oct. 2002.

Question: In patients who have post traumatic stress disorder (PTSD) and have responded to continuation sertraline treatment, does maintenance sertraline treatment reduce relapse?

The following article is briefly presented:
Efficacy of sertraline in preventing relapse of post traumatic stress disorder: results of a 28-week double-blind, placebo-controlled study. Davidson, J., Pearlstein, T., Londborg, P. *et al.*
Am. J. Psychiatry. **158**: 1974-1981, Dec. 2001

This was a randomised blinded placebo controlled trial carried out with 28 weeks follow up at 24 centres across the United States.

Almost 100 patients with post traumatic stress disorder were given 50-200 mg of sertraline or a placebo daily. No other intervention was permitted.

Results:
- Sertraline reduced relapse rates, study drop-out rates and acute exacerbation rates.
- Dizziness was reported as a significant side effect, in the placebo group.

Commentary

This study appears to be better quality than previous studies investigating the role of standard antidepressant treatment in the management of post traumatic stress disorder. Several other factors need to be considered however when interpreting the results:
- The small patient numbers actually included and completing the trial.
- Male patients were over-represented.
- The 40% of patients with criteria for diagnosis of secondary depressive disorder.
- Some patients had been taking sertraline prior to commencing the study.

Even taking into account the above, there is still undeniable evidence from this trial to support the use of sertraline for at least a year in the management of post traumatic stress disorder. Further work will clarify more specific management regimes.

It was noted that those who responded most quickly in the acute phase had reduced relapse rates upon discontinuation of therapy.

Assessment of independent effect of olanzapine and risperidone on risk of diabetes among patients with schizophrenia: population based nested case-control study. Kovo, C.E., Fedder, D.O. and LItalien, G.J. *et al.* Pharmaceuticals Health Services Research Department, School of Pharmacy, University of Maryland, Baltimore, MD, USA. **BMJ, 325**(7358): 243-246, 3 August 2002.

This population based nested case-control study aimed to quantify the association between olanzapine and diabetes. It was carried out in the UK using the General Practice Research Database for the years 1987-2000. Nearly 20 000 patients with a diagnosis of, and treatment for schizophrenia were included. Each incident case of diabetes was age and sex matched with six controls (with no diagnosis or treatment of diabetes). On analysis, it was shown that:
- The incidence rate of diabetes among all the schizophrenic patients using antipsychotics was 4.4/1000 person years, as compared with 10/1000 for olazapine, 5.4/1000 for risperidone and 5.1/1000 for conventional antipsychotics.
- The risk of diabetes was greatest among olanzapine users (odds ratio 4.4) which was significant. Risperidone also slightly increased the risk (odds ratio 1.6), but this was not significant.

Olanzapine use has been consistently associated with an increased risk of diabetes. This study has quantified this clinically important risk as significant in a large cohort of patients with schizophrenia.

Incidence of schizophrenia in ethnic minorities in London: ecological study into interactions with environment. Boydell, J, van Os, J and McKenzie, K. *et al.* Division of Psychological Medicine, Institute of Psychiatry, Denmark Hill, London, UK.
BMJ, **323**(7325): 1336-1338, 8 December 2001.

Some studies have reported an increased incidence of schizophrenia in ethnic minority groups in the UK. The reasons for this increased incidence remain unexplained. The aim of this retrospective study was to find out if the incidence of schizophrenia among non-white ethnic minorities is greater in neighbourhoods where they constitute a smaller proportion of the total population. Study participants were individuals over 16 who had contact with psychiatric services during 1988-1997 in 15 electoral wards in Camberwell, South London.

- The incidence of schizophrenia was highest in areas where ethnic minorities made up the smallest proportion of the population (incidence rate ratio 4.4).
- The incidence of schizophrenia was lowest in areas were ethnic minorities made up the largest proportion of the population (incidence rate ratio 2.38).

These results agree with those found in US studies. An explanation for these findings may be that a higher proportion of an ethnic minority in an area may provide greater protection to individuals against stresses such as discrimination and isolation.

EDITORIAL – Reducing violence in severe mental illness. Tilman, Steinert Head of Research Department and Clinical Department for General Psychiatry Centre of Psychiatry, University of Ulm, Weissenau, Germany.
BMJ, **323**(7321): 1080-1081, 10 November 2001.

The increase in forensic psychiatric patients and suicides associated with a reduction in the number of psychiatric hospital beds.
The author highlights a number of points:

- Assertive community treatment and intensive intervention need modifying to be more effective in patients prone to violent behaviour.
- Hospitalisation remains one proven effective treatment for violence in seriously mentally ill people. Schizophrenic inpatients show a continuous reduction in violent behaviour, with very low rates achieved after some weeks of treatment.
- Hospitalisation minimises factors such as substance abuse, non-compliance with medication, association with criminal peers and poor living conditions.
- Predictors for violent behaviour in mentally ill people are nearly the same as those in people without such disorders: Criminal history, age,

substance abuse, deviant lifestyle, family problems and anti-social personality disorder.

- Further research is needed to evaluate the clinical effectiveness of compulsory outpatient treatment combined with psychological support for violent psychiatric patients.

Reducing violence in severe mental illness: randomised controlled trial of intensive case management compared with standard care. Walsh, E, Gilvarry, C and Samele, C, *et al.* Section of Forensic Mental Health, Guy's, King's and St Thomas's School of Medicine, London, UK.
BMJ, **323**(7321): 1093, 10 November 2001.

This RCT aimed to assess whether intensive case management in the community, over a 2 year period, could reduce violence amongst patients with psychotic disorders. Case management involves a key worker assessing the needs of patients and drawing up care plans to ensure that the patient receives the services they require. Intensive case management involves case managers having 10-15 cases as opposed to approx. 30 cases for standard case management. Around 350 patients were randomised to the intervention group and around the same number received standard care. They found:

- Patients in the intervention arm received twice as much care as control patients; specifically they received more contacts related to finance, medication and the criminal justice system.
- A previous history of violence, learning disability, younger age and drug misuse predicted violent acts by psychotic patients.
- During the trial 22 % of participants committed a physical assault.
- There was no significant difference in the number of violent patients in the intervention and control groups.

They conclude that intensive patient management does not reduce violence among psychotic patients.

Perspectives of people with enduring mental ill health from a community-based qualitative study. Kai, J. and Crosland, A. Department of Primary Care and General Practice, University of Birmingham Medical School, Edgbaston, Birmingham, UK.
Br. J. Gen. Pract., **51**(470): 730-737, 1 September 2001.

The National Service Framework highlights the requirement for Primary Care Groups and Mental Health Services to work together to improve the standard and provision of services for those with mental illness.

This interview based study conducted across four general practices in disadvantaged areas explored patients individual perspectives and experiences of management. The aim was to effectively restructure services based on patients needs. They found the following:

- Full explanations of their condition and management by the doctor was seen as invaluable by patients.

- Continuity of care by the same healthcare professional prevented the feeling of always having to start form scratch at each visit.

- The social stigma and isolation experienced by patients prevented them from fully engaging in management.

- Some patients found contact with others experiencing mental health problems frightening. Others found it a great source of support and encouragement.

Continuity of care and social stigma experienced by patients are issues which must be dealt with comprehensively before optimal care can be achieved.

Patients with chronic mental ill health need to be reassured that they are not wasting GPs time many feel that this is the case. Equally, healthcare professionals need to be encouraged and reminded that feelings of inadequacy and frustration are common when dealing with patients suffering long term mental ill health.

How general practice patients with emotional problems presenting with somatic or psychological symptoms explain their improvement. Cape, J. Head of Psychology Camden and Islington Mental Health Trust, St Pancras Hospital, London, UK.
Br. J. Gen. Pract., **51**(470): 724-729, 1 September 2001.

Somatic presentations of psychological problems often prevent GPs from diagnosing emotional problems. This questionnaire based study was carried out across nine GP practices across North and East London. It compared patients perspectives and clinical outcomes in cases where presentations were either somatic, emotional, or both. They found the following results:

- There was no difference in outcome between groups presenting with emotional problems as compared to those presenting with somatic problems.

- Patients attribution for improvement differed. Those with somatic symptoms felt improvement was due to treatment of their physical complaints. Those with emotional problems felt improvement was the result of counselling by their GP.

- Patients with psychological symptoms and somatic symptoms attributed improved emotional health at least in part to improvement in their physical condition.

- Social support and time passing were implicated in the successful outcome of many cases.

Improvement in emotional disorders can still occur even in the absence of psychological symptoms being mentioned by either patient or doctor. The GPs role as a counsellor was heavily emphasised, as was the well recognised yet complex relationship between physical and psychological health.

EDITORIAL – Physical health of people with severe mental illness. Phelan, M., Stradins, L. and Morrison, S. Department of Psychiatry, Charing Cross Hospital, London, UK. **BMJ, 322**(7284): 443-444, 24 February 2001.

The national service framework states that patients with mental health problems should have an assessment of their physical needs. The physical needs of mentally ill patients often go unnoticed. People who are mentally ill are twice as likely to die as the general population. Neglect, smoking substance misuse, side effects of long term antipsychotic medication, inadequate diets and lack of exercise are some of the reasons for their poor health. Health professionals need to be more aware of the physical needs of people with mental illness and attention to physical needs should be part of routine care.

MUSCULOSKELETAL

- Expensive and time-consuming referrals for electrodiagnostic testing in patients with clear clinical signs of carpal tunnel syndrome should be curtailed as they do not contribute to diagnosis and management
- A 3 month graded aerobic exercise regimen is beneficial to fibromyalgia patients. This can be implemented effectively in the community by personal trainers with no previous experience of managing those with ill health.
- Editorial reviewing the use of Cyclo-oxygenase-2 specific non-steroidal anti-inflammatory drugs in treatment of acute gout
- Mortality is much higher in patients after fractured neck of femur compared to the general population and risk remains much higher for many months
- COX 2 inhibitors are gastrointestinally safer than traditional NSAIDS, but more research is needed to aid appropriate prescribing
- Celecoxib is as effective as other NSAIDs, but shows significantly greater tolerability and gastrointestinal safety
- Acute compartment syndrome must be identified and treated quickly to avoid permanent myoneural damage
- Patient education programmes for rheumatoid arthritis confer a small, short-lived benefit, with unclear clinical implications
- Rofecoxib is more effective than celecoxib or acetaminophen in the treatment of osteoarthritis of the knee
- Systematic Review finds no clear evidence to support the use of orthotic devices for tennis elbow
- New findings are emerging in arthritis treatment as work with cyclo-oxygenase inhibitors continues to progresses.
- The suggestions that selective COX 2 inhibitors are less likely to cause GI complications than traditional NSAIDs, made by authors of the CLASS trial, may be incorrect.
- Etoricoxib is an alternative treatment to indometacin in the treatment of acute gouty arthritis.
- Fluoroquinolone antibiotics increase risk of Achilles tendonitis or rupture
- Physiotherapy or a wait and see policy were found to be the best options for lateral epicondylitis at 1 year

EDITORIAL – Treating acute gouty arthritis with selective COX-2 inhibitors. Fam, A.G. Division of Rheumatology, Sunnybrook and Womens College Health Sciences Centre, University of Toronto, Toronto, Canada, UK.
***BMJ,* 325**(7371): 980-981, 2 November 2002.

Treatment options for the acute crystal arthropathies gout, pseudogout and calcific periarthritis include colchicine, non-steroidal anti-inflammatory drugs (NSAIDs) and corticosteroids. Colchicine is no longer first line therapy, and is reserved for patients without renal, hepatic or bone marrow disease who, for other reasons, can not tolerate NSAIDs. Intra-articular (methyprednisolone), systemic (prednisolone) or corticotrophin corticosteroids are effective and safe treatments for crystal arthropathies in patients with renal, hepatic or cardiac failure who can not tolerate NSAIDs or colchicine. However, the current treatment of choice is non-salicylate NSAIDs. No NSAID is clearly better than another, but a suitable initial therapy would be e.g. indomethacin 150-200 mg per day or naproxen 1000 mg per day. These conventional NSAIDs exert their effect by inhibiting both cyclo-oxygenase-1, (an enzyme producing housekeeping prostanoids which maintain renal blood flow and gastric mucosal health), and cyclo-oxygenase-2, (an enzyme producing inflammatory mediators which contribute to the symptoms of acute crystal arthropathies). Hence, conventional NSAIDs produce problems of renal impairment and gastric ulceration. New generation NSAIDs (e.g. etoricoxib) are cyclo-oxygenase-2 selective and hence have an anti-inflammatory effect with minimal side effects due to inhibition of cyclo-oxygenase-1. A recent study has shown etoricoxib 120 mg daily to be as effective as indomethacin 50 mg three times a day in management of acute gout, with a better safety profile of etoricoxib. Thus, the new cyclo-oxygenase-2 specific NSAIDSs may have a valuable role in treating acute gout.

Mortality after admission to hospital with fractured neck of femur: database study. Goldacre, M., Roberts, S. and Yeates, D. Department of Public Health, University of Oxford, Oxford, UK.
***BMJ*, 325**(7369): 868-869, 19 October 2002.

The death rate within 1 year for fractured neck of femur is around is around 30%. League tables based on mortality after admission have been promoted as a measure of performance. However, the only routine hospital statistic is death during the initial admission for the fracture. The authors looked at patients who had been admitted to one of eight hospitals with fractured neck of femur. Standardized mortality ratios (SMR) and case fatality rates were calculated for in-hospital deaths within 30 days and for all deaths within 30, 90 and 180 days of admission. Deaths certified as fractured neck of femur were calculated separately to other deaths.

- The SMR ratios show mortality is much higher in patients with fractured neck of femur compared to the general population and it remains higher many months after fracture.
- Only a minority of cases (16%) were certified as fractured femur being the underlying cause of death.

The mortality ranking of hospitals varies with whether death was in-hospital and time interval of death after admission. However this is again affected by information on the death certificate and whether information regarding the death is included at all.

Physiotherapy or a wait and see policy were the best options for lateral epicondylitis at 1 year. Kreder, H. University of Toronto, Sunnybrook and Womens College Health Sciences Center, Toronto, Ont., Canada.
***Evidence-based Medicine, 7**(5): 153, Sept./Oct. 2002.

Question: In patients with lateral epicondylitis, what is the effectiveness of a wait and see policy, physiotherapy or corticosteroid infections?

The following article is briefly presented.
Corticosteroid injections, physiotherapy or a wait-and-see policy for lateral epicondylitis: a randomised controlled trial. Smidt, N., van der Windt, D.A., Assendelft, W.J. *et al.*
Lancet **359**: 657-662, 23 Feb. 2002

This RCT was conducted in the Netherlands and involved 185 patients with lateral epicondylitis. They were offered either 9 sessions of physiotherapy, 3 corticosteroid injections or a wait and see policy.
- At 6 weeks follow up more people in the corticosteroid group reported success than the other two groups.
- At 1 year more people in the physiotherapy and wait and see group reported success compared with the corticosteroid group.

Commentary
A wait and see policy plus NSAIDs may be more cost effective than any of the other treatments for lateral epicondylitis.

EDITORIAL – Efficacy and safety of COX 2 inhibitors. Jones, R. Department of General Practice and Primary Care, Guys, Kings and St Thomas' School of Medicine, London, UK.
***BMJ, 325**(7365): 607-608, 21 September 2002.

In recent years, much debate has surrounded the issues of efficacy and gastrointestinal safety of specific COX 2 inhibitors, compared to traditional non-steroidal anti-inflammatory drugs (NSAIDS). This editorial describes the current evidence on this topic, with particular attention to two newly published papers. These papers (one a systematic review, one a cohort study) find comparable efficacy between COX 2 inhibitors and traditional NSAIDS, but lower rates of gastrointestinal side effects in the COX 2 inhibitors.

The author suggests that while these findings are of comfort to prescribers, more research is needed to guide appropriate prescribing, in particular to determine which groups of patients will benefit most from the newer COX 2 inhibitors.

Efficacy, tolerability, and upper gastrointestinal safety of celecoxib for treatment of osteoarthritis and rheumatoid arthritis: systematic review of randomised controlled trials. Deeks, J.J., Smith, L.A. and Bradley, M.D. Centre for Statistics in Medicine, Institute of Health Sciences, Oxford, UK.
BMJ, **325**(7365): 619-623, 21 September 2002.

Celecoxib was developed as a specific cyclo-oxygenase 2 (COX 2) inhibitor to relieve inflammation without the gastrointestinal complications of traditional non-steroidal anti-inflammatory drugs (NSAIDS). However, concerns remain over the efficacy and gastrointestinal safety of this drug. This systematic review and meta-analysis addresses the issue. Nine randomised controlled trials (with a total of 15 187 patients) were included in analysis. All nine studies compared celecoxib with traditional NSAIDs in the treatment of osteoarthritis and rheumatoid arthritis, with respect to efficacy, tolerability and gastrointestinal side effects. Overall:

- Celecoxib and NSAIDs were equally effective in the treatment of both osteoarthritis and rheumatoid arthritis
- The rate of withdrawals from studies due to adverse gastrointestinal events was 46% lower amongst patients taking celecoxib compared to those taking traditional NSAIDs
- The incidence of ulcers detected by endoscopy was 71% lower in those taking celecoxib compared to traditional NSAIDs

The author concludes that the tolerability and gastrointestinal safety of celecoxib are substantially superior to those of other NSAIDs, despite equivalent efficacies.

EDITORIAL – Acute compartment syndrome of the leg. Pearse, M.F., Harry, L. and Nanchahal, J. Department of Musculoskeletal Surgery, Imperial College School of Medicine, London, UK.
BMJ, **325**(7364): 557-558, 14 September 2002.

This article concerns acute limb compartment syndrome, a surgical emergency in which there is raised pressure in an unyielding osteofascial compartment. The pressure reduces capillary perfusion, resulting in permanent nerve or muscle damage.

The condition causes severe pain, out of proportion to any apparent injuries, and aggravated by passive muscle stretching. It is important to diagnose the condition and decompress quickly. Diagnosis can be exclusively from clinical signs; measurement of intracompartmental pressure is only necessary in equivocal cases and uncooperative patients.

The authors emphasise the importance of accuracy when decompressing, and give guidelines for those performing the procedure.

Fasciotomy may impair the calf muscle pump, causing chronic venous insufficiency. After 8 hours, an established myoneural deficit is unlikely to recover

A systematic review of the utility of electrodiagnostic testing in carpal tunnel syndrome. Jordan, R., Carter, T. and Cummins, C. Institute of Child Health, University of Birmingham, Whittall Street, Birmingham, UK.
***Br. J. Gen. Pract.,* 52**(481): 670-672, 1 August 2002.

Electrodiagnostic tests are considered to be beneficial in the diagnosis and management of carpal tunnel syndrome. Waiting lists are long and resources limited yet GPs and surgeons continue to refer. In order to establish the true cost effectiveness of these many referrals, electro-diagnosis was evaluated in it's role as a diagnostic tool. A range of tests including nerve conduction studies and electromyography were investigated in patients with good clinical signs of carpal tunnel syndrome.

- Electrodiagnosis was found to be highly specific in diagnosing carpal tunnel syndrome but not so highly sensitive thus resulting in patients suitable for surgery missing out as a result of falsely negative conduction studies.
- The evidence available for electrodiagnosis as a tool for predicting outcome of surgery in carpal tunnel syndrome is scarce and poor quality. There is no available evidence to support the use of electrodiagnosis as a tool for predicting likely successful outcome of surgery for carpal tunnel syndrome.

GP and surgeons should curb their referrals for electrodiagnostic testing in patients with good clinical signs of carpal tunnel syndrome. No evidence exists to support electrodiagnostic testing in patients with less obvious clinical presentations and further studies should focus on this.

Prescribed exercise in people with fibromyalgia: parallel group randomised controlled trial. Richards, S.C.M. and Scott, D.L. Poole Hospital NHS Trust, Poole, Dorset, UK.
***BMJ,* 325**(7357): 185-188, 27 July 2002.

This RCT evaluating the merits of prescribed community-based exercise programmes for fibromyalgia patients. Just over 130 men and women, aged 18-70 and suffering fibromyalgia, were allocated to either graded aerobic exercise or relaxation classes. These met twice weekly for an hour, over a period of 12 weeks. The personal trainers for each group were blinded to study hypotheses. Subjects continued medication, and received standard advice and encouragement for fibromyalgia.

- At 3 months, and 12 months significantly more of the exercise group were "better" or "very much better" compared to the relaxation group.
- At 3 and 12 months, tenderness at 18 sites had fallen in both groups, but with the exercise group doing better than the relaxation group.
- At 12 months, fewer patients in the exercise group, were classified as having fibromyalgia.
- The exercise group showed greater improvement in the fibromyalgia impact questionnaire and McGill pain scores.

This is the first published study confirming the effectiveness of "Healthy Living Centres" funded by the National Lottery. The authors conclude "a

3 month programme of prescribed graded aerobic fitness exercise" improves participants overall rating of fibromyalgia, and reduce tender-point scores. Many beneficial effects lasted 12 months.

Rofecoxib, 25 mg/day, was more effective than rofecoxib, 12.5 mg/day, celecoxib, or acetaminophen in osteoarthritis of the knee. Meyerhoff, J. Sinai Hospital of Baltimore, Baltimore, MD, USA.
Evidence-based Medicine, 7(4): 123, July/Aug. 2002.

Question: In patients with symptomatic osteoarthritis (OA) of the knee, are rofecoxib, celecoxib, and acetaminophen effective and safe?

The following article is briefly presented
Efficacy of rofecoxib, celecoxib, and acetaminophen in osteoarthritis of the knee. A randomised trial. Geba, G.P., Weaver, A.L., Polis, A.B. *et al.* Merck and Co Inc., West Point, Philadelphia, PA, USA.
JAMA **287**: 64-71, 2 Jan. 2002

This study was a RCT conducted in 29 clinical centres in the USA. Three hundred and eighty-two patients with symptomatic OA of the knee were randomised to either rofecoxib 25 mg per day, rofecoxib 12.5 mg per day, celecoxib 200 mg per day, or acetaminophen 4000 mg per day. They used standardised outcome measures after 6 weeks of treatment.
• Better global responses and symptomatic relief were experienced by the rofecoxib 25 mg per day group than any other group.
• Rates of adverse events were similar across all groups.

Commentary
Meyerhoff comments that as OA is a chronic condition requiring long term treatment, 6 weeks follow up is not long enough to predict long term treatment results. In addition, he notes that this study does not test a higher than usual dose of celecoxib (as it does for rofecoxib). Finally, he suggests that pharmacological treatment of OA should be individually tailored to each patient, on the basis of their gastrointestinal, cardiac and risk factors.

EDITORIAL – Potential alternatives to COX 2 inhibitors. Skelly, M.M. and Hawkey, C.J. Division of Gastroenterology, University Hospital Nottingham, Queen's Medical Centre, Nottingham, UK.
BMJ, **324**(7349): 1289-1290, 1 June 2002.

This editorial reflects on the potential substitutes of non-steroidal anti-inflammatory drugs (NSAIDs), cyclo-oxygenase inhibitors in the management of arthritis. It has been generally understood that NSAIDS were cyclo-oxygenase inhibitors which reduced prostaglandin synthesis in joints to good effect. This same effect caused gastroduodenal toxicity. Attempts were made to get around this with the selective use of cyclo-oxygenase inhibitors. Cyclo-oxgenase 2 (COX 2) inhibitors act mainly on joints and duodenal toxicity is avoided. Whereas cyclo-oxygenase 1 (COX 1) is the main source of prostaglandin in the stomach.

Safer and more potent rival preparations with wider usage are becoming increasingly recognised:

- Nitric oxide donating NSAIDS-Cyclo-oxygenase inhibiting nitric oxide donors.
- Dual inhibitors of cyclo-oxygenase and 5-lipoxygenase-licofelone. Studies showed that part of the duodenal toxicity was caused by an increase in leukotrine production by the 5-lipo-oxygenase enzyme. Licofelone inhibits both by acting as a "substrate competitor".

Although some human data is becoming available for these two classes of drug more work is needed such as efficacy studies, particularly of cyclo-oxygenase inhibiting nitric oxide donors.

EDITORIAL – Are selective COX 2 inhibitors superior to traditional non steroidal anti-inflammatory drugs. Juni, P., Rutjes, A.W.S. and Dieppe, P.A. Departments of Rheumatology and Social and Preventative Medicine, University of Berne, Switzerland. **BMJ, 324**(7349): 1287-1288, 1 June 2002.

The CLASS study (Celecoxib Longterm Arthritis Safety Study, JAMA, September 2000), suggested that use of selective COX 2 inhibitors had a lower risk of GI complications than using conventional NSAIDs. The trial was funded by the pharmaceutical company who manufacture celecoxib, a COX 2 inhibitor. Criticisms have been raised that contradict the conclusions of the original published study.

CLASS intended to measure the incidence of symptomatic ulcers and clinically relevant upper GI ulcer complications, in the first 6 months of treatment with either celecoxib or a traditional NSAID.

- It concluded that celecoxib was associated with a lower incidence of both symptomatic ulcers and ulcer complications.

However, the published study actually referred to a combined analysis of two separate longer trials with different protocols to CLASS.

The CLASS protocol stated that celecoxib would only be declared superior to traditional NSAIDs if both combined and separate comparisons with ibuprofen and diclofenac showed statistically significant reductions in ulcer complications.

- Analysis using the pre-defined protocol showed similar numbers of ulcer-related complications in the comparison groups.
- Almost all complications in the second half of the trial were in users of celecoxib.

Two concerns have been raised

- Firstly, that the authors failed to adequately justify the changes in the design, outcomes and analysis of the study, and their use of only 6 month follow-up data when longer term data was available.
- Secondly, the flawed findings have become widely accepted, and are cited by many other studies. This coincides with significant increases in celecoxib sales.

Independent meta-analysis is needed of all large scale, long-term COX 2 inhibitor trials, using the original protocols. The results of this must be distributed on a large scale, to prevent reliance by physicians on the results of the original flawed study. If this is not done, pharmaceutical companies will feel less obliged to correct discrepancies such as these in future.

Randomised double blind trial of etoricoxib and indometacin in treatment of acute gouty arthritis. Schumacher, Jr. H.R., Boice, J.A. and Daikh, D.I. *et al.* Division of Rheumatology, University of Pennsylvania School of Medicine and Department of Veterans Affairs Medical Center, Philadelphia, USA.
BMJ, 324(7352): 1488-1492, 22 June 2002.

This randomised, double-blind controlled trial compared the safety and efficacy of etoricoxib and indometacin in the treatment of acute gouty arthritis. Nearly 150 men and 8 women who presented with clinically diagnosed acute gout within 48 hours of onset were included in the study. Etoricoxib 120 mg was administered orally once daily, compared with indometacin 50 mg, administered orally three times daily, both for 8 days. They assessed pain over days 2 to 5.
  • Etoricoxib and indometacin showed comparable efficacy in the treatment of acute gouty arthritis over the entire treatment period.
  • Etoricoxib was associated with a lower incidence of all four pre-specified categories of adverse experiences than indometacin.
Etoricoxib is an effective alternative treatment to indometacin and one which is only required once daily.

Fluoroquinolones and achilles tendon disorders: a case control study. Van der Linden, P.D., Sturkenboom, M.C.J.M., Herings, R.M.C., Leufkens, H.G.M. and Stricker, B.H.C. Pharmaco-epidemiology Unit, Deparment of Epidemiology and Biostatistics and Internal Medicine, Erasmus Medical Centre Rotterdam, Rotterdam, Netherlands.
BMJ, 324(7349): 1306-1307, 1 June 2002.

It is unresolved whether fluoroquinolone antibiotics are associated with tendon disorders. This nested case control study, utilising the UKMediPlus database, reviewed the case records of almost 45000 fluoroquinolone users and randomly selected 10000 controls from the cohort. Of the fluorqionolone users 704 developed Achilles tendonitis while 38 had Achilles tendon rupture. Among patients with Achilles disorders, four categories of fluoroquinolone use were defined:
1. Current, tendon disorder occurred between start of treatment and 30 days after cessation)
2. Recent, tendon disorder occurred 30-90 days after drug cessation
3. Past, drug ceased more than 90 days before tendon disorder
4. No use.
The authors concluded:
  • Current use of fluoroquinolones nearly doubles the risk (relative risk 1.9) of Achilles tendon disorders. But this adverse effect is rare, with an absolute excessive risk of 3.2 cases per 1000 patient years.

- Increased risk of Achilles tendon disorders is restricted to patients older than 60 (relative risk of 3.2 compared with 0.9 in patients under 60).
- In patients over 60, fluoroquinolones and corticosteroids interact to further increase risk of Achilles tendon disorders (relative risk of 6.4) such that 87 of Achilles disorders in this group are due to this drug interaction.

Orthotic devices for tennis elbow: a systematic review. Struijs, P.A.A., Smidt, N. and Arola, H. *et al.* Academic Medical Centre, Department Of Orthopaedic Surgery, Amsterdam, The Netherlands.
Br. J. Gen. Pract., **51**(472): 924-929, 1 November 2001.

The authors performed a systematic review of the literature to examine the evidence for use of orthotic devices in the management of tennis elbow (lateral epicondylitis) condition. Five RCTs met the inclusion criteria. They found:
- No significant differences between use of orthotic device and corticosteroid injection, physiotherapy or anti-inflammatory cream.
- Studies comparing orthotic device plus anti-inflammatory cream/ manipulation/ ultrasound and these treatments alone found no benefit of adding an orthotic device.
- One trial comparing elbow band and splint found now significant difference between the two.

The authors conclude that there is no clear evidence to support the use of orthotic devices for tennis elbow.

FURTHER READING

See 'Back pain' for

EDITORIAL - X-rays for back pain? Community Clinical Sciences, University of Southampton, Southampton.
Br. J. Gen. Pract., **52**(480): 534-535, July 2002.

MYOCARDIAL INFARCTION

PRE-HOSPITAL MANAGEMENT
- Pre-hospital thrombolysis reduces all-cause in-hospital mortality but does not effect mortality at 2 years follow up

OTHERS
- Nurse-initiated thrombolysis decreases "door to needle times" in acute myocardial infarction
- A qualitative study found that patients often had problems relating symptoms to a heart attack
- Public access defibrillators may not be cost-effective. It may be better to improve response times and provision of CPR by bystanders
- Epidemiological analysis is needed to ensure that programs to maximise survival following cardiac arrest are fully effective
- Glycoprotein inhibitors reduce death and myocardial infarction in acute coronary syndrome, but increase the risk of major bleeding
- Including troponin in the diagnostic criteria for myocardial infarction would result in a major increase in its incidence

BACKGROUND

PRE-HOSPITAL MANAGEMENT

The aim of treatment is to reduce morbidity and mortality. British Heart Foundation guidelines suggest that:
- 'call to needle time' should be within 90 minutes;
- GPs should be prepared to give oxygen, aspirin and nitrates as well as having other drugs available such as adrenaline, atropine and lignocaine;
- those giving thrombolysis should be fully familiar with its use.

The GREAT study (*BMJ*, 1996) found that pre-hospital thrombolysis was associated with an 11% reduction in mortality at one year. The pre-hospital approach is much more useful when journey times to hospital are long. But pre-hospital treatment requires a co-ordinated system of care with good protocols, trained staff and audit of results. In addition pre-hospital thrombolysis is associated with increased side effects e.g. hypotension, bradycardia, tachycardia and irregular rhythms (*BJGP*, April 1995).

PRE-HOSPITAL MANAGEMENT

Potential impact of public access defibrillators on survival after out of hospital cardiopulmonary arrest: retrospective cohort study. Pell, J.P., Sirel, J.M. and Marsden, A.K. *et al.* Department of Medical Cardiology, University of Glasgow, Glasgow, UK.
BMJ, 325(7363): 515-519, 7 September 2002.

This study intended to estimate the effect of public access defibrillators on survival, following cardiac arrest outside hospital. Data was obtained retrospectively from an electronic register.

- The number of patients receiving defibrillation in sites judged unsuitable, possibly suitable and suitable for defibrillator deployment was 56%, 68% and 73%, respectively.
- Everyone receiving defibrillation was more likely to survive, with the highest survival in areas suitable for public defibrillators.

The authors argue that the provision of widespread public access defibrillators may not be cost-effective. They conclude that public access defibrillators may increase survival by just over 1% if put in public places such as shopping centres and airports. However, they suggest that is would be better to improve defibrillation given by first responders and to improve CPR given by bystanders.

Review: Pre–hospital thrombolysis for acute myocardial infarction decreases short term hospital mortality. Commentator, Mirle Kellet, Maine Medical Center, Portland, Maine, USA.
Evidence–based Medicine, 6(1): 12, Jan./Feb. 2001.

Question: Is pre-hospital thrombolysis more effective than in-hospital thrombolysis for decreasing short term mortality in patients with acute myocardial infarction (MI)?

The following article is briefly presented
Mortality and pre–hospital thrombolysis for acute myocardial infarction. A meta–analysis. Morrison, L.J., Verbeek, P.R., McDonald, and A.C., *et al.* *JAMA,* **283:** 2686–2692, 24 May 2000.

The aim of this meta-analysis was to examine the effectiveness of pre-hospital thrombolysis. Six RCTs and three follow up studies were analysed.

- Pre-hospital thrombolysis was associated with a lower all-cause hospital mortality than in-hospital thrombolysis.
- Mortality at 2 years did not differ between the two groups.

Commentary
The pre-hospital approach is much more useful when journey times to hospital are long; but pre-hospital treatment requires a co-ordinated system of care with good protocols, trained staff and audit of results.

OTHERS

Review: glycoprotein IIb/IIIa inhibitors reduced death or myocardial infarction in acute coronary syndromes not routinely scheduled for revascularization. Bates, E.R. University of Michian, Ann Arbor, MI, USA.
Evidence-based Medicine, 7(4): 108, July/Aug. 2002.

Question: In patients with acute coronary syndromes not routinely scheduled for early coronary revascularization, what is the efficacy and safety of glycoprotein (GP) IIb/IIIa inhibitors?

The following article is briefly presented
Platelet glycoprotein IIb/IIIa inhibitors in acute coronary syndromes: a meta-analysis of all major randomised clinical trials. Boersma, E., Harrington, R.A., Moliterno, D.J., *et al.* University Hospital Rotterdam, Rotterdam, The Netherlands.
Lancet 189-198, 19 Jan. 2002

RCTs from 1990-2002 examining the use of GP IIb/IIIa inhibitors in acute coronary syndrome not scheduled for early revascularization were analyzed. The main efficacy outcome was a composite of death and non-fatal MI, and the main safety outcome was major bleeding. Six RCTs were included in meta-analysis.
- Patients who received GP IIb/IIIa inhibitors had a lower risk of death or MI. Further analysis showed that men had a reduced risk and women an increased risk.
- The groups did not differ for mortality.
- Patients who received GP IIb/IIIa inhibitors had a higher risk of major bleeding

Commentary
The acute coronary syndrome refers to people with unstable angina (UA) and those with non-ST elevation MI (NSTEMI). Subgroup analysis in this study suggests that people that did well had positive troponin values. Positive troponin values are suggestive of NSTEMI. Hence, it may be more appropriate to limit treatment to this group. However, many patients who are labelled as having UA actually have NSTEMI and therefore would also benefit from treatment.

EDUCATION AND DEBATE SECTION – Quality improvement report. Safety and efficacy of nurse initiated thrombolysis in patients with acute myocardial infarction. Qasim, A., Malpas, K., O'Gorman, D.J. and Heber, M.E. Cardiology Department, Princess Royal Hospital, Apley Castle, Telford, UK.
BMJ, **324**(7349): 1328-1331, 1 June 2002.

The national service framework for coronary heart disease set a goal that by April 2002, 75 of eligible patients should receive thrombolysis within 30 minutes of arriving at hospital. This paper reports audit results of "door to needle times" in one hospital, and describes the initiation of thrombolysis by a "coronary care thrombolysis nurse" to achieve this goal. Three separate 1-year periods ("phases") were audited.

- In phase 1, all patients were seen by a doctor prior to thrombolysis, 38 of patients were treated within 30 minutes.
- In phase 2, a nurse assessed each patient, and a doctor started treatment, 47 were treated within 30 minutes.
- In phase 3, a "coronary care thrombolysis nurse" assessed each patient and initiated thrombolysis if appropriate, 80 of patients were treated within 30 minutes.
- There were no cases of inappropriate administration of thrombolysis by a nurse.

The authors conclude that thrombolysis can be safely and effectively initiated by nurses. This is one way in which door to needle time targets can be reached.

Decision making processes in people with symptoms of acute myocardial infarction: qualitative study. Pattenden, J., Watt, I. and Lewis, R. Department of Health Sciences, University of York, York, UK.
BMJ, **324**(7344): 1006, 27 April 2002.

Treatment for acute MI needs to be administered as soon as possible. Questions have been raised whether a patients' knowledge of heart attack symptoms reduces delays. The aim of this qualitative study was to identify the factors that influence a patients' decision to seek medical help and also those that delay them. The study included 22 patients, all of whom had had at least one previous MI. Six themes emerged including the following findings:

- Patients had problems relating their symptoms to a heart attack and confused them with things like indigestion. Some patients who had modified their lifestyle or undergone bypass surgery in the past felt they were no longer at risk and delayed seeking medical help when symptoms arose.
- Most of the patients interviewed mentioned that the symptoms were not similar to previous MIs. This delayed patients contacting help as well as some patients experience of false alarms when their feelings of a heart attack were subsequently unfounded.
- Some patients did not want to admit they were having a heart attack, which delayed matters as well as the fear of creating false alarms.
- Other patients didn't want to waste NHS time or feel like they were bothering people. If patients had another person with them at the time then this tended to cut down the time taken to seek help as the other person usually took action first.

The decision to seek help in patients is a complex interaction of factors. Efforts to reduce delay should cover all themes found. This may lead to reductions to morbidity and mortality.

EDITORIAL – Was it a heart attack? Troponin positive acute coronary syndrome versus myocardial infarction. McKenna, C.J. and Forfar, J.C. Department of Cardiology, John Radcliffe Hospital, Oxford, UK.
BMJ, **324**(7334): 377-378, 16 February 2002.

The WHO requires that strict criteria are met before a patient can be defined as having had a heart attack. The more recent development of the use of cardiac troponin, a serological marker that enables detection of very small amounts of cardiac necrosis, is not included in these criteria. This editorial discusses the merits and problems associated with a proposed redefinition of myocardial infarction (MI) suggested in a consensus document from the European Society of Cardiology, and the American College of Cardiology. It reports that:

• Troponin levels are prognostic and can be carried out at the bedside; levels of less than 0.4 ng/ml are associated with a 42 day mortality of 1%, compared with 7.5% when the value is increased to 0.9 ng/ml or more.

• A typical rise and fall in either troponin or creatinine kinase (MB) accompanied by one of either ischaemic symptoms, pathological Q waves, ischaemic ECG changes, or coronary intervention would be used to classify an MI as being acute, evolving or recent.

This suggested redefinition would identify more candidates for aggressive secondary prevention as more patients would be included in the MI category. It could also have major implications for individual patients (psychologically, and affecting life insurance) and on research (inclusion criteria) and society in general.

EDITORIAL – Outcome after cardiac arrest outside hospital. Engdahl, J. Division of Cardiology, Sahlgrenska University Hospital, Gothenberg, Sweden.
BMJ, **325**(7363): 503, 7 September 2002.

In spite of the huge effort to combat mortality from cardiac arrest outside hospital, this still accounts for many deaths.

The author suggests plans for widespread public deployment of automated external defibrillators may have limited success, according to current epidemiological evidence. Various studies have shown a minimal impact of previous such schemes; reasons for this include cardiac arrests occurring in private rather than public places, and the low number of arrests in which defibrillation is likely to be useful.

Engdahl acknowledges the proven worth of defibrillators in situations such as in aircraft, but says careful epidemiological evaluation is necessary for such programmes to be implemented where they will be most successful. He suggests numerous strategies, other than defibrillators, that are likely to be useful. These include prophylactic CABG or angioplasty, pharmacological treatments, and increased public awareness of how to deal with cardiac arrests.

Engdahl also questions whether modern treatment is prolonging patients lives to the extent that treating cardiac arrest at such an advanced stage of disease is more likely to be futile anyway.

NHS

- Private Funded Initiatives in the NHS does not necessarily offer "value for money"
- The Budget promises to almost double NHS expenditure over 5 years
- New regulatory agencies, such as NICE could mark the start of a new approach to improved performance and management in the NHS. This will depend on politicians being prepared to empower these agencies and relinquish centralised control
- To prevent "Bristol" from happening again, there needs to be improved communication between doctors and patients
- A single centre study concludes that providing patients with a confirmatory phone call and /or detailed written information prior to their appointment, can considerably reduce non-attendance rates
- US-style physician assistants may not be ideal for the NHS
- Equality of access in the NHS may compromise quality of care
- The peaks of negative reporting appearing in UK newspapers, suggests that editors respond to incidents rather than deliberately campaigning against doctors
- Public safety and professional integrity are threatened by a lack of regulation of health informatics services
- Measurements of quality in healthcare are important, but it is vital to account for different contexts when comparing individuals or organizations
- Doctors interpersonal skills are very important in gaining patients trust and patient involvement in decision making processes improves their satisfaction
- Medical education should aim to integrate the best qualities of the medical scientist with those of the medical humanist
- An editorial argues that the teaching of continuous quality improvement skills should be part of undergraduate medical education.
- An editorial argues that the Department of Healths proposals for monitoring and improving doctors performance are sound and based but based on limited evidence.
- Using educational interventions/model in general practices as a lever for improvement will enable clinical governance objectives to be met.
- Efficiency and quality of care provided by NHS walk-in centres still requires research.
- The Kaiser permanente health care system in California costs about the same per capita as the NHS, but performs much better.
- The performance and efficiency of health systems can be measured and compared across different countries and over time.
- Walk-in centres provide adequate and safe clinical care compared to general practice and NHS Direct.
- There is currently no conclusive evidence as to the cost effectiveness of telemedicine as a means of delivering healthcare.
- Non-linear approaches to education will best equip doctors of the future with the ability to adapt their skills to meet the changing demands placed on NHS services.

BACKGROUND

THE DEVELOPING NHS

From the very inception of the NHS in 1948 there has been a long-running debate concerning whether or not the NHS should be managed locally or nationally. Although the NHS eventually won the day, the local authority view was not dismissed lightly by Aneurin Bevan. Bevan initially favoured the idea of local authorities controlling local care. However he was sceptical of the local authorities ability to provide uniform care. Financial considerations would also affect the uniform provision of care provided locally. The same issues arose again in 1974 with the reorganization of the NHS. The local authority idea was again rejected but not as strongly as in 1948. Health and social care are closely related and both sectors need to work together. Local authority policies will affect the health of the local community; it is therefore important that the two co-operate.

Concentrating our efforts and resources into primary care is seen to be the main way we can reduce spiralling NHS costs. Primary care also provides a comprehensive and co-ordinated package of care.

ASSESSMENT OF NEED

An analysis of practice-level mortality data to inform a health needs assessment.
Webb, R. and Esmail, A. University of Manchester School of Primary Care, The Robert Darbishire Practice, Rusholme Health Centre, Manchester, UK.
Br. J. Gen. Pract., **52**(477): 296-299, 1 April 2002.

This paper aimed to assess whether a practice-level mortality analyses could provide data for a health needs assessment in the local population. Specifically, the authors examined the association between premature deaths and alcohol misuse, drug misuse and severe mental illness in an inner city Manchester general practice. The authors examined the case records of all deaths, in those aged 1–75 years, occurring between 1994 and 1998. The proportions of life years lost associated with alcohol, drug misuse or severe mental illness was calculated. The results were then compared with the mortality data for a general practice in Norwich. The authors found:

- The age standardised mortality rates were 5.7/1000 for the study practice and 3.2/1000 for the reference practice.
- In the study practice 42 of all years of life lost (YLL) were associated with alcohol or drug dependency, compared with 11 in the reference practice.
- There were no differences in the proportion of YLL associated with severe mental illness in the two practices.

They conclude that practice-level mortality analysis is able to provide a useful picture of local health care needs, which can help with service planning and monitoring health inequalities.

QUALITY OF CARE

EDUCATION AND DEBATE SECTION – Measuring goodness in individuals and healthcare systems. Pringle, M., Wilson, T. and Grol, R. Division of General Practice, University of Nottingham, Nottingham, UK.
BMJ, **325**(7366): 704-707, 28 September 2002.

Healthcare professionals must constantly compare their performance with that of their peers, in order to maintain and improve standards.

Difficulties arise when comparing people or organizations that work in different contexts. Incorrect conclusions can be drawn and inappropriate recommendations made, demotivating staff, and reducing patients trust. It is thus important to present data along with the context in which it was gathered.

The authors suggest certain attributes be used to measure the quality of data used in such comparisons, to maximise the validity of any conclusions. Data analysis should allow for the expected normal variation between different working environments, while identifying any unacceptable deviation from standards.

Measuring healthcare professionals performance is an important and valuable process, so long as the data is adjusted to account for the context in which it was gathered. This allows service users to make informed choices about their care, and facilitates identification and promotion of good clinical practice.

EDITORIAL – Patients views of the good doctor. Coulter, A. Chief Executive Picker Institute Europe, Oxford, UK.
BMJ, **325**(7366): 668-669, 28 September 2002.

Most doctors are viewed highly by patients, particularly by those who have recently experienced medical care. The medical profession has, however, attracted criticism due to the paternalistic model of medicine practised by some doctors.

Doctors and patients often have differing priorities. Patients place great value on both clinical ability and interpersonal skills, but prefer detailed information regarding their condition and consultations of adequate length at relatively short notice, contrasting with doctors tendency to focus on continuity of care and home visits, as the main priorities.

Patients trust strongly depends on their opinion of the doctors interpersonal skills. They want their doctor to give clear, honest information about their condition, and to listen to, and act upon, their wishes and concerns. The author suggests some doctors may require training in the shared decision making process, and cites studies illustrating such training to benefit patient satisfaction.

Other healthcare professionals can share the extra work generated by including patients in the decision making process, a step that is imperative to maintaining their trust for doctors in the long term.

EDITORIAL – Whats a good doctor, and how can you make one? Hurwitz, B. and Vass, A. School of Humanities, Kings College London, London, UK.
***BMJ,* 325**(7366): 667-668, 28 September 2002.

This editorial explores different definitions of what makes a good doctor. This is a contentious issue due to increased litigation and calls for greater transparency and accountability of the medical profession.

There are two approaches to defining a good doctor. One focuses on the doctors scientific knowledge and clinical ability, while the other has more to do with desirable personal qualities. Respondents to a BMJ debate on this topic tended to focus on the latter, however the authors point to increasing practitioner assessment and audit as evidence that personal qualities are no longer seen as a guarantee of being a good doctor.

There is a difference between a poor and a bad doctor. The former refers more to a lack of clinical ability, while the latter is concerned with undesirable motives.

The authors conclude that good, bad and poor qualities are diverse, and may be present in the same individual. Medical education should aim to maximise doctors good qualities, by bringing together the best aspects of the medical scientist and medical humanist.

EDITORIAL – Putting improvement at the heart of health care. Wilcock, P. Visiting Fellow In Healthcare Improvement and Lewis, A. Community Clinical Teacher, Peninsula Medical School, Plymouth, UK.
***BMJ,* 325**(7366): 670-671, 28 September 2002.

The authors of this editorial argue that, given our consumerist culture and increasing complaints against the medical profession, the need to monitor and improve the quality of healthcare has a central role in medical practice. However, resistance to quality assurance measures from physicians is commonplace, hampering attempts to improve healthcare. This editorial suggests that making the teaching of quality assurance/improvement a part of undergraduate medical education would help create a medical profession receptive to use of quality assurance measures. It is proposed that Kolbs plan-do-study learning framework could be applied to teach quality assurance/improvement to undergraduates. The authors claim that teaching quality assessment to undergraduates is essential to maintain the relevence of medical education and prepare students adequately for medical practice.

EDITORIAL – How can good performance among doctors be maintained? West, M. Professor of Organizational Psychology Aston Business School, University of Aston, Birmingham, UK. *BMJ,* **325**(7366): 669-670, 28 September 2002.

The Department of Health has recently proposed that physicians should practice continuing professional development, have annual appraisals and revalidation. This editorial discusses the evidence that these measures will improve health care. Appraisal is defined as setting physicians performance targets and providing feedback on their ability to meet these targets. This article reports that such methods of appraisal are associated with improvements in performance and a reduction in error rates in non-medical employment settings, and a reduction in patient mortality in a medical setting. The author points out that the effectiveness of such appraisals in healthcare will depend upon the goals that are set i.e. they must be attainable and relevant otherwise the appraisal process will have less impact. Moreover, the skill of the individual performing the appraisal is also critical, as badly conducted appraisals can have a negative impact on physicians performance. The author concludes by highlighting the lack of direct evidence for the effectiveness of revalidation.

EDUCATION AND DEBATE SECTION – The rise of regulation in the NHS. Walshe, K. Centre for Healthcare Management, University of Manchester, UK. *BMJ,* **324**(7343): 967-970, 20 April 2002.

Regulation is defined as "sustained and focused control exercised by a public agency over activities which are valued by a community". The author highlights a number of points.

- The last 20 years have seen a considerable increase in the use of regulators in the private and public sectors in an attempt to help manage performance and achieve social goals.
- In the last 4 years the government created five new national agencies to regulate the NHS.
- Accountable to the Department of Health the new agencies currently have little independence and, taken together, represent a significant strengthening of central government control of the NHS.
- In contrast to existing regulatory agencies the new NHS regulators are focused on the clinical quality of healthcare. They are well resourced and have the potential to deliver real improvements for patients.

Clinical governance in Scotland: an educational model. Lough, M., Kelly, D. and Taylor, M. *et al.* Department of Postgraduate General Practice, Glasgow, UK. *Br. J. Gen. Pract.,* **52**(477): 322-328, 1 April 2002.

This discussion paper evaluates the educational model for clinical governance in general practice. Though the ideas underlying clinical governance throughout the United Kingdom do not differ greatly, the modes of delivery differ. This model aims to raise awareness on practical ways of assessing quality assurance. It advocates the use of the practice governance plan to highlight areas of practice need which require attention. The authors feel that by using education as a lever for improvement, good practice will be embraced by all practice staff and continuous learning will ensue. The Scottish model utilises an educational construct and it is based on four domains:

- clinical effectiveness;
- risk management;
- delivery of patient services;
- continuous professional development.

and three levels of attainment. These levels are versatile and can be used for all stages of development at practice level through a staged approach.

For each domain Level 1 provides a benchmarking exercise, while levels 2 and 3 provide a framework for measuring progress towards explicitly set standards. The model also incorporates the means to acknowledge achievement at an individual level.

Successful clinical governance is defined as the practice achieving clearly stated standards developed by general agreement. The standards in the model were taken from the Scottish Intercollegiate Guidelines Network.

Primary Care: After Bristol: putting patients at the centre. Coulter, A. Chief Executive Picker Institute Europe, Oxford, UK.
BMJ, **324**(7338): 648-651, 16 March 2002.

Key recommendations from the public inquiry into the serious performance failures of children's cardiac surgeons in Bristol in the 1980s and 1990s included:

- Active involvement of patients and parents in decision-making.
- Improving communication.
- Keeping patients and parents informed.
- Encouraging feedback and listening to patients' views.

Responding to patients' views has been a long-term goal of UK health policy. However, despite good intentions, NHS staff find that such patient involvement often takes second place to coping with the continued financial, staffing and management pressures of daily work.

This paper looks at both the need for, and benefits of, increasing responsiveness to patients.

- The 2000 NHS Plan aims to incorporate patient feedback into its star-rating system for performance indicators.
- Patients have become less satisfied with inpatient care over the last decade despite increased public spending and increasingly available effective treatments.
- Well-informed patients are more likely to comply with treatment and have better outcomes. They are also likely to make more rational,

more conservative and less risky choices than their doctors. Failure to seek or act on their views could lead to inappropriate health care.

- Informing patients may encourage self-reliance.
- For maximum benefit clinical management decisions need to be shared between doctors and patients, who should be considered 'experts' based on their own experience.
- The incidence of formal complaints, legal action, medical errors and adverse events could be reduced with improved communication and increased acknowledgement of the patients' perspective.

Implementation of these achievable recommendations requires:

- Tools to empower patients.
- Training in communication skills for doctors.
- Good quality surveys to assess patients' and carers perspectives with a focus on specific events and processes.
- Clear leadership from the clinical professions.
- Willingness to change established ways of working.

EDUCATION AND DEBATE SECTION – Quality improvement report. Information given to patients before appointments and its effect on non-attendance rate. Hardy, K.J., O'Brien, S.V. and Furlong, N.J. Diabetes Centre, Whiston Hospital, Prescot, Merseyside, UK. **BMJ, 323**(7324): 1298-1300, 1 December 2001.

Non-attendance occurs in all healthcare sectors and specialities. It is a common source of inefficiency, wasting time and resources. Non-attendance is recorded throughout all age groups, social, cultural and ethnic backgrounds and inevitably results in increased waiting times. The author highlights a number of points.

- Non-attendance rates for outpatients at a diabetes clinic were reduced from 15% to 7% when patients were told by post what to expect, who they would see, what to bring and where to park.
- When, in addition to the written information, patients were telephoned 1 week before their appointment, the rate of non-attendance fell to around 1%.
- The costs associated with the issuing of postal information and telephone calls prior to appointments, was more than offset by the more effective use of existing appointments, together with reductions in the number of letters concerning non-attendance, cancellations and rescheduled appointments.

EDITORIAL – Equity versus efficiency: a dilemma for the NHS. Sassi, F., Le Grand, J. and Archard, L. Department of Social Policy and LSE Health and Social Care, London School of Economics and Political Science, London, UK. **BMJ, 323**(7216): 762-763, 6 October 2001.

Health policy analysts have voiced concerns about the lack of just distribution and funding of health care in the NHS. Policies to overcome health inequalities are still elusive. Policies that promote health equality but compromise efficiency are still not addressed. The authors reflected the equity-equality conflict on three NHS scenarios that showed that:

- There are inconsistencies between NHS policies and the absence of guiding principles that promote equity.
- In the cervical screening programme which uses financial incentives for GPs, the cost-effectiveness of this programme can be improved by targeting of resources for high risk, low socio-economic groups of women with high mortality rates.
- In a renal transplant programme where donor organs are in short supply, prioritising younger recipients of kidneys from young donors is not necessarily an effective, efficient or even equitable measure.
- In an attempt to promote societal equity, offering universal screening for sickle cell disease to the UK population may not be cost-efficient.

There are inconsistencies observed in many previous NHS policies due to the lack of information offered to decision makers to formulate an acceptable equity-equality compromise. Researchers and policymakers are equally responsible for these inconsistencies.

Wrong SIGN, NICE mess: is national guidance distorting allocation of resources?
Cookson, R., McDaid, D. and Maynard, A. School of Health Policy and Practice, University of East Anglia, Norwich, UK.
BMJ, 323(7315): 743-745, 29 September 2001.

The Health Technology Board for Scotland, the Scottish Intercollegiate Guidelines Network (SIGN), and the soon to be set-up Scottish Medicines Consortium are the three Scottish committees that produce national guidance on NHS practice. SIGN has been reluctant to consider resource issues, and economic considerations have also been limited. This approach does nothing at all to increase efficiency in the allocation of resources; being efficient does not equate to being cheap.

In England and Wales, the National Institute for Clinical Excellence (NICE) produces national guidance on individual technologies ("apprai-appraisals"), the management of specific conditions ("clinical guide-lines"), and clinical audit. The decisions of NICE are not mandatory, but advisory. NICE has concluded that all of the new pharmaceuticals it has appraised are cost effective and has refused to rank them in any form of hierarchy. It has effectively become an advocacy mechanism by which lobbies of specialists and their supporters in the pharmaceutical industry extract more public money from the NHS.

To remedy these problems, NICE needs to become a national healthcare-rationing agency, and SIGN and the other Scottish agencies should complement this activity; elementary economic principles have already been carefully and clearly set out in many introductory texts on economic evaluation in health care. As an aid to decision making, NICE should publish information on cost effectiveness in a format that makes it readily comparable across appraised technologies, including league tables of incremental cost effectiveness whenever possible.

INFORMATION IN PRACTICE: Verifying quality and safety in health informatics services. Rigby, M., Forsström, J. and Roberts, R. J. Wyatt TEAC-Health Partners, Centre for Health Planning and Management, Keele University, Keele, UK.
BMJ, 323(7312): 552-556, 8 September 2001.

Information and its handling and transmission form an essential part of health care. The European accreditation and certification of telematics services in health group (TEAC-Health) has recently concluded a study into health informatics services; its strategic proposals have now been welcomed by the European Commission.

- Health informatics services were classified into three categories: software and related services, telemedicine, and internet sites.
- In the health sector, precedents have been set in the regulation of drugs and medical devices, but neither of these is directly applicable to health informatics services.
- TEAC-Health have proposed the development of a new European system and standard, entitled the EuroSeal, would be a seal supplied to a website by an accredited agency. A scheme like CE marking of electrical goods is recommended for software, national regulatory bodies should be identified for telemedicine, and a European certification of integrity scheme developed for websites.
- This project has demonstrated that public safety and professional integrity are threatened by the lack of regulation of health informatics services; these risks will increase rapidly as services expand and as telecommunications and globalisation radically change attitudes to and delivery of health care.

EDITORIAL – Commission for Health Improvement invents itself. Day, P. and Klein, R.
BMJ, 322(7301): 1503-1504, 23 June 2001.

The editorial evaluates the Commission for Health Improvement's (CHI) first year. This year has been about CHI developing its strategy for implementing its goal of assuring, monitoring and helping to improve quality of care.

- There is conflict between the expectations of government ministers and CHIs own expectations of itself. Ministers would like CHI to be 'quality police'. CHI like to promote continuous improvement rather than heavy handed policing.
- Assessing quality is a difficult area. The article looks at the importance or otherwise of statistical indicators such as waiting times and patient's perceptions of their experiences.
- CHI will be responsible for the traffic light system for trusts. A green light is for trusts who are doing well with their indicators. A red light is for those ranked at the bottom for indicators.
- Review teams (doctor, nurse, lay person, manager and one other clinical professional) assess clinical governance and audit, as well as

staffing levels and delivery of care. Consistency between different review teams is an additional challenge.

- Whether or not CHI will actually improve patient care remains to be seen.

EDUCATION AND DEBATE SECTION – THE WHITE PAPER
From command economy to demand management.
BMJ, **316**(7126): 212-216, 17 January 1998.

Encouraging responsibility: different paths to accountability.
BMJ, **316**(7127): 296-301, 24 January 1998.

From specialist services to special groups.
BMJ, **316**(7128): 378-381, 31 January 1998.

The above three set of commentaries deal with the white paper on the NHS, called '*The New NHS*'. Various professionals, e.g. public health doctors, clinicians, policy analysts were asked to comment on various aspects of the white paper. Some of the points highlighted in the commentaries are summarized below.

An NHS available to all

The government is committed to an NHS which is available to all on the basis of need and not ability to pay and funded through general taxation. The idea of rationing or charging for treatment is rejected.

Long-term planning

Rather than the short-termism of the recent past, the white paper suggests a 10 year programme of improvements.

Primary care groups as building blocks

GPs and their patients are set to be the building blocks of the new NHS. By April 1999, 500 new primary care groups, each representing 100 000 people will replace commissioning groups and fundholding practices. These groups will be made up of all local GPs and community nurses. The framework of these groups seems to resemble an extension of total purchasing very much like American HMOs. These new primary care groups will need public health skills. There has been some concern that the new groups will be neither 'small enough to walk' nor 'big enough to hurt'.

Information services for both patients and professionals: NHS Direct and NHSnet

The provision of information to both patients and professionals is set to improve. This involves the setting up of NHS Direct and NHSnet. NHS Direct will be a 24 hour nurse-led telephone helpline. This may be one of the most important developments of the new NHS, but some fear that increasing access to the NHS will increase demand. In order to counter this, the new NHS needs to emphasize self-care. The HMOs in America have a well developed telephone advice service which is integrated with patient-owned self-care manuals. There are some worries that NHS Direct will not be available to all those who really need it. It is estimated that around 600 000 people will have difficulty using a telephone advice service because they neither speak English nor have access to an interpreter. NHSnet will be an information superhighway that links GP surgeries to any specialist centre in the country.

Health and not just health care

The government aims to provide 'an NHS that does not just treat people when they are ill but works with others to improve health and reduce health inequalities'. The government will therefore need to look closely at services for black and ethnic minority groups.

Quality of care and accountability

The government will also focus on quality of care and accountability issues. Two new national bodies are to be set up, a National Institute of Clinical Effectiveness and a Commission for Health Improvement. The role of the National Institute of Clinical Effectiveness will be to develop and implement national evidence-based guidelines. The Commission for Health Improvement will focus on quality and clinical accountability or 'clinical governance'.

The 50th anniversary of the NHS was commemorated by devoting an entire issue to '50 years of the NHS'.

THE DEVELOPING NHS

Information in practice: Systematic review of cost effectiveness of studies of telemedicine interventions. Whitten, P.S., Mair, F.S. and Haycox, A. *et al.* Department of Telecommunications, Michigan State University, USA.
***BMJ,* 324**(7351): 1434-1437, 15 June 2002.

This study examines whether or not conclusions regarding the cost-effectiveness of telemedicine can be drawn from existing literature. Twenty-four (out of approx. 600) studies met the inclusion criteria.
  • None of the studies adequately approached the issue of the degree to which telemedicine would need to be used in order that it became more economical than traditional healthcare.
  • Most ignored the impact on patients when examining the financial benefits of telemedicine.
  • Many papers failed to clearly define the boundaries and context of their analyses, and used analytical techniques inappropriate to the task.
  • Telemedicine services vary depending on local circumstances, so it is difficult to apply the results of an individual cost effectiveness analysis to a wider area.
  • Studies generally covered too short a period to give a good view of long-term costs and benefits of an established telemedicine service.

The authors state that it is impossible to assess the cost effectiveness of telemedicine using current literature, owing to a lack of uniformity in data analysis. Current claims that telemedicine is highly effective are not based on strong evidence, as there is little to say decisively whether or not telemedicine is a valuable means of healthcare delivery. There is a need for better designed and better executed trials examining the efficacy of telemedicine.

EDUCATION AND DEBATE SECTION – The physician assistant: would the US model meet the needs of the NHS? Hutchinson, L., Marks, T. and Pittilo, M. University Hospital Lewisham, London, UK.
BMJ, 323(7323): 863-864, 24 November 2001.

The NHS is facing a potential shortage of staff to deliver primary care. One possible solution is the introduction of a new group of staff, "physician assistants", similar to those already working in the United States. This article describes the US physician assistant, and discusses the potential creation of such healthcare professionals in the NHS.

- In the United States, physician assistants perform equivalent roles to junior doctors, but for their entire careers. They do not perform "nursing" tasks.
- Physician assistant training is typically 24 months duration, and is similar to a shortened traditional medical course.
- Wider use of nurse practitioners is one possibility to combat staffing problems in the NHS. However, nursing staff is already depleted, with major recruitment and retention problems.
- Introduction of the physician assistant as a new career pathway might aid recruitment of healthcare staff to the NHS, including individuals who might not otherwise have pursued healthcare careers.
- However, there is concern that the introduction of a new group of professionals could exacerbate rivalries between different staff within the healthcare system.
- Overall, an introduction of US-style physician assistants to the NHS would reduce medical staffing problems, but also create new problems in health care.

FUNDING

EDUCATION AND DEBATE SECTION – Private finance and value for money in NHS hospitals: a policy in search of a rationale? Pollock, A.M., Shaoul, J. and Vickers, N. Health and Policy and Health Services Research Unit, School of Public Policy, UCL, London, UK.
BMJ, 324(7347): 1205-1209, 18 May 2002.

In this article the authors examine the extra cost to NHS trusts of Private Finance Initiatives (PFI) as compared to public funding. They also question the "value for money" argument cited in favour of PFI on the grounds of assumption of risk by the private sector. (PFI is a loan raised by the private sector used to fund the building and running of hospitals.) Some issues discussed by the authors were as follows:

By looking at the structural costs for some PFI schemes in England the authors have identified the extra costs incurred when using PFI. They found it does not necessarily offer "value for money" as:

- PFI projects cost approximately twice as much as similar public funded projects.
- Increased annual capital costs occur with PFI.
- Higher cost partially due to financing costs which account for just over a third.
- An affordability shortfall in the NHS as it has to generate additional money required.

EDITORIAL – Gold For The NHS. Robinson, R. LSE Health and Social Care, London School of Economics and Political Science, London, UK.
BMJ, **324**(7344): 987-988, 27 April 2002.

The current budget statement is highly focussed on the issue of NHS funding. The special 5 year settlement for the NHS will raise the NHS budget from sixty five billion pounds in 2003 to one hundred and five billion pounds in 2008. The planned increase in expenditure will also mean that the percentage of gross domestic product spent on the NHS will rise from 7.7 to 9.4, bringing us closer into line with other European nations. However, there are some concerns with these expenditure plans:

- It is uncertain whether economic growth will be sufficient to support NHS spending.
- It is unclear how the Government will reconcile increased NHS spending with decreased spending in other sensitive areas such as education.
- Extra money may not be able to solve all the problems facing the NHS, e.g. difficulty in recruiting nurses.
- The new inspectorates for Health and Social services may merely result in added bureaucracy and wastage of money.

EDUCATION AND DEBATE SECTION – Should NHS patients be allowed to contribute extra money to their care. Richards, C., Dingwall, R. and Watson, A. Nottingham Health Authority, Nottingham, UK.
BMJ, **323**(7312): 563-565, 8 September 2001.

The NHS was founded on the principle that "the best that science can do is available for the treatment of every citizen at home and in institutions, irrespective of his personal means ". However it is felt that widespread access as provided by the NHS may compromise quality and this is thought to explain poor cancer survival rates in the UK.

A recent case was put forward to the Nottingham ethics of clinical practice committee where a cancer patient wished to pay for additional treatment which was not available on the NHS due to its effect being reported as 'marginal'.

The committee's discussions included:

- Current literature does not address this issue. The literature also does not apply to supplementation of state provided health care.
- Committee decided to approach the case from first principles, autonomy vs. justice.

Arguments for allowing supplementation:

- Any restriction on an individual infringes on their autonomy and their right to use their financial facilities to aid their health.
- Supplementation is present in today's NHS: private seldinafil (Viagra) prescription for erectile dysfunction, infusion pumps, purchase of some expensive drugs (beta-interferon for multiple sclerosis), private screening leading to NHS care, and NHS antenatal care following self-funded infertility treatment.

Arguments against supplementation:

- NHS provides care by citizenship, and clinical need is the only way to rank individual claims for care.
- Nursing staff have expressed concern at caring for individuals with access to different levels of treatment.
- NHS duty towards taxpayers collides with rights of individuals.
- Seldinafil prescription is not a NHS decision, but a government decision on the use of funds.

Conclusions: The committee was unable to reach a consensus. Further discussion on this complex issue will be required.

COMPLEXITY SCIENCE

EDUCATION AND DEBATE SECTION – The challenge of complexity in health care. Plsek, P.E. and Greenhalgh, T.
BMJ, **323**(7313): 625-628, 15 September 2001.

and

EDUCATION AND DEBATE SECTION – Complexity science and clinical care. Wilson, T. and Holt, T.
BMJ, **323**(7314): 685-688, 22 September 2001.

This is a series of articles looking at the new science of complex adaptive systems. Traditional models of looking at any organisational structure have tended to take a mechanistic or reductionist viewpoint. For example, the body is viewed as a machine, protocols for care lead us in a step by step fashion to the desired endpoint. Complexity science admits that organisations, be it the body or the stock market, do not work like machines in a predictable, linear fashion. A complex adaptive system is made up of individual parts which may not always act in a predictable way. These individual parts also interact together so that changing one part effects the others. For example, human behaviour is governed by internal 'rules' or 'ideas, concerns and expectations'. Changing behaviour is more likely to be successful if the action is in agreement with these 'rules'.

The zone of complexity is described as the situation whereby there is insufficient knowledge or certainty to take an obvious next step. When there is a high level of certainty e.g. concerning a surgical procedure a mechanistic approach may be more appropriate. But, for example with the control of diabetes, a mechanistic, reductionist approach can be detrimental. Predicting the interaction between blood glucose levels and insulin is very difficult and often strict control results in hypoglycaemic episodes. Complexity science would view these interactions as complex, unpredictable and non-linear, which means that additional strategies need to be utilized. This would involve the patient having a good knowledge of their blood glucose profiles, but also of their own body rhythms and having confidence to experiment to reach "good enough control" of their blood glucose.

Strategies for dealing with situations of uncertainty include using intuition. Doctors have been shown to be good at making the 'right' decisions in such situations. Other techniques involve chunking which involves sorting out one or two of the issues rather than trying to tackle them all. Using metaphors is another strategy. A metaphor may encapsulate the situation and promote shared understanding. Provocative questions may also promote insight into a situation.

An individuals view of health is shaped by social relationships and information taken from alternative sources. These are described as **'shadow systems'**. We need to work alongside these 'shadow systems' rather than challenge them, if we want to effect positive change.

Change can also be facilitated by substituting 'attractors'. For example for someone who smokes what keeps them smoking e.g. work, partner, intake level. The new attractor has to be as important as the old one. For example for a smoker who is pregnant for the first time, the alternative to smoking and the benefits to her offspring may be a powerful 'attractor'.

EDUCATION AND DEBATE SECTION – Complexity science: Complexity, leadership, and management in healthcare organisations. Plsek, P.E., Wilson, T. and Paul, E. Plsek and Associates, Roswell, GA, USA.
***BMJ,* 323**(7315): 746-749, 29 September 2001.

This study is a comparison between the NHS and one of the integrated health care systems in the USA (Californias Kaiser Permanente).

- After making various adjustments, they found that costs per capita expenditure were similar in the two systems.
- However, the Kaiser system performed much better than the NHS especially in terms of access to specialists and hospital waiting times. Some reasons for this are thought to include the following:
  1. Kaiser has a much higher level of integration between services than the NHS;
  2. care is more cost effective in the Kaiser system e.g. patients spend a third less time in hospital;

3. competition from other health maintenance organisations drives efficiency and good performance;
4. information technology is put to much better use in the Kaiser system.

The NHS is moving towards better performance levels with increased integration and the use of information technology. More efficient use of hospitals would improve the situation still further.

EDUCATION AND DEBATE SECTION – Coping with complexity: educating for capability. Fraser, S.W. and Greenhalgh, T., Dinton, Aylesbury, UK. **BMJ, 323**(7316): 799-803, 6 October 2001.

For the NHS to meet with public expectations, medical education must address "capability" as well as "competency"; that is the ability to adapt to changing circumstances, as well as basic skills and knowledge.

Traditional education focuses on knowledge acquisition rather than understanding the interconnections between disciplines; however there is now so much information available for a given subject that it is more important to understand how facts relate to one another, rather than attempting to learn every fact.

Clinical guidelines and care pathways are useful once a problem is defined, but practitioners require the ability to recognise problems in the context in which they present. Capability allows effective application of skills and knowledge in unfamiliar environments, such as in these situations.

It is important that people recognise the efficacy of non-linear approaches to learning rather than traditional fact acquisition methods. More research is needed into the use of clinical stories and such like in medical education, rather than teaching independent facts.

Learning is most effective when the learner is aware of the topic's contextual relevance. To maximise capability, educators must provide feedback about the learner's performance, allowing them to adapt their behaviour as appropriate.

The new NHS University will have to adopt such teaching methods, to reflect the dynamic nature of modern healthcare. Learning should focus on the actual learning processes. By using process techniques, learning is driven by the individual needs of the learner, with tutors acting as facilitators rather than lecturing or training.

Small group learning is effective, as social interaction raises productivity by motivating and raising the confidence of group members. This may be ineffective, however, if group members are incompatible or the facilitator fails to set clear guidelines regarding the session objectives. In non-linear learning, learning objectives relate to capability in addition to competence of the learners. The tutor's expertise in the learning process is fundamental to the success of such techniques.

An observational study comparing quality of care in walk-in centres with general practice and NHS Direct using standardised patients. Grant, C., Nicholas, R. and Moore, L. *et al.* Division of Primary Health Care, University of Bristol, Bristol, UK. *BMJ,* **324**(7353): 1556 1561, 29 June 2002.

Walk in centres offer assessment, advise and treatment for minor illness and injury. Most consultations are with nurses who use care protocols and clinical software. The aim of this observational study was to determine whether walk-in centres provide adequate and safe clinical care, by comparing them to general practice and NHS Direct. The study assessed clinical consultation of standardised patients (professional role players) in 20 walk-in centres, 20 general practices and 11 NHS Direct sites (297 consultations). The role players provided five clinical scenarios; post-coital contraception, chest pain, sinusitis, headache and asthma. Assessment was via checklists for the management of each scenario from which mean scores were derived.

- Walk-in centres had significantly higher mean scores, when all the scenarios were combined, than general practice and NHS Direct.
- Walk-in centres scored particularly highly for the management of post-coital contraception and asthma.

The author concludes that walk-in centres provide 'adequate' and 'safe' clinical care compared to general practice or NHS Direct. But their cost-effectiveness and impact on workload of other care providers needs further investigation.

PRIMARY CARE – What is the role of walk-in centres in the NHS? Salisbury, C., Chalder, M. and Scott, T.M. *et al.* Division of Primary Health Care, University of Bristol, Bristol, UK. *BMJ,* **324**(7334): 399-402, 16 February 2002.

This report studies the structure and activities of walk-in centres. It is a description based on monthly monitoring returns from the centres, including numbers of visits, waiting times and referrals and anonymised patient data. Twelve of the 36 centres opened by January 2001 were investigated. Information was also collected by questionnaires from and semi-structured interviews with walk-in centre managers. Some of the findings found were that:

- There has been a gradual but steady increase in the number of visitors to these walk-in centres, with an average of 81 per day in August 2001.
- A high proportion of young adults used the centres, as compared with relatively few elderly visitors.
- The median waiting time was 10 minutes, and the average length of consultation was 14 minutes.

- In May 2001, approximately 78% of consultations were managed entirely at the walk-in centres, with no referral to other healthcare providers.

Walk-in centres are especially attractive to young men. The pattern of use of walk-in centres suggests that they are providing an accessible service to those finding it less convenient to use existing healthcare options. However, it has not been determined to date whether these services are more efficient or cost-effective than traditional systems of healthcare. Further studies will need to assess the efficiency of walk-in centres and the competency of nurses who run nurse-led clinics.

Getting more for their dollar: a comparison of the NHS with Californias Kaiser Permanente. Feachem, R.G.A., Sekhri, N.K. and White, K.L. Institute for Global Health, University of California, San Francisco and Berkeley, USA.
BMJ, 324(7330): 135-143, 19 January 2002.

Implementation of change in the health service has traditionally been viewed by managers to require rigid protocols and targets. This article suggests that an alternative strategy, the complex adaptive system (CAS), could improve both productivity and relationships within the health sector. The Army have undertaken such a strategy in recent years, moving from a system of generals to facilitators.

- The CAS entails abolishing the introduction of separate targets and budgets for different areas of the NHS. It advocates pooled budgets and minimum specifications to enable a system of creativity and best practice to evolve.
- The healthcare system is currently a set of discrete parts which would run more smoothly if they were to work together; setting different targets for different subgroups of the healthcare system does not necessarily benefit the patient.
- A system of minimum specifications should be implemented, given population variation between practices, it is no longer appropriate to enforce blanket protocols. Healthcare delivery can still be effective in the absence of detailed targets.
- Managers often feel that there is resistance to the changes they are trying to implement; the CAS aims to reduce resistance to change because it takes into account the natural attractor patterns that clinicians have.

Bad press for doctors: 21 year survey of three national newspapers. Ali, N.Y., Lo, Y.S. and Auvache, L. St Bartholomew's and the Royal London School of Dentistry, Queen Mary College, London, UK.
BMJ, 323: 782-783, 6 October 2001.

Many doctors believe that the media portrays a negative image of their profession. The authors in this study aimed to discover if newspapers have published more negative stories in past 21 years. They examined the Daily Telegraph, Guardian and Daily Mail. They found that:

- Medical reports in general increased over time, with no change in the ratio of positive to negative stories in the time scale examined.
- Peaks in negative reports were found in 1986-1989 and 1996-2000, coinciding with high profile cases such as HIV-positive doctors and the Shipman enquiry.
- Overall, they found that the newspapers examined contained twice as many negative stories as positive ones. However the peaks of negative reporting suggest that UK newspapers respond to incidents rather than deliberately campaigning against doctors.

PRIMARY CARE SECTION – Comparative efficiency of national health systems: cross national econometric analyses. Evans, D.B., Tandon, A., Murray, C.J.L. and Lauer, J.A. Global Programme on Evidence for Health Policy, WHO.
***BMJ,* 323**(7308): 307-310, 11 August 2001.

This paper aims to estimate the relation between levels of population health and the inputs used to produce health. It uses one of WHO World Report 2000 intrinsic goals Improving health. The authors seek to analyze the methods used for measuring and monitoring performance of health systems. They look at performance of 191 countries. Performance is defined as "the current level of population health, in excess of the estimated minimum compared with, the maximum achievable level of health given the inputs". They found that:

- performance varies widely, some countries are close to their potential while others are very far from reaching the maximum levels of health;
- performance is positively related to health expenditure per capita, particularly lower expenditure. An apparent minimum level exists at which a health system would cease to function;
- performance in low performing countries is hindered by civil unrest or high prevalence of HIV/AIDS;
- healthy life expectancy is reduced by between 511 years across the 191 countries in study;
- current resources could be better deployed to bring about health improvement.

The ability to measure inputs and outputs of a health system is critical and this study provides evidence that the performance of a health system can be measured and compared over space (countries) and time.

FURTHER READING

EDUCATION AND DEBATE SECTION - Equity in the new NHS: hard lessons from implementing a local health care policy on donepezil.
Doyle, Y., Merton, Sutton and Wandsworth Health Authority London.
***BMJ,* 323**(7306) 222-224, 28 July 2001.

EDUCATION AND DEBATE SECTION - Implementing clinical governance: turning vision into reality. Halligan, A. and Donaldson, L., NHS Clinical Governance Support Team Millstone Lane, Leicester.
BMJ, **322**(7299)1413-1417, 9 June 2001.

OBESITY

- A school based intervention to tackle obesity was largely ineffective
- Adult obesity is related to birth weight and growth in early childhood
- The Newcastle thousand families study showed that those who were thin children and fat adults had the highest risk of disease in adulthood.
- The STORM study showed that sibutramine is useful for maintaining weight loss after an initial period of weight reduction.
- It has been suggested that the waist circumference measurement should be regarded as a "vital sign" and should be recorded in the medical records
- In the Swedish multimorbidity study, Orlistat was associated with significantly greater reductions in weight, serum cholesterol and LDL cholesterol, fasting glucose and HBA1c levels compared with placebo.
- Population strategies are needed to control obesity; the most effective are likely to be those incorporating a multidisciplinary approach with a range of actions aimed at the individual, community and environment.

EDITORIAL – Population strategies to prevent obesity. Crawford, D. Faculty of Health and Behavioural Sciences, School of Health Sciences, Deakin University, Victoria, Australia. *BMJ,* **325**(7367): 728-729, 5 October 2002.

Although obesity has long been recognised as increasing individual risk of ill health, the need for population interventions has only recently been recognised.

The obesity epidemic in most developed countries has been attributed to greater availability and marketing of foods, coupled with an increase in sedentary pastimes.

Various environmental strategies have been proposed to counter obesity, including improving access to stairs, making food labels clearer, and encouraging walking and healthy eating. None of these interventions have yet been subjected to analysis in proper scientific trials.

Few studies have looked directly at the impact of preventing weight gain; those that do involve educational and behaviour interventions. None involving adults have been shown to be effective in the long term. Studies with children have shown strategies reducing sedentary behaviour, and increasing physical activity, are likely to reduce childhood obesity.

The author concludes obesity is a risk to the populations health, requiring urgent action, and calls for more research into its determinants, and the best places to intervene.

EDITORIAL – Adult obesity and growth in childhood. Law, Catherine senior lecturer MRC Environmental Epidemiology Unit, Southampton, UK.
BMJ, **323**(7325): 1320-1321, 8 December 2001.

Heavy mothers tend to have heavy babies who tend to grow into heavy adults. However, Parsons *et al.*, reporting in the same issue of the *BMJ*, noted an association between thin mothers, low birth weight and rapid childhood growth. The study involved around 10 600 births in England, Scotland and Wales, followed to age 33 (and controls for confounders). Law suggests that thin mothers are usually those from poor socio-economic backgrounds. In developed countries, the small babies are usually those who suffered intrauterine growth retardation or who were born prematurely. A change in socio-economic circumstance results in rapid postnatal growth, especially in the Western environment with its low levels of physical activity and high levels of fat and sugar. It is suggested that there are critical periods *in utero* and in early childhood which determine future morbidity.

Implications of childhood obesity for adult health: findings from thousand families cohort study. Wright, C.M., Parker, L., Lamont, D. and Craft, A. Donald Court House, University of Newcastle upon Tyne, Gateshead, UK.
BMJ, **323**(7324): 1280-1284, 1 December 2001.

This is an analysis of data from the Newcastle thousand families study; a prospective study of 1142 children born in 1947. The aim of the study is to examine the relationship between childhood and adult obesity.
- Body mass index (BMI) as a child was correlated with BMI as an adult but not percentage body fat.
- Children who were obese at age 13 were twice as likely to become obese adults.
- Most obese adults had not been obese children
- The leanest children had significantly higher adult percentage body fat.
- Those who were thin children and fat adults had the highest risk of disease in adulthood.The authors suggest that the relative change in size may be an important predictor of future health. Others have suggested that there is a critical period of influence in the perinatal period. This present study suggests that this period should be extended to later childhood.

Randomised controlled trial of primary school based intervention to reduce risk factors for obesity. Sahota, P., Rudolf, M. C. J. and Dixey, R. *et al.* School of Health Sciences, Metropolitan University, Leeds, UK.
BMJ, **323**(7320): 1029-1032, 3 November 2001.

Reports have shown that over 17% of 11 year old children are obese and 30% are overweight. The aim of this RCT was to assess whether school

based intervention can reduce the risk factors for obesity? It involved just over 630, 7-11 year olds from 10 primary schools in Leeds. The intervention schools received an active programme promoting lifestyle education in schools, involving teacher training, school meal changes and action plans designed to promote healthy eating and physical activity.
- The only clinically important positive outcome was a moderate increase in vegetable consumption.
- There was, a small increase in global self-worth for obese children in the intervention schools.

The authors were disappointed with the results and highlighted concern over both the increasing prevalence of obesity in this entire school population and the struggle between public health initiatives and antagonistic social and environment.

EDITORIAL – Drug treatment for obesity. Després, J.-P. Professor Quebec Heart Institute, Laval Hospital Research Center, Sainte-Foy, Canada.
BMJ, **322**(7299): 1379-1380, 9 June 2001.

Després discusses the impact of the STORM (sibutramine trial of obesity reduction and maintenance) study (Lancet 2000). This showed that sibutramine was successful for 43% of people (16% in the placebo group) in maintaining at least 80% of the weight loss by individuals who had already used it to lose 5% of their body weight. In addition favourable changes in cardiovascular risk factors were seen:
- reduced triglycerides;
- increased HDL;
- reduced insulinaemia;
- reduced C peptide levels;
- reduced uric acid concentrations.There was no effect on blood pressure. Further long term studies need to confirm these findings.

EDITORIAL – Abdominal obesity and the hypertriglyceridaemic waist phenotype.
Little, P. and Byrne, C. Southampton University, Southampton, UK.
BMJ, **322**(7288): 687-688, 24 March 2001.

and

Treatment of obesity: need to focus on high risk abdominally obese patients.
Després, J.-P., Lemieux, I. and Prudhomme, D. Quebec Heart Institute, Laval Hospital Research Centre, Sainte-Foy, Quebec, Canada.
BMJ, **322**(7288): 716-720, 24 March 2001.

Abdominal obesity is a better predictor of CHD than body mass index. It is also a major risk factor for type 2 diabetes, as it is associated with glucose intolerance and insulin resistance.

People with abdominal obesity tend to have high triglycerides levels and low HDL levels. The low HDL gives them a high cholesterol: HDL ratio, which is a powerful predictor of CHD. Even with normal LDL levels.

These individuals often have increased small, dense LDL particles and increased apolipoprotein B giving them a very atherogenic profile. This profile is associated with increased risk of CHD, even in the absence of traditional risk factor such as type 2 diabetes, hypercholesterolaemia and high blood pressure.

THE NEW 'TRIAD' OF METABOLIC RISK FACTORS

- Increased fasting insulin levels.
- Increased small dense LDL particles.
- Increased apolipoprotein B levels.Have been associated with a 20 fold increased risk of CHD, in asymptomatic middle aged men over a 5 year period.

WAIST CIRCUMFERENCE AND FASTING TRIGLYCERIDES AS SCREENING

Waist circumference is a good measure of abdominal obesity and it is also useful to measure the change in this over time. Useful screening markers are waist circumference and fasting triglycerides levels, with cut off points of 90 cm and 2 mmol/l, respectively (in men). Using these two cut off points will identify 80% of men with the atherogenic metabolic triad and only 10% of men below these levels will be positive for the triad. Even in the absence of the triglycerides measurement, using a waist cut off measurement of 100–102 in men (and 88–90 cm in women) is likely to identify those at high risk of chronic metabolic diseases. These cut-off levels may be different in other ethnic groups.They suggest that the waist circumference measurement should be regarded as a "vital sign" and should be recorded in the medical records

The editorial agrees with the findings of significant associations between waist circumference and the metabolic syndrome. They note that a fasting triglycerides > 2.3 doubles the risk of MI. However, they highlight some unanswered questions:
- many people who go on to develop type 2 diabetes have no risk factors;
- how reliable is waist circumference and were do you put the tape measure?
- most patients who are overweight, know that they are at increased risk for CHD;
- weight reduction methods work in clinical trials, but may not be so good in 'real life'. They conclude that there is insufficient evidence to support the recording of waist circumference in medical notes.

Orlistat with diet was effective and safe for weight loss and coronary risk reduction in obesity. Commentator, Paul Levinson, Memorial Hospital of Rhode Island, Rhode Island, USA.
Evidence-based Medicine, **6**(2): 54, March/April 2001.

The following article is briefly presented
The effect of orlistat on body weight and coronary heart disease risk profile in obese patients: the Swedish Multimorbidity study. Lindgärde, F. on behalf of the Orlistat Swedish Multimorbidity Study Group.
J. Intern. Med., **248:** 245–254, Sept. 2000

The Swedish Multimorbidity study is a randomized controlled trial with a 1 year follow up period and involving around 370 patients from over 30 primary care centres in Sweden. Subjects had a body mass index between 28 and 38 kg/m^2. They received orlistat 120 mg three times a day. All subjects were encouraged to maintain a mildly hypocaloric diet and advised to walk daily.
- Weight loss in the orlistat group was significantly higher than in the placebo group (nearly 6% vs. just under 5%, P = 0.05).
- Orlistat was associated with significantly greater reductions in serum cholesterol and LDL cholesterol, fasting glucose and HBA1c levels.
- Blood pressure and waist hip circumference did not differ between the groups.

Commentary
The difference in mean weight loss amounts to about 1.3 kg, which is not great. However, it is known that a 5–10% reduction in body weight can have health benefits.

OSTEOPOROSIS

> • Debate continues over the usefulness of bone densitometry.
> • Dutch researchers recommend screening for patients aged 71 and over.
> • Hip protectors reduce fractures in those at risk of falling.

BACKGROUND

Osteoporosis is a situation characterized by low bone mass, decreased bone strength and a resulting increased risk of fractures. It represents a major cause of morbidity and mortality in the population over the age of 50. Osteoporosis causes more than 150 000 fractures a year at considerable cost to the health service. Population based screening for low bone mass in peri-menopausal women cannot be justified; however dual energy X-ray absorptiometry (DEXA) scans should be performed on those at high risk of osteoporosis. At present the health service does not have the resources for this.

Smoking is a major risk factor for osteoporosis. A meta-analysis involving 48 studies (*BMJ*, 1997) found that:
- in pre-menopausal women, smoking had no appreciable effect on bone density;
- in postmenopausal women, smoking had an effect on bone density and risk of hip fracture which increased with age;
- in all women one in eight hip fractures can be attributable to smoking;
- there is a dose-response relationship between risk of hip fracture and number of cigarettes smoked. In former smokers the effect on bone density and risk of fracture lies between that seen in never and current smokers.

MANAGEMENT

Available treatments include:
- oestrogen;
- calcium and vitamin D;
- bisphosphonates. Alendronate can be used as an alternative to oestrogen and may have fewer side effects (*EBM*, July/Aug. 1998).
- SERMS. Raloxifene is a selective oestrogen receptor modulator (SERM). It has many features in common with oestrogen:
  - positive effects on bone (reduced vertebral fractures);
  - positive effects on LDL;
  - increased risk of venous thromboembolism;

Unlike oestrogen raloxifene:
- does not affect the endometrium;
- has no effect on climacteric symptoms.

EDITORIAL – Hip protectors. Cameron, Ian D. Associate Professor of Rehabilitation Medicine Rehabilitation Studies Unit, Department of Medicine, University of Sydney, Ryde, NSW, Australia. **BMJ, 324**(7334): 376-377, 16 February 2002.

Several studies have shown that hip protectors can reduce hip fractures. They should be used at all times in those at risk of falling. They can be modified to be used as underwear with or without incontinence pads. The cost of the hip protectors may prohibit use. In addition some may need help when dressing and using the toilet whilst wearing hip protectors.

EDUCATION AND DEBATE SECTION – For and against, bone densitometry is not a good predictor of hip fracture. Wilkin, T.J., Devendra, D., Dequeker, J. and Luyten, F.P. Department of Medicine, Postgraduate Medical School, Derriford, UK. **BMJ, 323**(7316): 795-799, 6 October 2001.

Bone densitometry is frequently employed in osteoporosis clinics to predict patients' risks of fractures. However, opinion is divided on the usefulness of densitometry for this purpose. In this article, both sides of the argument are presented. The following points are made.

Against bone densitometry:
- Age-related decline in bone density contributes little to the increased risk of fractures.
- There is a poor relationship between gain in bone mass and fracture protection.
- Age is a better predictor of hip fracture risk than bone density.
- The epidemiological evidence used to support densitometry is flawed.

In support of bone densitometry:
- Bone densitometry is currently the best validated method for predicting fragility fractures.
- Although hip fractures are very strongly correlated with age, fractures at other sites are not, thus other ways of predicting risk (such as densitometry) are necessary.
- Bone densitometry is a valuable tool for reassuring low-risk patients that long term antiresorptive treatments are not necessary.

Clinical risk factors as predictors of postmenopausal osteoporosis in general practice. Verluis, R.G.J.A., Papapoulos, S.E. and de Bock, G.H. *et al.* Department of General Practice, Leiden university Medical Centre, The Netherlands. **Br. J. Gen. Pract., 51**(471): 806-810, 1 October 2001.

Expert committees in the UK and other countries have suggested case-finding strategies to identify those at high risk of osteoporosis. This study evaluates such a strategy in one general practice in the Netherlands. Of just over 700 women aged 55–84 who were randomly selected, around 450 actually took part in the study. They were interviewed, completed a questionnaire and had a bone mineral density scan.

- Three risk factors were significantly associated with osteoporosis: previous osteoporotic type fracture, low body mass index and loss of height or kyphosis.
- The three risk factors identified 60% of those with osteoporosis (but missed 40%).
- Addition of spinal X-ray to the screening procedures increased accuracy of case-finding.
- The prevalence of risk factors increased with age.
- Fifty three percent of women without osteoporosis had at least one risk factor.

They recommend screening for patients aged 71 and over. Those below this age should be investigated based on strong clinical indicators. They cannot recommend pharmacological interventions based on risk factors alone.

OUT-OF-HOURS CARE

- To maximise the efficacy of services available out-of-hours for elderly patients, their long standing falsely held beliefs must be addressed.
- Daytime frequent attenders account for a large proportion of all contacts within general practice (both daytime and out-of-hours).
- A N. Ireland study showed that the home visit rate varied according to which PCC had been contacted, age of patient and where the patient lived (with patients living furthest away been least likely to get a home visit).
- The introduction of NHS Direct had no effect on the rate of GP consultations for influenza-like and other respiratory infections.

BACKGROUND

MORALE

Out-of-hours work is, for most GPs, an unwelcome part of general practice. One study (Lattimer, *BMJ*, 1996) found that 50% of GPs wanted to cut their on-call commitment and 25% wanted no on-call at all. The introduction of co-operative services has been a positive step forward for many GPs and their families. Studies have found that their introduction has been associated with an increase in morale amongst GPs and their spouses and an increase in the health status of GPs (*BJGP*, March 1999 and Oct. 2000).

A request for an out-of-hours visit can present a difficult dilemma for a GP, particularly if it is thought that the visit is not required. One study (Court, *BMJ*, 1996) found that although most visits are performed because of the perceived urgency of the condition, many were performed because patients demanded it, or the need to avoid a complaint.

NURSE TRIAGE

Nurse triage for out-of-hours calls is becoming increasingly popular. Nurses have been found to be effective at handling up to 50% of calls normally handled by GPs (*BMJ*, Jan 1997, Oct 1998 and Nov 1999). One study using nurse triage during the day (for house call requests) found that nurse triage was able to reduce home visits by a half and free up an extra 3 hours of doctor consulting time (*BJGP*, June 1998).

There seems to be a difference between the care and advice given by deputizing doctors as compared with practice doctors. However the differences in health outcomes between the groups do not differ. An RCT (*BMJ*, 1997) found the following:

- Practice doctors were more likely to offer telephone advice than were deputizing doctors. Deputizing doctors were more likely to make a home visit than were practice doctors.
- Practice doctors wrote fewer prescriptions compared with deputizing doctors and had a higher rate of generic prescribing.

- Practice doctors visited sooner than deputizing doctors.
- Overall patients were more satisfied with care received from their own practice doctor than from deputizing doctors. They were most dissatisfied by the time delay, but were also more dissatisfied about communication and the attitude of the deputizing doctors compared with practice doctors.
- There was no difference in the number of patients referred to hospital, number of admissions or duration of admission, or other use of health services between the two groups.

TELEPHONE CONSULTATIONS

Impact of NHS Direct on general practice consultations during the winter of 1999-2000: analysis of routinely collected data. Chapman, R.S., Smith, G.E. and Warburton, F. *et al.* Royal College of General Practitioners, Birmingham Research Unit, Harborne, Birmingham, UK. **BMJ, 325**(7377): 1397-1398, 14 December 2002.

This study assessed the impact of the introduction of NHS Direct on cases of influenza-like illness and other respiratory infections seen by General Practitioners. Data was gathered for the winter of 1999-2000, using routine RCGP weekly returns. Data was also gathered for the three winters preceding the introduction of NHS Direct.

- Analysis of the data suggests that the introduction of NHS Direct had no effect on the number of GP consultations for influenza-like illness and other respiratory infections.

OTHERS

A qualitative study of older peoples views of out-of-hours services. Foster, J., Dale, J. and Jessopp, L. Guys, Kings and St Thomas School of Medicine, Division of Primary Care and Public Health Sciences, Department of General Practice and Primary Care, Weston Education Centre, London, UK.
Br. J. Gen. Pract., 51(470): 719-723, 1 September 2001.

This study conducted in Lambeth, Southwark and Lewisham (multi-ethnic, socio-economically challenged areas of South London) qualitatively assessed elderly patients views of out-of-hours services with the aim of making services more user friendly.

Patients who had and had not used services were questioned. The results were as follows:

Reluctance to utilize services was found to be mainly to long-standing beliefs such as:

- The doctor was not to be consulted unless you were desperately ill.

- It is always appropriate to wait and see if it is better in the morning
- A fear of what the true nature of the illness may be.
- Advice is not appropriate unless offered by your own GP.
- Nurses are insufficiently qualified to offer advice.
- GPs today are generally less caring and more reluctant to carry out home visits.
- Diagnoses made over the phone cannot be accurate.

Experiences of out of hours services ranged from very good to very poor.

These barriers need to be addressed in order to satisfactorily restructure out-of-hours services so that they provide more effectively for the needs of the elderly population. The cost to the NHS and to society as a whole of ignoring these views will only be met later on in terms of increased morbidity, both physical and psychological.

General practice out-of-hours service, variations in use and equality in access to a doctor: a cross-sectional study. O'Reilly, D., Stevenson, M., McCay, C. and Jamison, J. Health and Social Care Research Unit, the Queens University of Belfast, UK. **Br. J. Gen. Pract., 51**(469): 625-629, 1 August 2001.

This cross-sectional study analyses the variation in use and access to primary care centres (PCCs). They analyze over 100 000 calls received by one of the largest co-operatives in the UK (situated in N. Ireland and utilizing around 230 GPs).

- Just over 50% of patients received telephone advice only.
- Patients living furthest away from the call centre were least likely to call the centre. These patients were also least likely to get a fact-to-face consultation with a GP, if they did call.
- Up until the age of 15 years, males and females had the same chance of seeing a GP. After this age females were 20% more likely to receive telephone advice only.
- People aged over 65 years were 40 times more likely to receive a home visit than those aged under 15 years.
- Patients from deprived backgrounds were more likely to get home visits.
- The home visit rate varied according to which PCC had been contacted, age of patient and where the patient lived.

Some of these findings may represent inequality of service provision particularly for those living furthest away from the PCC.

The association between daytime attendance and out-of-hours frequent attendance among adult patients in general practice. Vedsted, P., Sorensen, H.T., Nielsen, J.N. and Olsen, F. The Research Unit and Department of General Practice, University of Aarhus, Denmark.
***Br. J. Gen. Pract.,* 51**(463): 121-124, 1 February 2001.

This Danish population based, cross sectional study sets out to determine the association between daytime frequent attendance and out-of-hours frequent attendance. They define out-of-hours as being GP consultations after 4.00 p.m. during the week, weekends and public holidays.

Danish GPs have similar working arrangements to U.K. GPs. Frequent attendance was defined as the 10% of most frequent attenders amongst all attenders during the 12 months. They found:

- a strong association between daytime attendance and out of hours frequent attendance;
- patients who are frequent attenders both in the day and out of hours, make up 10% of the day time frequent attenders and 42% of the out of hours frequent attenders. This was more so for women than men;
- more than half of the frequent attenders during the daytime had no out of hours contacts.

They conclude that daytime frequent attenders account for a large proportion of all contacts within general practice.

POSTNATAL DEPRESSION

- Postnatal depression is associated with the risk of sudden infant death syndrome
- One study has found that depression is more likely in the antenatal period than postnatally.

Is postnatal depression a risk factor for sudden infant death? Sanderson, C.A., Cowden, B., Hall, D.M.B. and Taylor, E.M. University Department of Paediatrics, Sheffield Children's Hospital, Sheffield, UK.
Br. J. Gen. Pract., 52(481): 636-640, 1 August 2002.

A previous study in New Zealand has shown an association between postnatal depression and sudden infant death syndrome (SIDS). This study aimed to determine whether this association could be observed in Sheffield, UK. A case-control study design was employed, using prospectively collected data from all live births in Sheffield from 1988-1993. The Sheffield Child Development Study database was used, in addition to demographic and obstetric data collection from birth notification forms, and administration of the Edinburgh Postnatal Depression Scale (EPDS) at 1 month after delivery. During the study period there were 33000 live births. Forty two babies died with the cause registered as SIDS.

- High maternal EPDS score was associated with the risk of SIDS (Odds ratio 3.20)

The authors concluded that postnatal depression may be associated with unexpected infant death. They suggested that further work is needed to determine whether the observed association is causal.

Cohort study of depressed mood during pregnancy and after childbirth. Evans, J., Heron, J. and Francomb, H. *et al.* on behalf of the Avon Longitudinal Study of Parents and Children Study Team.
BMJ, 323(7307): 257-260, 4 August 2001.

The aim of this prospective cohort study was to follow mood changes in pregnant women. Around 14 500 women were recruited for the Avon longitudinal study of parents and children. They were sent a series of four postal questionnaires (including the Edinburgh postnatal depression scale) throughout pregnancy and the postnatal period. Just over 9000 (65%) women returned all four questionnaires.

- Higher depression scores were more likely during pregnancy rather than after pregnancy.
- The proportion of women with probable depression at 18 weeks pregnancy was 11.8%: at 32 weeks was 13.5%: at 8 weeks postpartum was 9.1% and 8 months postpartum was 8.1%. Further studies need

to investigate the effect of depression during the antenatal period on the child. The benefits of treatment antenatally should also be explored.

PRACTICE NURSE

- Nurses seem to be able to provide quality of care similar to that of doctors
- Nurse triage systems in Primary Care may not be as effective as originally thought

Primary Care: Nurse telephone triage for same day appointments in general practice: multiple interrupted time series trial of effect on workload and costs.
Richards, D., Meakins, J. and Tawfik, J. *et al.* School of Nursing, University of Manchester, Manchester, UK.
BMJ, 325(7374): 1214-1220, 23 November 2002.

This study conducted in Yorkshire compared the costs and workloads for doctors and nurses of dealing with requests for same day appointments either by nurse telephone triage or standard routine management. The setting was a large general practice with a study population of around 20 800. Standard management involved adding the same day appointment to the end of GP surgeries. The triage system involved practice nurses assessing the request and seeing whether telephone advice or, routine or emergency appointment was necessary. The study was conducted over 12 months with the first 3 months allocated to standard management and the remaining 9 months used for triage management.

- Overall around 5000 patients were included with around 3500 of these managed by triage and the remainder by standard management.
- Patients in the triage group had more presenting complaints and in particular a higher proportion of respiratory and skin complaints.
- Triage resulted in fewer patients receiving a GP appointment than standard management.
- More patients in the triage system returned for follow up practice based care within one month than standard management patients.
- Triage was associated with an increased number of patients attending out-of-hours and accident and emergency departments.
- Triage system resulted in around 30% fewer same day appointments with nurses alone handling around 40% of requests.

However triage was no cheaper than standard management as savings in GP time were offset by increases in nursing and follow up time.

Systematic of whether nurse practitioners working in primary care can provide equivalent care to doctors. Horrocks, S., Anderson, E. and Salisbury, C. Division of Primary Health Care, University of Bristol, Bristol, UK.
***BMJ, 324**(7341): 819-823, 6 April 2002.*

The aim of this systematic review was to compare care given by doctors with that given by nurse practitioners (nps). Forty-six studies were analysed. They found:
- No difference in health outcomes between doctors and nps.
- Nurses had longer consultations by about 3 and a half minutes and ordered more investigations.
- Nurses were better at record keeping and identified more physical abnormalities.
- Nurses were as accurate as doctors at interpreting x-rays.

Nurses seem to be able to provide quality of care similar to that of doctors. However they discuss some of the limitations of this analysis.
- Many of the trials were old.
- There was considerable heterogeneity between studies and outcomes.
- Nurses often did not work under the same conditions as doctors.
- Research needs to include more complex psychosocial conditions and chronic diseases.

FURTHER READING

See 'Elderly' for

Effectiveness and economic evaluation of a nurse delivered home exercise programme to prevent falls. 1: Randomised controlled trial. Department of Medical and Surgical Sciences, Otago Medical School, Dunedin, New Zealand.
***BMJ, 322**(7288): 696-701, 24 March 2001.*

PRESCRIBING

- A cross-sectional survey found that financial rewards did not influence prescribing
- Prescribing initiatives at PCG/T level can have an impact on prescribing costs in general practice.
- A qualitative study has confirmed that pharmaceutical companies are a major influence on the prescribing of new drugs.
- An RCT found that educational outreach by community pharmacists increases the number of patients treated within national guidelines.
- Prescribing behaviour may be based on experience, attitude, and perceptions of GPs.

BACKGROUND

PACT (PRESCRIBING ANALYSIS AND COST) DATA

The PPA (Prescription Pricing Authority) collects information on prescriptions made by GPs. Drugs are categorized by their *British National Formulary* section. Information is available at practice, health authority and national levels. GPs receive the standard printed version of PACT whereas health authorities receive this version and have access to PACTLINE, which supplies computerized PACT data. The PPA has developed HEAPACT (health authority electronic PACT), which allows health authority pharmaceutical advisors to obtain information on prescribing of specific drugs directly, using a modem link. Some practices also have access to HEAPACT but many practices are still unaware of it.

HOW PACT IS USED

Budget setting
The NHS executive has begun to use PACT data to develop formulae for setting health authority budgets. Health authorities can monitor general practice prescribing budgets.

Research
PACT can be used for research and audit. It can be used to develop prescribing indicators e.g. the inhaled corticosteroid:bronchodilator ratio.

Expensive drugs
Expensive drugs can be identified and health authorities can take this information into account when setting budgets. PACT, however, cannot identify 'expensive patients', i.e. patients requiring multiple low-cost drugs.

LIMITATIONS OF PACT

- It can only supply a narrow range of information
- The data cannot be linked to demographic or clinic data. They cannot be used to calculate age and sex specific prescribing rates or look at prescribing rates for specific conditions. Using a unique patient identifier with each prescription would allow the calculation of age- and sex-specific prescribing rates. Including diagnostic data with the prescription would enable the analysis of prescribing rates for specific conditions.
- PACT data does not include private prescriptions or prescriptions issued but not dispensed.
- The number of items prescribed is not always an accurate measure of the amount of drug prescribed.
- PACT does not tell us about prescribing activities in hospitals.

The **number-of-'items'** prescribed is often used to analyse prescribing activity. This is supposed to measure the volume of drug prescribed; however, no account is made of the quantity of drug present in an item. Some have concluded that the 'item' is unsuitable as a measure of drug volume and should be replaced by a standardized measure such as the 'defined daily dosage'.

The **prescribing unit** is another term used in the analysis of prescribing activity. One prescribing unit represents any patient under the age of 65. Patients over 65 count as three prescribing units.

The **ASTRO-PU** has been described. It incorporates 18 age-sex groups and one temporary resident group. It is generally accepted as a better way of controlling for demographic features when looking at a practice's overall prescribing. When practices are compared with local populations or local averages, the old prescribing unit is used. Some have suggested that comparisons should be made for specific therapeutic groups and should take into account that practices have different age-sex structures. Hence a prescribing unit has been developed called the **STAR-PU**. Its age-sex bands are the same as those used for the ASTRO-PU. The STAR-PU can be calculated using an aggregation of data from computer systems such as General Practice Research Database (formerly known as VAMP) and Intercontinental Medical Statistics (IMS).

Prescribing incentive schemes in two NHS regions: cross sectional survey. Ashworth, M., Golding, S. and Shepard, L. *et al.* Guy's, King's College and St Thomas's School of Medicine, Department of General Practice and Primary Care, London, UK.
BMJ, 324(7347): 1187-1188, 18 May 2002.

This study was a cross-sectional survey investigating the associations between prescribing indicators and financial rewards in 66 London and 79

South East primary care groups. Prescribing indicators included 'quality' based indicators and 'cost' based indicators.

- The prescribing costs, as an indicator, ranged from 7% underspend to 14% overspend across the primary care groups. The size of financial rewards also varied from maximum payments of £3000 to £45000.
- The authors did not find a significant relation between the magnitude of the financial rewards and the prescribing overspend of the primary care groups.

The authors suggest that the lack of an association between the financial incentives and the prescribing overspends implies an 'inefficient system, in which large rewards are not clearly connected with either cost or quality based prescribing achievements'.

COMMENTARY – Prescribing incentive schemes-more evidence is needed of how they work. Sullivan, F. Professor of Research and Development in Primary Care, Tayside Centre for General Practice, University of Dundee, Dundee, UK.
BMJ, **324**(7347): 1188, 18 May 2002.

Sullivan explains that in theory incentives should help change prescribing behaviour, but the evidence base to guide this is 'scant'. The reasons given for this, illustrated by the study conducted by Ashworth *et al.*, include:

- Opportunistic research often provides 'mixed' evidence with positive and negative effects. Planned investigations are preferred.
- Ashworth *et al.* were not able to incorporate into their studies other factors which influence prescribing costs e.g. pharmacists attached to the practices.
- Ashworth *et al.* only describe incentive schemes in London and the South East.

In conclusion, Sullivan suggests that 'firing silver bullets' may change the behaviour of practices, but a 'richer evidence base' is required to help them.

A qualitative comparative investigation of variation in general practitioners' prescribing patterns. Jaye, C. and Tolyard, M. Department of General Practice, Dunedin School of Medicine, University of Otago, New Zealand.
Br. J. Gen. Pract., **52**(478): 381-386, 1 May 2002.

In New Zealand, changes in funding strategies for primary care and also in costs of pharmaceuticals has prompted research into variation in prescribing behaviour between GPs. Previous studies have taken a quantitative approach, examining variations in drugs prescribed, the volumes prescribed and costs. This study investigates the qualitative aspects of 30 GPs that may help explain variations in their prescribing behaviour. Ten GPs from each of three prescribing categories (Low-, medium- and high-cost prescribers) participated in a 60-minute interview.

- Low-cost prescribers reported more experience in practice. They found it easier to refuse patients prescriptions, and offered more education and counselling.

- High-cost prescribers showed higher motivation towards medicine. They felt that patients view prescriptions as representing provision of a service.

The authors conclude that differences exist between GPs with different prescribing behaviours. These include differences in experience, attitudes towards medicine, and perceptions of their roles as GPs.

A randomised controlled trial of the effect of educational outreach by community pharmacists on prescribing in UK general practice. Freemantle, N., Nazareth, I. and Eccles, M. *et al.* Department of Primary Care and General Practice, The Medical School, University of Birmingham, Edgebaston, Birmingham, UK.
Br. J. Gen. Pract., **52**(477): 290-295, 1 April 2002.

Educational outreach visits by community pharmacists are commonly utilised in primary care to improve use of guidelines in prescribing practice. This RCT aimed to assess the effect of such outreach programmes on utilisation of prescribing guidelines in General Practice. Seventy-five practices participated in the trial, these practices were offered educational outreach visits covering two of four guidelines (Aspirin therapy, ACEI in heart failure, NSAIDS in osteoarthritis and anti-depressants in depression). The trial examined to what extent prescribing guidelines were followed before and after the outreach visit. Six of the 75 practices refused follow up. The study found that:

- After intervention 5.2 more patients were treated according to prescribing guidelines.
- Smaller practices improved their prescribing more after outreach than large practices.

The authors suggest that larger practices may have a more entrenched organisational system and so be less amenable to change prescribing.

The impact of a general practice group intervention on prescribing costs and patterns. Walker, J. and Mathers, N. University of Sheffield, Institute of General Practice and Primary Care, Sheffield, UK.
Br. J. Gen. Pract., **52**(476): 181-186, 1 March 2002.

The aim of this study was to assess whether prescribing initiatives at the PCG/T level can reduce prescribing costs in general practice. Nine practices (36 GPs) in south Derbyshire were part of an initiative to cut prescribing costs. This involved input from the health authority pharmaceutical advisor, peer review and prescribing recommendations. Nine practices from the same health authority, who were not part of the initiative were used as a comparison group.

After the initiative, the study group made greater savings than the comparison group. The study groups costs fell whereas the comparison groups costs continued to rise. The reduction in costs in the study group were noted one month after the initiative was started.

Reductions in costs were marked for gastrointestinal drugs and for drugs used to treat infections.

They conclude that prescribing initiatives at PCG/T level can have an impact on prescribing costs in general practice.

Prescribing new drugs: qualitative study of influences on consultants and general practitioners. Jones, M.I., Greenfield, S.M. and Bradley, C. Department of Primary Care and General Practice, Medical School, University of Birmingham, Birmingham, UK. **BMJ, 323**(7309): 378-381, 18 August 2001.

The aim of this qualitative study is to assess what influences GPs and consultants to prescribe new drugs. They interview 56 GPs and 38 consultants from Birmingham hospitals and general practices.

- Consultants tended to prescribe a narrower range of new drugs than GPs and these were related to their specialty.
- Pharmaceutical companies were a major influence on the prescribing of new drugs
- Consultants asked drug reps for additional literature on new drugs. GPs tended to prescribe new drugs based on 'drug rep' information only.
- GPs tended to be vague about which journals they read and there was little evidence of critical appraisal of these sources.
- *Drug and Therapeutic Bulletin* was highly rated amongst GPs.
- Cost of drugs tended to be secondary to other factors in terms of prescribing priorities.
- If a drug worked well during the first few experiences of the drug, GPs and consultants were more likely to continue using it.

In hospitals, new drugs are introduced via a drug and therapeutics committee. This could be extended to include the community. Data from NICE could also be used.

PRIMARY CARE

- Gallagher *et al.*, found that appointment making is a process involving complex interactions between patient and receptionist
- The ATTRACT project suggests that doctors 'want summaries of evidence rather than the skills to produce them themselves'
- As up to 80% of diagnoses can be made on the basis of history, the telephone may be an appropriate medium for some consultations
- No single practice type has a monopoly on high quality care, different practices have different strengths
- Most patients would like to be given the choice of having a chaperone present. Women prefer a female nurse, but men are less likely to want a female chaperone, and there are few male alternatives
- Soft toys in GPs waiting rooms show higher levels of bacterial contamination than hard toys and are more difficult to clean and keep clean than hard toys.
- One study found that there is no evidence that single-handed practices are under performing clinically.
- Material deprivation may need to be addressed rather than practice factors when dealing with missed appointments Payments to GPs, for giving antismoking advice is unlikely to yield any positive outcomes
- Payments to GPs for giving antismoking advice is unlikely to yield any positive outcomes
- Targeted strategies may reduce hospital non-attendance.
- Informal carers needed to be included as members of the primary health care team.
- The Health Act 1999 made it mandatory for NHS organizations to work in partnership
- Larger merged PCGs do not necessarily perform better than smaller ones
- Pollock argues that the 1999 Health Act and the Health and Social Care Bill move the UK towards a US-style health care system
- Primary care research should involve patient input after careful evaluation.
- 'Manage or be managed' is the message for GPs today
- Personal medical services are proving popular but still dont address all the primary healthcare concerns today.
- A computerised support system did not significantly aid the implementation of evidence based guidelines in the management of asthma and angina in adults in primary care

EDITORIAL: The new contract: renaissance or requiem for general practice. Marshall, M. and Roland, M. Professor of General Practice. National Primary Care Research and Development Centre, University of Manchester, UK.
Br. J. Gen. Pract., 52(480): 531-532, 1 July 2002.

A radical new contract demanded by general practitioners has arrived. A welcome change is the allocation of 30–50% of income to be in the form of quality payments rather than quantity. A comprehensive approach to rewarding quality has been chosen, with particular focus on chronic disease management.

The authors recommend that GPs should not underestimate the changes in their practices that will be required to achieve these quality payments: comprehensive computerisation and specialisation within practices. However, the authors comment that the specialised, clinic-based model may not provide patients with the same continuity of care making general practitioners into 'partial' practitioners.

The new contract allows GPs to opt out of providing certain services so that they can limit demands made on them. However, this will force primary care trusts to seek other providers causing fragmentation and reducing co-ordination of care.

A proportion of the quality payments will be 'upfront' allowing practices to invest in their infrastructure.

In the authors' view the new contract offers a renaissance of general practice. They claim that appropriate pricing and GPs responding to the challenges of the new contract will make British primary care the 'envy of the world'.

Managing patient demand: a qualitative study of appointment making in general practice. Gallagher, M., Pearson, P., Drinkwater, C. and Guy, J. Department of Primary Care, University of Newcastle upon Tyne, UK.
Br. J. Gen. Pract., 51(465): 280-285, 1 April 2001.

This was a qualitative study analysing the process of appointment making in general practice. Three practices in the North of England participated in the study. Observers watched the appointment making process and conducted interviews with patients, receptionists, nurses, managers and doctors.

- They found that appointment making is a complex process involving:
- patient illness behaviour;
- patient expectations;
- receptionists actions and attitudes;
- appointment availability;
- negotiation.
- Certain groups were labelled as consulting inappropriately:
- middle aged employed people;
- patients allocated by the health authority;
- patients who did not comply with appointment making rules.

Just in time information for clinicians: a questionnaire evaluation of the ATTRACT project. Brassey, J., Elwyn, G., Price, C. and Kinnersley, P. ATTRACT Wales, Mamhilad House, Pontypool, UK.
BMJ, 322(7285): 529-530, 3 March 2001.

The ATTRACT project was introduced in Gwent in 1997 to allow GPs to request quick evidence-based information. The information was summarized and faxed back to the GP within 6 hours. A questionnaire was given to 50 ATTRACT users.

- Nearly 70% rated the service as 'very useful' and just over 30% as 'useful'.
- Many had changed their practice as a result of the information received.

They conclude that doctors 'want summaries of evidence rather than the skills to produce them themselves'.

RESEARCH

EDITORIAL – Participating in primary care research. McKinley, R., Dixon-Woods, M. and Thornton, H. Department of General Practice, University of Leicester, Leicester, UK.
Br. J. Gen. Pract., **52**(12): 971-972, 1 December 2002.

GPs should encourage a partnership between those people that perform research and also those for whom the research is intended. GPs may have felt that researchers have merely used their patient lists without the courtesy of asking them for their opinions of study design and patient recruitment. This editorial explores the issue of primary care research from a patient, GP and researcher perspective.

- Major research organisations have made it a priority for patients to have a role in the formulation of research agendas. This idea has been used in recent stroke and HRT clinical trials, which has led to benefits for both participants and investigators.
- However for primary care research there are disparities in what patients and researchers expect for research agendas. Patients must be involved in deciding what research outcomes are measured.
- However there needs to be careful evaluation of involving patients in research projects. There is a danger of over emphasizing patients priorities and ignoring the initial legitimate research objectives.
- Research impacts on GPs as well as patients hence, there should be discussion among all parties involved in the research.

PRIMARY CARE GROUPS/TRUSTS

Primary care in Bradford: from group to trust and beyond. Small, N. and Proctor, S. School of Health Studies, University of Bradford, Bradford and Bradford Health Authority, Shipley, UK.
BMJ, **323**(7322): 1161-1163, 17 November 2001.

This paper describes the decision-making and process involved in the four primary care groups (PCG) in Bradford changing to primary care trust (PCT) status in October 2000. The authors used observations from the main staff involved in the process (mostly GPs). They also use analysis and quotes from discussions at Bradford Universitys conference 'Primary care groups one year on' in April 2000, and questionnaires sent to 40 professionals looking at research in the trusts.

- Views on the decision to change varied from a sense of innovation, to a loss of independence and having no other option in the current political climate.
- The achievements of the PCGs were recognized to include providing local services for local people, gaining significant extra healthcare resources and offering innovative services such as GP specialists.
- The consultation process was helped by all four PCGs applying together and involved meetings with professional groups, voluntary sector organizations, patient groups and neighbourhood groups. Although preparation of the submission documents required much work, sometimes detracting from everyday work, it had the benefit of accelerating change.
- The timetable for change presented the major challenge in transfer to trust status.
- The differing organisation and responsibility of the trust compared with group status became more apparent in the first few months after the transfer. The authors comment that it is difficult to assess which of the current simultaneous changes in primary care (PCTs, clinical governance, re-accreditation, and development of personal medical services) will have the most importance in the long-term.

PRIMARY CARE SECTION – Will primary care trusts lead to US–style health care?
Allyson, Pollock, Health Policy and Health Services Research Unit, School of Public Policy, University College London, London, UK.
BMJ, 322(7292): 964-967, 21 April 2001.

- The 1999 Health Act saw the introduction of PCGs and primary care trusts (PCTs). The government's aim is that PCTs will hold 70% of the entire NHS budget. The Health and Social Care Bill allows for PCTs to also become care trusts, where they have budgets for social care. Social and personal care in England is part funded from charging individuals. The two acts together make it easier to integrate health and social care, but also for the first time, the NHS will be able to charge for services. Scotland has decided against introducing charges.
- PCTs are set to face increasing cost pressures. By 2007, trusts will have to start repaying £4.5 bn of private finance.
- Pollock discusses ways of reducing costs e.g. reducing expenditure on premises, increased income from commercial and retail projects.
- Pollock argues that the NHS plan and the Social Care Bill move us further towards a US style managed health care with user charges and time limited care. She states that there are four ways that this can be prevented:
    1. reaffirm the old NHS principles of universal care. Reimburse trusts on the basis of population size and not practice list sizes;
    2. make social care free at the point of delivery as recommended by the Royal Commission on Long Term Care;

3. prevent the sale of health insurance and private health care within the NHS;
4. remove financial duties from trusts. Remove the contracting system which encourages internal market behaviour.

EDUCATION AND DEBATE SECTION – Is bigger better for primary care groups and trusts? Bojke, C., Gravele, H. and Wilkin, D. National Primary Care Research and Development Centre, Centre for Health Economics, University of York, York, UK.
BMJ, **322**(7286): 599-602, 10 March 2001.

• This article discusses the reasons and implications of PCG mergers. Two thirds of trusts have considered merger. Many feel that the optimum size of population is 200 000. Many mergers have been encouraged by health authorities, who are hard pressed to provide management support to PCGs with inadequate staffing levels.
• Although merger may be an answer to the management problem, it may not be beneficial for other PCG functions. Evidence from US groups suggests that mergers do not work and they can have a damaging effect on staff morale. The NHS executive needs to look at the provision of resources, so that mergers do not happen simply because of lack of management resources.
• Dealing with conditions that have varying prevalence in different populations is difficult in larger groups.
• An already merged unit may benefit from forming smaller commissioning units or locality groups for specific tasks.
• Non-merged units may benefit from forming alliances with other groups to give a larger combined group for specific tasks.

TELEPHONE CONSULTATIONS

The effect of GP telephone triage on numbers seeking same-day appointments.
Jiwa, M., Mathers, N. and Campbell, M. Institute of General Practice and Primary Care, University of Sheffield, Sheffield, UK.
Br. J. Gen. Pract., **52**(478): 390-391, 1 May 2002.

Previous studies have suggested that telephone consultations with GPs do not effectively reduce the demand for face-to-face consultations. This study examines the introduction of a telephone triage system in a four-doctor practice. Over a 1-year period, all patients requesting same-day appointments were told that a GP would telephone them later. GPs recorded the outcomes of these telephone consultations, and patients completed satisfaction surveys. Numbers attending out-of-hours were compared with previous years.
• Demand for face-to-face appointments fell by 39
• The majority of the patients were satisfied with the outcome of the telephone consultation
• Use of out-of-hours services dropped in the study period

The authors conclude that telephone consultations are a potentially useful alternative to face-to-face consultations for patients requiring same-day contact with a doctor.

EDITORIAL – Using telephones in Primary Care. Toon, P. Department of Primary Care and Population Sciences, University College London, London, UK.
***BMJ*, 324**(7348): 1230-1231, 25 May 2002.

Much of the debate surrounding Britain's NHS Direct telephone advice system has focussed on its effectiveness and value for money; however little work has been done regarding the wider role of teleconsultations in Primary Care.

Previous assessments of telephone use have examined its impact on the workload of healthcare staff, without looking into the benefits for patients. Up to 80% of diagnoses can be made on the basis of history, so the telephone may be an appropriate medium for some consultations. While this may not save time for healthcare staff, it can be advantageous to patients in many ways, as they don't have to arrange for childcare, take time off work, or worry about transport to and from the GP surgery.

Attitudes towards consultations by telephone are generally negative; indeed the GMC appears to discourage the practice. There is a need for systematic, controlled trials to measure the telephone's potential for monitoring chronic illnesses, and educating patients. It is important that the benefits and limitations of teleconsultation, to GPs and to patients, are quantified to maximise the efficacy of its use.

In addition to more research, Toon suggests that commercial organisations and charities that have already implemented telephone advice systems be consulted, so that their experiences can be used to assist in implementing such facilities for use by NHS patients.

OTHERS

EDITORIAL – Personal medical services; Have made steady, if unspectacular progress. Lewis, R. Visiting Fellow Kings Fund, London, UK.
***BMJ*, 325:** 1126-1127, 16 November 2002.

Personal medical services are now in their fourth year as a pilot. Their rapid growth has led to over a fifth of GPs in England working in these schemes. Personal medical services now enable local contracts between the provider and primary care trusts. This has led to a rise in the number of salaried General Practitioners and in theory allows Primary Care Trusts to use alternative providers if targets are not met.

Politicians are enthusiastic about these changes. Employers feel salaried GPs are cheaper and there is greater productivity with no detriment on quality of care. People also feel that personal medical services are serving people such as refugees and the homeless who traditionally had poor access to medical care. However the number of GPs overall has not increased with most salaried GPs having joined from a previous post.

The overall effect of personal medical services is difficult to measure with some evaluations seeing little difference between them and traditional practices. There is still no formal accountability of GPs. Ministers support both types of contract and it seems that GPs will have a choice of what to choose in the future for some time.

PRIMARY CARE – Effect of computerised evidence based guidelines on management of asthma and angina in adults in primary care: cluster randomised controlled trial. Eccles, M., McColl, E. and Steen, N. *et al.* Centre for Health Services Research, University of Newcastle, Newcastle upon Tyne, UK.
***BMJ,* 325**(7370): 941, 26 October 2002.

This cluster randomised controlled trial across 60 practices in the north of England aimed to define the role of a computerised support system to aid implementation of evidence based guidelines for management of asthma and angina in adults in the primary care setting.

Outcome was documented in terms of adherence to the guidelines and it was measured by condition specific features and a review of the patients case records.

It was found that:

- Consultation rates, processes of management (such as prescribing) and patient reported outcomes in both angina and asthma were not significantly affected by the use of a computerised protocol support system.
- The level of use of the software package was poor despite maximal efforts to ensure it was user friendly.

Patient, hospital, and general practitioner characteristics associated with non-attendance: a cohort study. Hamilton, W., Round, A. and Sharp, D. Public Health Medicine North and East Devon Health Authority, Exeter, UK.
***Br. J. Gen. Pract.,* 52**(462): 317-319, 1 April 2002.

The aim of this prospective cohort study was to examine the factors which affect hospital out patient clinic non-attendance. They looked at new referrals from 26 GPs (13 practices) in Exeter. They found:

- No significant difference in non-attendance rate between specialties.

The main predictive factors were patient, hospital and GP characteristics.

- Patient factors were male sex, younger age group (16–35 years), high levels of deprivation.
- The single hospital factor was the interval between referral and appointment date.
- The single GP characteristic was a high referring GP. GP status e.g. fund holding or having an MRCGP was not significant.

The authors suggest that GPs should consider when making referrals

- that patients may fail to attend the appointment and

• that there may be potential benefit in mentioning the non-attendance issue when referring to a young male patient.

Toys are a potential source of cross-infection in general practitioners waiting rooms. Merriman, E., Corwin, P. and Ikram, R. Department of Public Health and General Practice, Christchurch School of Medicine, New Zealand.
Br. J. Gen. Pract., **52**(475): 138-140, 1 February 2002.

This study assesses the bacteria contamination level of toys in GP waiting rooms, in six practices in New Zealand.
• Hard toys showed much lower contamination levels than soft toys.
• Cleaning hard toys by soaking them in hypochlorite solution for an hour was an effective means of decontamination. Soft toys need to be soaked as for hard toys, but also washed in the washing machine.
• After 2 days for soft toys and 1 week for hard toys, contamination levels returned to pre-cleaning levels.More research needs to evaluate whether these contamination levels constitute an infection risk

Variance in practice emergency medical admission rates: can it be explained. Duffy, R., Neville, R. and Staines, H. Tayside Centre for General Practice, University of Dundee, Scotland.
Br. J. Gen. Pract., **52**(474): 14-18, 1 January 2002.

This study analyzes the variation in emergency medical admission rates in practices in Dundee, Scotland. They use Scottish Morbidity Record 1 (SMR 1), which had details of all hospital admission rates.
• They found a nearly two-fold variation in admission rates between practices.
• Much of the variation was explained by age and level of deprivation.
• Doctor factors such as training status or holding MRCGP were not associated with the variation in admission rates.

Informal carers and the primary care team. Simon, C. Department of Primary Care, Aldermoor Health Centre, University of Southampton, Southampton, UK.
Br. J. Gen. Pract., **51**(472): 920-923, 1 November 2001.

The Government policy of care in the community, ageing population and increasing numbers of people surviving acute illness has lead to increased numbers of disabled people in the community requiring care from an informal carer. There are currently 6 million carers in the UK, and caring for their friend or relative can damage these individuals physical and mental health. Forty percent report poor psychological health as a result of their caring and the all cause mortality rate is elevated by 60% in this group. Currently GPs believe they have a reactive role in assisting carers responding to problems as they arise. The main reasons GPs feel they cannot adopt a proactive role, helping to prevent problems and providing support, is lack of time and training. However, adopting a proactive role may help minimise the preventable problems carers suffer. Though evidence is limited, the author suggests the following measures:

- Treat carers as members of the formal care team and include them in discussions about patient management.
- Give carers a choice in which tasks they are prepared to perform.
- Provide information about support groups, benefits and the patients condition.

PRIMARY CARE – Identifying predictors of high quality care in English general practice: observational study. Campbell, S.M., Hann, M. and Hacker, J. National Primary Care Research and Development Centre, University of Manchester, Manchester, UK. ***BMJ*, 323:** 784-787, 6 October 2001.

The authors in the study aimed to assess the variation in quality of care in general practice and identify factors associated with high quality care. They recruited 60 general practices from a stratified random sample from six areas in England, and used the following outcome measures to assess quality of care;

1   Chronic disease (angina, asthma, type 2 diabetes)
2   Preventative care (uptake rates for immunisations and cervical smears)
3   Access and interpersonal aspects.

They found the following,

- Quality of care varied substantially, and access to care and interpersonal care varied moderately
- Scores of asthma, angina and type 2 diabetes were 67%, 21%, and 17% higher in practices with 10 minute booking intervals compared to 5 minute intervals
- Diabetes care was better in larger practices and in practices with better team climate
- Access to care was better in smaller practices and in practices where staff reported better team climate
- Preventative care was worse in practices located in socio-economically deprived areas

Missed appointments in general practice: retrospective data analysis from four practices. Neal, R.D., Lawlor, D.A. and Allgar, V. *et al.*
Br. J. Gen. Pract., 51(471): 830-832, 1 October 2001.

The aim of this study was to examine the type of patients that miss appointments. They performed a retrospective analysis of computer records of missed appointments covering a 1 year period in four practices in Yorkshire.

- Overall nearly 8% of patients missed appointments
- Six percent of patients missed three or more appointments
- The likelihood of missing an appointment was associated with being female, living in a deprived area (associated with three times increased likelihood of missing an appointment), being a young adult.They suggest that material deprivation may need to be addressed rather than practice factors when dealing with missed appointments.

Use of risk adjustment in setting budgets and measuring performance in primary care I: how it works. Majeed, A., Bindram, A.B. and Weiner, J.P. School of Public Policy, University College London, UK.
BMJ, 323(7313): 604-607, 15 September 2001.

and

Use of risk adjustment in setting budgets and measuring performance in primary care II: advantages, disadvantages and practicalities. Majeed, A., Bindram, A.B. and Weiner, J.P. School of Public Policy, University College London, UK.
BMJ, 323(7313): 607-610, 15 September 2001.

PCGs and PCTs are to be funded through capitation based payments. These are based on the number of patients registered with their constituent practices and other factors such as age, sex, socio-economic status and community rates of chronic disease. They take no account of prevalence and severity of disease, which may discourage GPs (working with fixed and inflexible budgets) from taking on "expensive" patients.

In the US, risk adjustment methods are being employed as a more prospective method for predicting health service use. Different models exist but essentially the patients health status and likely use of health services is predicted from their medical history.

Uses of risk adjustment methods

Risk adjustment methods can be applied to individual patients as well as groups of physicians or providers working for Health Maintenance Organisations or health plans. Hence as well as predicting use of services, it can also be used to measure the performance of doctors.

It can also be used to provide a better comparison between practices, because it gives a better indication of case-mix. This is particularly important for smaller practices, which may show wide variations in spending, which at times may be due to a small number of "expensive" patients.

Some of the problems with risk adjustment methods

They are relatively new even in the USA, hence it is difficult to assess whether they really will be useful.

'Upcoding' is a problem in the US, whereby, physicians assign patients more serious diagnoses than they actually have in order to benefit from more funding.

The NHS is committed to a fully computerized healthcare system, which will be essential for risk adjustment methods to function. One of the fundamental differences between the US and the UK health systems is that risk adjustment in the US is used in a competitive market place whereas in the UK it would be used to enhance fairness and equity.

Qualitative study of pilot payment aimed at increasing general practitioners antismoking advice to smokers. Coleman, T., Wynn, A.T., Stevenson, K. and Cheater, F. Department of General Practice and Primary Health Care, Leicester Warwick Medical School, Leicester General Hospital, Leicester, UK.
BMJ, 323(7310): 432-435, 25 August 2001.

and

Intervention study to evaluate pilot health promotion payment aimed at increasing general practitioners antismoking advice to smokers. Coleman, T., Wynn, A.T., Barrett, S., Wilson, A. and Adams, S. Department of General Practice and Primary Health Care, Leicester Warwick Medical School, Leicester General Hospital, Leicester, UK.
BMJ, 323(7310): 435-436, 25 August 2001.

These studies assess the effectiveness of GP payments for anti-smoking advice. Thirty one GPs participated in the qualitative study. They were initially invited to come for smoking cessation training. Clinical behaviour was then observed before and after the payment scheme was introduced.

There was no evidence of a change in anti-smoking advice after the payment scheme was introduced.

The aim of the qualitative study was to assess GPs and practice nurses attitudes towards the payments.

Most felt that the payments would not alter their anti-smoking interventions. GPs preferred to discuss smoking with patients only if it seemed appropriate and in context with the reason for the patients attendance.

Doctors who made the highest number of claims for the payment, simply changed their recording of anti-smoking advice rather than changing their consulting behaviour.

PRIMARY CARE SECTION – Do single-handed practices offer poorer care? Cross sectional survey of processes and outcomes. Hippisley-Cox, J., Pringle, M. and Coupland, C. *et al* Division of General Practice, University of Nottingham, UK.
BMJ, 323(7308): 320-323, 11 August 2001.

Carrying out a cross sectional survey this papers objective was to determine whether there are important differences in activity between multiple partner practices and single-handed general practitioners and the degree to which the differences can be accounted for by practice characteristics such as deprivation. Just over 200 single-handed practices and just over 600 group practices in the Trent region took part in the survey. Single-handed doctors were older, tended to be male, had larger list size per doctor, were less likely to have a practice nurse and were less likely to receive Continuous Professional Development and Training.

Comparing performance and outcome measures in the single-handed practices with the GP partnerships, they found:
- higher admission rates for asthma and epilepsy in single-handed practices;
- no significant difference for avoidable admissions;
- higher teenage pregnancy rate in single handed practices.

They conclude that there is no evidence that single-handed practices are under performing clinically.

Attitudes of patients towards the use of chaperones in primary care. Whitford, D.L., Karim, M. and Thompson, G. Newcastle upon Tyne, UK.
***Br. J. Gen. Pract.,* 51**(466): 381-383, 1 May 2001.

Guidelines suggest that patients undergoing intimate examination should be given the option of having a chaperone present. Previous studies indicate that females would welcome this opportunity; little is known about male patients' preferences. A questionnaire was posted to 404 females (261 respondents) response and 400 males (190 respondents) aged 16-65, taken from three research practices, none of which routinely use chaperones.
- Females were more likely than males to want a chaperone, and patients were less likely to want a chaperone with their usual doctor.
- Equal numbers of patients would like a chaperone to those who would prefer not to be chaperoned.

- Most respondents felt receptionists were unsuitable as chaperones, with females preferring female nurses. Males were less likely to want a female nurse chaperone.

Whitford suggests a relative lack of males to act as chaperones could pose problems in future as relatively more women become NHS employees.

PROSTATE DISEASE

- A qualitative study found that patients who advocate PSA screening follow different principles than those used to plan population screening programmes
- Doctors and politicians must better understand public opinion, to provide better information regarding screening programmes and other such matters

BACKGROUND

BENIGN PROSTATIC HYPERTROPHY (BPH)

For many years transurethral resection of prostate was the most commonly available treatment for this condition. It at least doubles urinary flow rates and symptom scores, but because of complications (retrograde ejaculation occurs in 70%), it is best reserved for those with severe BPH. There are now many more treatments available for the treatment of BPH.

Finasteride is a selective 5-α reductase inhibitor, which blocks the conversion of testosterone to dihydrotestosterone. The effects are limited to the prostate and scrotal skin. Two large studies using 5 mg/day for 12 months reported reduced prostate size (by 20%), increased peak urine flow rate (by 20%) and improved symptom scores (by 20%). Most of the changes took 3-6 months to develop. Improvements may continue for up to 3 years.

The newer α-adrenergic blockers reduce smooth muscle tone in the bladder neck, urethra and prostatic capsule. Symptoms are improved within weeks. (Doxasozin is also useful in hypertension.) Efficacy is maintained for up to 30 months.

Unwanted effects

Finasteride reduces libido and ejaculate volume and increases the incidence of impotence. Gynaecomastia can occur. Prostate-specific antigen (PSA) can fall by 50%. This could mask a diagnosis of prostate cancer, which is important because finasteride is not indicated for the treatment of prostate cancer. It should be used with caution in those with obstructive symptoms because it takes weeks to work. Finasteride can be teratogenic to male fetuses, therefore women should be careful not to handle crushed or broken tablets. It is excreted in semen, therefore condoms should be worn for sexual intercourse. Osteoporosis is reported as a possible side effect. The α-blockers can cause hypotension, dizziness and sedation. They cause tiredness and nasal stuffiness in 10% of users.

In conclusion, surgery is appropriate for those with severe BPH. Drug treatment with finasteride or the more expensive α-blockers is appropriate in those for whom surgery is contraindicated or who have milder symptoms.

PROSTATE CANCER

Prostate cancer is the second most common cancer in men. At autopsy, 30% of men over 50 are found to have latent prostate cancer; only 1% have clinically significant disease. The 5-year survival for prostate cancer is 43%. It is often diagnosed late, when 60% have metastases. Most men are over the age of 60 at diagnosis.

Screening problems

- There are few potential years of life to save. Most subjects who do not have metastases die of something else.
- There is no evidence that screening or treatment will decrease mortality.
- There is enormous scope for over-diagnosis, for example detection of very mild disease which may have no impact on life except psychological and physical morbidity.
- There is as yet no valid test.
- There is no consensus on the most appropriate treatment.
- The side effects of treatment are problematic.
- The financial costs need to be taken into consideration.

Tests

- Digital;
- PSA;
- transurethral ultrasound.

Test sensitivity increases from the first to the third, but all still have a low sensitivity. PSA has high false-positive rates because of BPH. The way forward may be to use digital examination together with PSA and send for an ultrasound scan if one or both of these tests is abnormal. However, cancers will still be missed with this regime.

Two reviews commissioned by the NHS Health Technology Assessment programme and a summary by the NHS Centre for Reviews and Dissemination have recommended that routine screening for prostate cancer is not appropriate and they have discouraged purchasers from paying for it.

Why men with prostate cancer want wider access to prostate specific antigen testing: qualitative study. Chapple, A., Ziebland, S. and Shepperd, S. *et al.* DIPEx, Department of Primary Health Care, Institute of Health Sciences, University of Oxford, Oxford, UK. **BMJ, 325**(7367): 737-781, 5 October 2002.

This study qualitatively examined the views of 52 men, with suspected or confirmed prostate cancer, to prostate specific antigen testing.

- Most candidates were given little information about the test prior to having it, and the implications were only discussed following a positive result. Almost all participants discussing the concept of routine PSA testing were in favour of it. This was mainly due to a perceived better chance of a positive outcome if the cancer was found early, and to avoid regret at a later date that they were unaware of the cancer and could have had it diagnosed.

• Screening was generally viewed as a right, and a responsible behaviour similar to smear testing in women. Those favouring screening were of the opinion that poor advice, lack of funding, and shortage of resources to treat identified cancers, were the reasons a PSA screening programme does not exist. The four interviewees against screening thought such programmes would cause undue anxiety, and that no treatment could be provided for identified cancers, in any case.

The authors do not consider those advocating screening programmes to be uninformed; rather they follow different principles from those guiding screening programme planning. They conclude that politicians and doctors need to understand the reasons that men want access to screening, to allow better communication of the associated risks. This will allow those patients to make informed choices about whether or not to participate.

EDITORIAL – Prostate specific antigen testing for prostate cancer. Thornton, H. and Dixon-Woods, M. Department of Epidemiology and Public Health, University of Leicester, Leicester, UK.
***BMJ,* 325**(7367): 725-726, 5 October 2002.

Screening programmes are often futile; using ineffective tests to diagnose diseases that medicine is, as yet, unable to cure.

The public is keen for such initiatives to continue, and attempts to stop them are suspiciously viewed as being financially motivated or discriminatory. Traditionally, the medical community has considered this behaviour irrational; the authors suggest there is a need for greater understanding of the public by scientists, in order to allay these fears.

While the public retain their unshakeable faith in screening programmes, intensive screening appears to be of no benefit in the context of prostate cancer.

Medicalisation of those with positive results is the major disadvantage of such programmes. In addition to the financial costs, there may be loss of patients trust where doctors invite them for screening tests, diagnose an illness, and are then unable to provide an effective treatment.

The authors say engaging with the public will allow reconciliation between risk conscious citizens and cautious authorities. Investigating public concerns and beliefs, and responding appropriately, will result in better solutions for the interaction of individual concerns and public health spending.

They conclude better public engagement will ensure satisfactory outcomes for issues such as screening, which can have such far-reaching consequences.

RESPIRATORY INFECTIONS

COMMON COLD
• Well-conducted larger studies are required to answer the zinc question

OTITIS MEDIA AND GLUE EAR
• An α-streptococcal nasal spray may reduce recurrence of otitis media in children
• An analysis by John Bain has found that children with otitis media recruited to clinical trials are not representative of the cases we normally see in practice
• A study by Little *et al.* found that a delayed antibiotic prescribing strategy was associated with a 76% reduction in antibiotic use

INFLUENZA
• Vaccination should still be the mainstay of influenza management but the neuraminidase inhibitors may form a useful adjunct to this
• One study reports that zanamivir is unlikely to work in elderly patients unless better delivery systems are developed

COUGH
• A systematic review of the natural history of acute cough in children showed that for most children cough had resolved by 7 days

OTHERS
• Most cases of LRTi are treated with antibiotics but this does not seem to alter outcome
• A study by Dowell *et al.* found that delayed antibiotic prescribing can reduce antibiotic use. It may deter patients from consulting but these patients are less satisfied with their care and are less 'enabled' to deal with their illness
• Supplementation of verbal advice with an information leaflet decreased patients use of antibiotics in acute bronchitis
• Intranasal fluticasone might be a useful addition to cefuroxime in the treatment of acute rhinosinusitis, especially in patients with a known underlying allergy
• Oral dexamethasone is more effective than nebulized dexamethasone in the treatment of mild croup
• A literature review demonstrates which symptoms and clinical signs can be used to make a diagnosis of purulent sinusitis in General Practice
• Antibiotics are moderately beneficial in acute rhinitis, but should only be used in patients with persistent infection

BACKGROUND

SORE THROATS

A Cochrane review (18 trials, over 9000 patients: *EBM*, March/April 1998) looked at the efficacy of antibiotics for sore throats. They found that antibiotics reduce the incidence of rheumatic fever and quinsy at 2 months,

sore throat at 3 days and otitis media at 14 days. Looking at these crude results, one would be tempted to prescribe antibiotics for sore throats, but they state that the absolute reduction in risk of complications is small and hence, the benefits derived from treatment is likely to be small. One must also add the usual arguments concerning antibiotic treatment for URTIs, namely:
- cost;
- antibiotic resistance;
- adverse effects;
- legitimization of illness. An RCT by P Little *et al.* (*BMJ*, Aug. 1997) found that immediate prescribing of antibiotics compared with delayed prescribing increased re-attendance rates. Off-course, re-attendance could also be due to new or recurrent infection, which may be caused by antibiotics wiping out the normal flora.

Alternatives to immediate antibiotic treatment
- Delayed prescribing strategies. (P Little *et al.*, *BMJ*, March 1997 and Aug. 1997). Antibiotic use was reduced by 70% in the delayed prescribing group.

Other strategies include:
- NSAIDs and paracetamol;
- good doctor-patient communication;
- vaccination against pneumococcus;
- supracolonization of the upper respiratory tract.

COMMON COLD

Zinc acetate lozenges reduced the duration and severity of symptoms of the common cold. Commentator, Paul Little, University of Southampton, Southampton, UK. *Evidence–based Medicine,* **6**(2): 46, Mar./Apr. 2001.

Question: In patients with a common cold, do zinc acetate lozenges reduce the duration and severity of symptoms?

The following article is briefly presented
Duration of symptoms and plasma cytokine levels in patients with the common cold treated with zinc acetate. A randomized, double–blind, placebo–controlled trial. Prasad, A.S., Fitzgerald, J.T. and Bao, B. *et al. Ann. Intern. Med.,* **133:** 245–252, 15 Aug. 2000.

This RCT involved 50 USA volunteers who were identified within 24 hours of developing a cold. They were given either 12.8 mg of zinc acetate 2/3 hourly whilst awake or placebo.
- The zinc group had cold symptoms for 4.5 days compared with 8.1 days in the placebo group.

The study is underpowered and uses university volunteers which makes it difficult to extrapolate the findings. Well conducted larger studies are required to answer the zinc question.

OTITIS MEDIA AND GLUE EAR

Pragmatic randomised controlled trial of two prescribing strategies for childhood acute otitis media. Little, P., Gould, C. and Williamson, I. *et al.* Community Clinical Sciences (Primary Medical Care Group), University of Southampton, Aldermoor Health Centre, Southampton, UK.
BMJ, **322**(7282): 336-342, 10 February 2001.

The author claims this to be the largest RCT of antibiotic use for acute otitis media in primary care. The aim of the study was to compare immediate with delayed prescribing in children aged 6 months to 10 years presenting with acute otitis media. The study includes around 300 children from practices in southwest England. They are either given an immediate prescription or asked to wait at least 3 days before collecting their prescription from reception.

- They found that the immediate group recovered around one day earlier than the delayed group with less discharge, paracetamol use and crying at night.
- There was no difference in pain scores or days off school.
- Eleven percent more children in the immediate group had diarrhoea compared with the delayed group.
- Parents in the delayed group were less likely to believe in the effectiveness of antibiotics.
- The delayed strategy was associated with a 76% reduction in antibiotic use.
- The majority (77%) of the delayed group were very satisfied with their care.

Treatment of acute otitis media: are children entered into clinical trials representative? Bain, J. Professor of General Practice, Tayside Centre for General Practice, University of Dundee, Dundee, UK.
Br. J. Gen. Pract., **51**(463): 132-133, 1 February 2001.

This study asks whether children entered into clinical trials with otitis media are representative of the cases that we actually see in practice. He analyses eight trials. He finds that when one considers the number of cases a typical GP would be expected to see, the recruitment of otitis media cases by doctors is low. Half of the exclusions in studies occur because the GP has judged that the child needs antibiotics. This would suggest that the children who are entered into trials are those with mild or moderate episodes of otitis media. This may account for the fact that meta-analyses show that antibiotics are not helpful in acute otitis media.

Effect of recolonisation with 'interfering' α–streptococci on recurrences of acute and secretory otitis media in children: randomised placebo controlled trial. Roos, K., Hakansson, E.G. and Holm, S. Ear, Nose and Throat Department, Lundby Hospital, Gothenburg, Sweden.
BMJ, **322**(7280): 210-212, 27 January 2001.

Children prone to otitis media have been found to have low levels of α-streptococci. This is the dominant (normal) flora found in the upper respiratory tract. This Swedish study is an RCT involving 108 children who are prone to otitis media. The aim of the study is to assess whether re-colonization with a mixture of five strains of normal (α-streptococci) flora will reduce recurrences of otitis media. Half the children were randomized to receive a α-streptococcal nasal spray and half to receive placebo spray. They used the spray for two 10-day episodes over 2 months.

• At 3 months 42% of children in the α-streptococcal group were healthy compared with 22% in the placebo group.
• Recurrence of secretory otitis media was significantly lower in the streptococcal group compared with the control group.

The authors point out that antibiotics wipe out normal flora, as well as the bacteria causing the infection. Multiple courses of antibiotics, not only increase drug resistance but also may promote further infections, by hampering the body's natural defence system.

INFLUENZA

Comparison of elderly people's technique in using two dry powder inhalers to deliver zanamivir: randomised controlled trial. Diggory, P., Fernandez, C. and Humphrey, A. *et al.* Department of Elderly Care Medicine, Mayday Hospital, Croydon, UK.
BMJ, **322**(7286): 577-579, 10 March 2001.

The aim of this RCT was to assess elderly people's technique in using the Diskhaler to deliver zanamivir. Just over 70 elderly patients recovering in hospital were allocated to either Diskhaler or Turbohaler. Patients were scored on their technique.

• Just under 60% of patients in the Turbohaler group achieved perfect scores for technique compared with around one quarter in the Diskhaler group.
• The biggest difference between the two groups was for loading and priming the device.
• Twenty-four hours after being shown, nearly 70% (24 of 37) of the Diskhaler group had poor loading and priming scores compared with only one person out of 32 in the Turbohaler group.

They conclude that zanamivir is unlikely to work in elderly patients unless better delivery systems are developed.

COUGH

The natural history of acute cough in children aged 0–4 years in primary care: a systematic review. Hay, A.D. and Wilson, A.D. Division of Primary Health Care, University of Bristol, Cotham Hill, Bristol, UK.
Br. J. Gen. Pract., **52**(478): 401-409, 1 May 2002.

Approximately £20 million of the annual NHS budget is spent on consultations and antibiotic prescription for cough in the pre-school age group. It is thought that uncertainty amongst doctors and patients about the natural history and complications of acute cough in pre-school children contributes to the high rate of antibiotic use and re-consultation. This systematic review aimed to clarify the natural history of acute cough. Eight RCTs and two cohort studies met the inclusion criteria. The meta-analysis found:

- At 1 day after consultation 60% of children have improved symptoms, this rises to 75% at 7 days and 100% at 28 days. However, 1 week after consultation 50% of cases have not completely resolved.
- Within 2 weeks of consultation, 12% of children experience a complication of acute cough.
- Earache (18%) and rash (20%) are the commonest complications, with no deaths occurring in any study.

OTHERS

EDITORIAL – Antibiotics for purulent rhinitis. Arroll, B. and Kenealy, T. Department of General Practice and Primary Health Care, University of Auckland, Auckland, New Zealand.
BMJ, **325**(7376): 1311-1312, 7 December 2002.

Antibiotics are prescribed for 60% of upper respiratory tract infections, despite efforts to lower this figure. Guidelines recommend against using antibiotics for mucopurulent rhinitis, for which they are generally ineffective. However, the colour of nasal discharge has been shown to double the likelihood of patients being given antibiotics.

The authors suggest these guidelines be re-examined, as recent trials have suggested a role for antibiotics in reducing the duration of purulent symptoms. They cite various studies showing the beneficial effects of antibiotics in treating rhinitis, and highlighting flaws in the logic of papers and guidelines stating the opposite.

They conclude there may be evidence to support using antibiotics in acute rhinitis, though is it unclear exactly which patients will benefit. Guidelines advising against antibiotic use may be incorrect in saying they are ineffective. Antibiotics have a modest beneficial effect, though guidelines correctly highlight valid reasons for minimising their use increased bacterial resistance, drug side effects and cost to the NHS in conditions such as rhinitis, which are rarely life threatening.

It is suggested that doctors should treat the symptoms of rhinitis. Antibiotics should be avoided in the early stages of illness, when they are less effective, and used only in those with persistent infection, where they are likely to be most useful.

Verbal advice plus an information leaflet reduced antibiotic use in acute bronchitis.
Becker, Lorne A. SUNY Upstate Medical University, Syracuse, NY, USA.
Evidence-based Medicine, 7(4): 119, July/Aug. 2002.

Question: In patients presenting with acute bronchitis, does verbal advice plus an information leaflet describing the uncertain value of antibiotics reduce antibiotic use more than verbal advice alone?

The following article is briefly presented

Reducing antibiotic use for acute bronchitis in primary care: blinded, randomised controlled trial of patient information leaflet. MacFarlane, J., Holmes, W., Gard, P. *et al.* Nottingham City Hospital, Nottingham, UK. *BMJ* **324:** 91-94, 12 Jan. 2002.

This study was a RCT conducted in three general practices in Nottingham. Two hundred and twelve patients with acute bronchitis not judged to require immediate antibiotics were included. All patients received a prescription for antibiotics and verbal advice regarding advantages and disadvantages of antibiotics. Further to this, patients were randomly allocated to control (no additional information) and intervention (given an additional antibiotic information leaflet) groups. The main outcome measures were use of the prescribed antibiotics within 2 weeks, and representation with the same symptoms within 4 weeks.

* Fewer patients of the leaflet group took their antibiotics than of the control group.
* The groups did not differ in rates of representation

The authors concluded that the supplementation of verbal advice with an information leaflet reduced antibiotic use for acute bronchitis.

Commentary

Becker comments that prescription with information is clearly not the final answer, as half of the patients ended up taking antibiotics that were not considered to be entirely necessary by the doctor. However, she suggests that such prescribing with both verbal and written information might be a useful strategy in patients who will not happily leave without a prescription for antibiotics.

Adding intranasal fluticasone to cefuroxime resolved acute rhinosintis.
Willett, L. Robert Wood Johnson Medical School, New Brunswick, NJ, USA.
Evidence-based Medicine, 7(4): 117, July/Aug. 2002.

Question: In patients with acute rhinosinusitis and a history of chronic or recurrent sinus symptoms, is the addition of intranasal fluticasone to cefuroxime more effective than the addition of placebo for prompting recovery?

The following article is briefly presented
Comparison of cefuroxime with or without intranasal fluticasone for the treatment of rhinosinusitis. The CAFFS Trial: a randomised controlled trial. Dolor, R.J., Witsell, D.I., Helkamp, A.S., *et al.*, for the Ceftin and Flonase for Dinusitis (CAFFS) Investigators. Duke Clinical Research Institute, Durham, North Carolina, USA.
JAMA **286**: 3097-105 26 Dec. 2001.

This study was a RCT conducted at 12 primary care and 10 otolaryngology sites in the USA. Ninety-two adult patients with recurrent or chronic sinusitis requiring antibiotic treatment were included. All patients received a 10-day course of cefuroxime axetil, and a 3-day course of xylometazoline hydrochloride per nostril. Following this, patients were randomised to receive either intranasal fluticasone propionate or placebo for 21 days. The main outcome measure was a 6-point scale of clinical success (whether the patients felt cured, improved, the same, or worse), as reported at telephone interview.
  • More patients who received fluticasone than placebo achieved clinical success.
  • More of the fluticasone group achieved improvement in fewer days than the placebo group.
The authors conclude that the addition of intranasal fluticasone to cefuroxime was more effective than placebo in achieving cure or improvement of acute rhinosinusitis, in patients with chronic or recurrent sinus symptoms.

Commentary
Willett comments that up to a half of patients included in this study had a known diagnosis of allergic addition in addition to recurrent or chronic sinusitis. For this reason, she does not believe that this study proves that fluticasone speeds the resolution of acute rhinosinusitis unrelated to allergy. However, given that atopy and rhinosinusitis frequently coexist, fluticasone might be a useful addition to cefuroxime, especially in patients with an underlying allergy or recurrent episodes of rhinosinusotis

Oral dexamethasone led to fewer treatment failures than did nebulised dexamethasone or placebo in children with mild croup. Paton, J. Royal Hospital for Sick Children, Glasgow, Scotland.
Evidence-based Medicine, 7(4): 113, July/Aug. 2002.

Question: In children with mild croup, does oral dexamethasone decrease the need for subsequent treatments and care and shorten symptom duration more than nebulised dexamethasone or placebo?

The following article is briefly presented
Effectiveness of oral or nebulised dexamethasone for children with mild croup. Luria, J.W., Gonzalez-del-Rey, J.A., DiGulio, G.A. *et al.* Childrens Hospital Medical Centre, Cincinnati, OH, USA.
Arch. Pediatr. Adolesc. Med. **155:** 1340-1345, Dec. 2001.

This study was a RCT conducted in Ohio, USA. Just under 270 children (6 months-6 years old) with symptoms of mild croup for less than 48 hours, were allocated to oral dexamethasone with nebulized placebo, oral placebo with nebulized dexamethasone, or oral and nebulized placebos. The main outcome was treatment failure requiring a further prescription of either corticosteroids or racemic epinephrine.
- There was lower risk of treatment failure with oral treatment, than with nebulized treatment or placebo only.
- Treatment failure did not differ between nebulized treatment and placebo groups

The authors conclude that in children with mild croup, treatment failure is decreased by the use of oral dexamethasone, compared to nebulized dexamethasone or placebo.

Commentary
Paton notes that this study confirms the effectiveness of oral dexamethasone in the treatment of croup. He suggests that the observed ineffectiveness of nebulized dexamethasone, which conflicts with the results of a meta-analysis, could result from inappropriately low doses of nebulized dexamethasone in this study. Finally, he suggests that more research is needed, in order to determine whether less potent steroids might also be effective, and whether combined oral and nebulized steroids might be useful in severe croup

Review: The clinical diagnosis of acute purulent sinusitis In general practice: a review. Lindbaek, M. and Hjortdahl, P. Department of General Practice, University of Oslo, Oslo, Norway.
Br. J. Gen. Pract., 52(6): 491-495, 1 June 2002.

Acute sinusitis, can present as a purulent or serous form. The purulent form benefits from antibiotic treatment. The gold standard for diagnosis of sinusitis is sinus puncture. In clinical practice diagnosis of uncomplicated cases is made by history taking and examination. Differentiating between the two presentations can be difficult, thus many patients who do not require antibiotic therapy receive treatment. This paper aimed to review the literature relating to the diagnosis of acute sinusitis, and propose historical findings and clinical signs which help differentiate serous from purulent sinusitis. The authors found:Purulent rhinnorhoea was associated with purulent sinusitis in three of the four studies.Pain in the teeth was associated with purulent sinusitis in two of the four studies.Clinical signs associated with purulent sinusitis were pain in the sinuses on bending forwards and purulent secretions in the nasal cavity.

Symptoms, signs and prescribing for acute lower respiratory tract illness. Holmes, W.F., Macfarlane, J.T., Macfarlane, R.M. and Hubbard, R. Department of Respiratory Medicine, Nottingham City Hospital, Nottingham, UK.
Br. J. Gen. Pract., **51**(464): 177-181, 1 March 2001.

This study examines GP prescribing for acute lower respiratory tract illness (LRTi). They describe LRTi as an illness where cough is the main feature, with at least one other lower respiratory tract symptom and with no other explanation for the cough e.g. cardiac, asthma, sinusitis. Just over 300 patients recruited by 40 GPs were seen and followed up at 10 days.

- Just over 70% of patients received antibiotics.
- One quarter had abnormal signs on auscultation.
- Abnormal chest signs increased the likelihood of the patient receiving a prescription.
- However 64% of patients who received antibiotics had no abnormal signs.
- At 10 days nearly two thirds of patients still had a cough.

They conclude that physical signs at presentation are not helpful at predicting outcome in patients presenting with LRTi. Other studies with longer follow up report cough persisting for 3 weeks.

A randomised controlled trial of delayed antibiotic prescribing as a strategy for managing uncomplicated respiratory tract infection in primary care. Dowell, J., Pitkethly, M., Bain, J. and Martin, S. Tayside Centre for General Practice, University of Dundee, UK.
Br. J. Gen. Pract., **51**(464): 200-205, 1 March 2001.

This RCT involved around 190 patients. The aim was to assess the effectiveness of delayed prescribing strategies for the management of 'cough' in general practice. Patients were randomized to receive either an immediate prescription or were asked to wait at least a week before collecting a prescription that had been left for them at reception.

- At 2 weeks there was no difference in clinical outcome between the two groups.
- Fifty-five percent of people in the delayed group did not pick up their prescription.
- People in the delayed arm were less satisfied with their care than people in the immediate group.

- Consultation rates in the following 6 months did not differ between the groups.
- Patients in the delayed arm were less likely to feel 'enabled' to manage their illness than people in the immediate group.
- People in the immediate group said that they intended to consult their GP for future episodes of cough.
- At 6 months, nearly 70% of the 92 GPs who took part said that they used delayed prescribing regularly.

They conclude that delayed prescribing can reduce antibiotic use. It may deter patients from consulting but these patients are less satisfied with their care and are less 'enabled' to deal with their illness.

SMOKING

- A re-analysis of the Hackshaw data on passive smoking shows a relative risk of lung cancer of 15% rather than the first published 24%
- Female smokers have a higher relative risk of MI than male smokers
- Intervention to cease/decrease smoking preoperatively reduces morbidity following joint replacement.
- One study found that self-help approaches to smoking cessation in pregnancy are ineffective when delivered by midwives as part of routine care.
- Most national smoking cessation guidelines are evidence based
- The media is a powerful influence on the publics perceptions of new pharmacological treatments, and should not be underestimated by doctors.
- Continuous promotion of smoking cessation amongst angina patients can be effective, and should be encouraged.

BACKGROUND

Lung cancer and CHD are the most common fatal conditions caused by tobacco, which is responsible for 30% of all deaths in the UK.

- A prospective study by Doll and Peto, which began in 1951 and involved 35 000 male British doctors (*BMJ*, Oct. 1994), found that smoking is associated with excess mortality from the following diseases: cancer of the mouth, oesophagus, larynx, pharynx and lung, chronic obstructive airways disease (COAD), and other respiratory and vascular diseases. Doctors who stopped smoking by the age of 35 reduced their risk to zero.
- Another prospective study (Rimm *et al.BMJ*, 1995) involving 40 000 men found that smoking over 15 cigarettes per day was associated with a doubled risk of developing type 2 diabetes. Having 2-4 alcohol containing drinks per day was associated with a decreased risk of developing diabetes.
- A study published in *JAMA* (Wannamethee *et al.* 1995) found that life-long smokers have a nearly four-fold increased risk of having a stroke. The risk in ex-smokers was found to be nearly twice that in non-smokers. Benefits from stopping smoking can be seen within 5 years.

The risks experienced by smokers are likely to affect those living in close proximity to the smoker. Also, smoking in pregnancy is known to be associated with low-birth weight babies.

- A study in *Pediatrics* (DiFranza, 1996) found that the use of tobacco products by adults increases childhood mortality and morbidity (otitis media, tonsillitis, asthma, coughs, etc).
- Breathing other people's smoke increases one's risk of IHD by up to 30% (Law *et al.,BMJ*, 1997; Hackshaw *et al.*, *BMJ*, 1997). Tobacco-specific carcinogens are found in the blood and urine of non-smokers exposed to environmental tobacco smoke.

Smoking cessation can be improved by brief intervention in general practice. Five per cent of people will stop smoking after receiving advice from their GP. Two meta-analyses showed that nicotine replacement therapy as an adjunct to brief advice was associated with a 10% cessation rate sustained for 1 year.

An advertising ban could cut consumption by 6%. This would prevent more deaths than the breast and cervical screening programmes combined. People are more likely to be successful at quitting if they:
- smoked for psychological reasons;
- smoked to be sociable;
- perceived more support from people around them.

People are more likely to fail if they:
- see smoking as a health risk;
- have tried multiple methods;
- experience withdrawal symptoms.

One study (Townsend, *BMJ*, 1994) found that price setting could be used as an effective preventive public health tool, especially in men and women from social class five, the very group with the highest prevalence of smoking.

MORTALITY AND MORBIDITY

A preoperative smoking intervention decreased postoperative complications in elective knee or hip replacement. Kozak, E. Spectrum Health Primary Care Partners, Grand Rapids, MI, USA.
Evidence-based Medicine, 7(4): 112, July/Aug. 2002.

Question: **In patients having elective knee or hip replacement, is a preoperative smoking intervention more effective than usual care for reducing post-operative morbidity and mortality?**

The following article is briefly presented
Effect of preoperative smoking intervention on postoperative complications: a randomised clinical trial. Moller, A.M., Villebro, N., Pederson, T. *et al.*
Bispebjerg University Hospital, Copenhagen, Denmark.
Lancet **359**: 114-117, 12 Jan. 2002.

This study was a RCT conducted in Copenhagen, Denmark. Just over 100 patients who were daily smokers and scheduled for primary elective hip or knee alloplasty were included. Sixty patients were randomly allocated to the smoking intervention. Six to 8 weeks before surgery, these patients were offered weekly meetings with the project nurse, involving testing of nicotine intake and dependence, encouragement to stop or reduce smoking, supply of nicotine substitution products, advice and education.

The remainder of patients received little or no information or counselling on smoking.

The main outcome measures were death and post-operative morbidity requiring treatment.

- No patients died before discharge.
- Rates of post-operative complications were lower in the smoking intervention group (18%) than in the non-intervention group (52%).

The authors conclude that a pre-operative smoking intervention reduced post-operative complications in patients undergoing elective knee or hip replacement.

Commentary

Kozak notes that certain features of the study design limit the ability to generalise these results. For example, the study was performed in Denmark, where the median hospital stay was 12 days (compared with 5 days in the USA). For this reason, it is suggested that the study should be replicated in other settings. Kozak also recommends that a cost-benefit analysis should be performed.

Reanalysis of epidemiological evidence on lung cancer and passive smoking.
Copas, J.B. and Shi, J.Q. Department of Statistics, University of Warwick, Coventry, UK.
BMJ, **320**(7232): 417-418, 12 February 2000.

A meta-analysis by Hackshaw *et al.* (*BMJ*, 1997) reported that inhaling environmental tobacco smoke could increase the risk of lung cancer by 24%. This present study is a reanalysis of the data to take publication bias into consideration. Publication bias arises when studies are not written up or selected for publication, usually because the results are negative or inconclusive.

- The re-analysis shows that there is a substantial reduction in the relative risk of lung cancer from 24% to 15%.

Mortality in relation to smoking: 40 years' observations on male British doctors.
Doll, R., Peto, R., Wheatley, K., Gray, R. and Sutherland, I. Imperial Cancer Research Fund Cancer Studies Unit, Nuffield Department of Clinical Medicine, Radcliffe Infirmary, Oxford, UK.
BMJ, **309**(6959): 901-911, 8 October 1994.

In two case-control studies performed in 1950, Doll and Wynder reported on the association between cigarette smoking and lung cancer. This current prospective study, which began 40 years ago in 1951, was largely in response to this evidence. Questionnaires were sent at intervals to 40 000 male British doctors. They report on the results of just over 34 000 of these subjects. Early results have not only confirmed the association between lung cancer and smoking but also found smoking to be related to deaths from other diseases.

- They found an excess mortality in the following diseases: cancer of the mouth, oesophagus, larnyx, pharynx, lung, pancreas, chronic obstructive airways disease and other respiratory and vascular diseases.
- They found a negative association between smoking and Parkinson's disease.
- Doctors who had stopped smoking by the age of 35 reduced their risk back down to zero.
- They also found excess mortality due to suicide, cirrhosis and poisoning.

The authors conclude that half of all cigarette smokers are eventually killed by their habit.

CESSATION

Self help smoking cessation in pregnancy: cluster randomised controlled trial.
Moore, L., Campbell, R. and Whelan, A. *et al*. Cardiff University School of Social Sciences, Cardiff, UK.
BMJ, **325**(7377): 1383-1388, 14 December 2002.

This cluster RCT evaluated the effectiveness of a self-help approach to smoking cessation in pregnancy, in 1527 women who smoked at the beginning of pregnancy. Subjects were from three hospital NHS trusts in England. Midwives distributed five self-help booklets to the intervention half of the cohort. This had a step-by-step programme to motivate them to stop smoking, supported by behavioural strategies to help them succeed. The control group received only normal pregnancy care.
- There was no significant difference in validated smoking cessation rates at the end of the second trimester, between the intervention and control groups (18.8% and 20.7% respectively).
- Qualitative findings revealed that the time spent introducing the intervention varied across the intervention group.

Lack of verbal reinforcement may have contributed to the interventions failure. The authors suggested that the context and audience of such interventions are also highly influential with regards to the success or failure of the initiative. Interventions may be more effective when delivered by dedicated staff.

Use of systematic reviews in clinical practice guidelines: case study of smoking cessation. Silagy, C.A., Stead, L.F. and Lancaster, T. Monash Institute of Health Services Research, Monash Medical Centre, Clayton, Victoria, Australia.
BMJ, **323**(7317): 833-836, 13 October 2001.

This study examined the extent to which national guidelines for smoking cessation are based upon evidence from systematic reviews (in particular those from the Cochrane library). The authors assessed the national smoking cessation guidelines for the United Kingdom, United States, Canada and New Zealand to determine what evidence there was to underpin each recommendation. It was found that:

- Fifty nine percent of UK, 56% of New Zealand, 47% of US and 60% of Canadian recommendations were based on evidence from systematic reviews (both Cochrane and non-Cochrane reviews).
- Cochrane reviews could have been utilised to formulate 39-73% of recommendations, but only 0–36% of recommendations were based upon Cochrane reviews.
- The US guidelines made least use of Cochrane reviews, performing 26 new meta-analyses to develop their guidelines, while the UK guidelines made most use of Cochrane reviews.

It is suggested that greater use of Cochrane reviews to underpin guidelines may save money by preventing duplication of research.

OTHERS

EDITORIAL – The power of the press in smokers' attempts to quit. Hyder Ferry, L. Associate Professor, Departments of Preventive Medicine and Family Medicine, Loma Linda University School of Medicine, Loma Linda, CA USA.
BMJ, 324(7350): 1346-1347, 8 June 2002.

Public opinion of new medical treatments is greatly influenced by their coverage in both print and television media. Recently, bupropion hydrochloride was heralded in the press as the new wonderdrug that would cure people of their smoking addiction. This prescription-only, non-nicotine agent was subsequently reported to be causally linked to the deaths of a number of smokers using it. Prescriptions declined from nearly 30 to just 20 in the space of a few months. This scenario is reminiscent of the media hype surrounding the suggested link between nicotine patches and myocardial infarctions in America a decade ago. In both cases, the Medicines Control Agency and the National Institute of Clinical Excellence, refuted the links, but the damage could not be undone. The media is a powerful influence on patients' perceptions of new medications, and doctors should be aware of this when deciding to prescribe new pharmacological treatments.

NICE have given clear guidance about the safety of both nicotine replacement and bupropion hydrochloride.

PRIMARY CARE SECTION – Quitting and restarting smoking: cohort study of patients with angina in primary care. Corrigan, M., Cupples, M.E. and Stevenson, M. Department of General Practice, Queen's University, Belfast.
BMJ, 324(7344): 1016-1017, 27 April 2002.

Much research has examined the smoking habits of patients with coronary heart disease following acute cardiac events. This study investigated smoking amongst a cohort of about 500 patients over a 5-year period. All patients were diagnosed as having angina at least 6 months previously, and were interviewed at baseline and at 2 and 5 years.

• More than half the participants changed their smoking habits over the 5-year period.
• About 5% of baseline non-smokers subsequently reported smoking.
• More than a third of baseline smokers reported quitting during the study.

These results suggest that promoting smoking cessation amongst cardiovascular patients can be effective.

STROKE

- A qualitative study found that that few people are able to recognize the symptoms of stroke and this is likely to delay presentation to medical services
- HOPE study found that ramipril reduced risk of fatal strokes by 61%.
- The presence of atrial fibrillation is associated with a significant increase in the prevalence of other risk factors for ischaemic stroke.

BACKGROUND

BLOOD PRESSURE AND STROKE

Fatal strokes tend to be haemorrhagic and there is a known association between increasing diastolic blood pressure and haemorrhagic stroke. A study by Rodgers *et al.* (*BMJ*, July 1996) found that:

- each 5 mmHg lower diastolic blood pressure was associated with 34% fewer strokes, and each 10 mmHg lower systolic blood pressure was associated with 28% fewer strokes;
- each 1 mmHg decrease in diastolic blood pressure was associated with one less stroke per 100 people over a 4-year period.

Another study, by Du *et al.* (*BMJ*, Jan. 1997) found that:

- the quality of the blood pressure control in the 5 years before the stroke was significantly associated with risk of stroke;
- controlling blood pressure to below 150/90 reduced the risk of stroke by 53%;
- in terms of NNT: 86 hypertensive patients would need to be controlled below 150/90 over a 5-year period to prevent one stroke.

ANTICOAGULATION FOR NON-VALVULAR ATRIAL FIBRILLATION

Anticoagulation with warfarin is recommended for patients aged 65-74 with non-valvular atrial fibrillation for the prevention of stroke. The target range for INR should be 2.0-3.0. The risk of stroke increases with INRs below and above this range. The use of aspirin with low-dose warfarin is not as effective as adjusted dose warfarin (Stroke Prevention in Atrial Fibrillation Investigators, *Lancet,* Sept. 1996).

Perceptions of stroke in the general public and patients with stroke: a qualitative study. Yoon, S.S. and Byles, J. Centre for Clinical Epidemiology and Biostatistics, Faculty of Medicine and Health Sciences, University of Newcastle, New South Wales, Australia.
BMJ, 324(7345): 1065-1068, 4 May 2002.

Studies have shown that stroke outcome is improved if the symptoms are recognised early. In this qualitative study a series of four focus group discussions were conducted, with a total of 35 participants in order to ascertain people's thoughts about stroke and to plan educational strategies in the community. Fourteen people had previously had a stroke, 10 were carers and 11 were members of the general public. The author highlights a number of points:

- Patients avoid thinking about any illness or other adverse events, regarding the thought of illness as an unnecessary additional worry.

- People were likely to seek urgent medical attention if they experienced difficulties with their speech, although they would not associate numbness, tingling sensations, weakness or paralysis of one side of the body with a need to seek urgent treatment.

- There were mixed feelings about the extent that patients felt involved in management decisions affecting their medical condition.

- People expected their general practitioner to be the primary source of information relating to stroke. This information should be simple and understandable.

Use of ramipril in preventing stroke: double blind randomised trial. Bosch, J., Yusuf, S. and Pogue, J. *et al* on behalf of the HOPE Investigators.
BMJ, 324(7339): 699-702, 23 March 2002.

and

EDITORIAL – Preventing stroke. Schrader, J. and Lüder, S. Medizinische Klinik, St Josefs Hospital, Cloppenburg, Germany.
BMJ, 324(7339): 687-688, 23 March 2002.

The aim of this part of the HOPE study was to evaluate the effect of ramipril on the secondary prevention of stroke. The HOPE study is a double blind RCT with a 2 x 2 design, whereby patients receive either 10 mg of ramipril, 400 IU of vitamin E or both or placebo. Just under 9300 patients (average age 66) from 19 countries take part in the study. All patients have vascular disease or diabetes plus one extra risk factor. Follow up was for 4.5 years.

- They found that fatal stroke was reduced by 61% and any non-fatal stroke by 24% in the ramipril group compared with placebo.

- Those who did suffer with a stroke were better off if they were taking ramipril. Cognitive and functional status, sleep and swallowing were better in the ramipril group.

- The effect on blood pressure was minimal (3.8 mmHg/2.8 mmHg)

- The reduced risk of stroke was seen across all blood pressure ranges, even in those with a normal blood pressure. The editorial highlights several points.
- The HOPE study is not a hypertension study. They excluded anyone with uncontrolled blood pressure. They point out that hypertension is still the primary risk factor for hypertension. The PROGRESS study (Lancet, 2001) using perindopril and indapamide, found that a 9/4 mmHg reduction in blood pressure resulted in a 28% reduction in risk of stroke.
- This and other studies suggest that ACE inhibitors have an effect on blood vessels which prevents the development of atherosclerotic plaques.
- The higher dose of 10 mg of ramipril worked better than the 2.5 mg dose.
- Patients taking aspirin or with a previous history of a cerebral event do less well on ramipril.
- It is unclear whether one would get the same effect from other ACE inhibitors. The HOPE authors suggest that ACE inhibitors be used for the primary and secondary prevention of stroke.

Comorbidity associated with atrial fibrillation: a general practice-based study.
Caroll, K. and Majeed, A. Office for National Statistics, London, UK.
Br. J. Gen. Pract., **51**: 884-891, 1 November 2001.

Although it is known that atrial fibrillation is an important risk factor for ischaemic stroke, little is known about the comorbidity associated with it. The objectives of this study were to determine the prevalence of known risk factors for ischaemic stroke in patients and the prevalence of contraindications to anticoagulant treatment among patients with atrial fibrillation. This was a 1 year prospective cohort study was set in 60 general practices in England and Wales with a total population of just over 500 000 people and is the largest population based study so far in the UK to examine the comorbidity associated with atrial fibrillation. The main results were:
- There was an increase in the prevalence of other risk factors for ischaemic stroke in patients with atrial fribillation with age, from 48% at 45-64 years to 64% at 75 years and over.
- Forty percent of patients with atrial fibrillation had at least one other risk factor for ischaemic stroke but no contraindications to anticoagulation.

The authors describe the papers strengths as its large population size and its rigorous data collection and validation procedures.

TEENAGERS

PREGNANCY AND CONTRACEPTION
• Teenage pregnancy rates in Scotland are associated with level of deprivation

OTHERS
• Teenagers having their second child are more at risk of adverse perinatal outcomes than older mothers.
• An Australian study has confirmed an association between bullying and onset of anxiety/depression in early teenagers.
• Young people (especially smokers) are actively involved in and receive benefit from tobacco marketing.
• Teacher-delivered sex education may be at the limit of its ability to influence sexual health among adolescents.
• Current primary interventions are ineffective at delaying first sexual intercourse, increasing use of contraceptives, and preventing unwanted teenage pregnancies.

BACKGROUND

Teenage pregnancy rates in the UK are amongst the highest in Europe. Strategies to reduce teenage pregnancies include:
• provision of services for teenagers;
• dealing with sexual education and peer group pressure;
• recognizing and dealing with the complex 'risky behaviour triangle', which includes mental illness, substance abuse and early age at first intercourse;
• recognizing and dealing with the socio-economic determinants of teenage pregnancies.

PREGNANCY AND CONTRACEPTION

Changing patterns of teenage pregnancy: population based study of small areas.
McLeod, A. MRC Social and Public Health Sciences Unit, University of Glasgow, Glasgow, UK.
***BMJ*, 323**(7306): 199-203, 28 July 2001.

This study uses hospital data to evaluate the effects of deprivation on teenage pregnancy rates in Scotland, over a 10-year period (1981-1985 to 1991-1995).
• For deprived teenagers aged under 18, pregnancy rates increased over the 10-year period, but did not change for teenagers from more affluent areas.

- For 18-19 year olds, pregnancy rates increased in deprived areas but decreased in more affluent areas.
- The proportion of pregnancies resulting in births was positively associated with deprivation level.
- In the 1990s, deprivation explained more than 50% of the variation in local pregnancy rates.

They discuss the bias inherent in using only hospital data. They point out that teenagers from affluent areas may have had a significant amount of care provided in the private sector compared with teenagers from deprived areas. It is likely that the reasons for the deprivation effect are complex, involving provision of contraceptive services, sex education as well as attitudes towards teenage pregnancy and job opportunities in the local area.

OTHERS

Limits of teacher delivered sex education: interim behavioural outcomes from randomised trial. Wight, D., Raab, G.M. and Henderson, M. *et al*. Medical Research Council Social and Public Health Sciences Unit, Glasgow, UK.
BMJ, **324**(7351): 1430-1435, 15 June 2002.

Sex education is believed to positively influence sexual behaviour; however few studies have illustrated this. This randomised trial investigated the effect of a new sex education program, "SHARE", aimed at 3rd and 4th year (13–15 year olds) in Scotland, during the period 1996-1999. The programme involved 20 academic sessions. Twenty-five non-Catholic state secondary schools in the East of Scotland were recruited and assigned to the intervention or control group, (who continued with any existing sex education programmes). Follow up data was collected by questionnaire, interviews, group discussion and classroom observation.

- There was no difference between the control and intervention groups in their use of contraception at the first and most recent sexual intercourse.
- There was no difference between the groups in regretting first intercourse or enjoyment of most recent intercourse.
- The intervention group were more knowledgeable about sexual health and had better coverage of practical sexual health issues.
- Students rated the new programme more positively than comparative courses.

The authors say that more subjects than had been expected already used condoms, so it may be more challenging for the intervention to further increase their use. They also suggest that school classes were too short to sufficiently develop skills that could be recalled at the appropriate time; skills-based classes required more motivation on the part of students; and that family, local culture and mass media had a more significant influence on the sexual health of adolescents.

It was pointed out that students having their first sexual intercourse during the study period were the least likely to respond to the intervention. Sex education programmes may have influenced students in control schools.

The authors conclude that conventional teacher-delivered sex education may have reached the limits of its ability to influence sexual behaviour in adolescents; other means of delivery should be investigated in future studies.

Interventions to reduce unintended pregnancies amongst adolescents: systematic review of randomised controlled trials. DiCenso, A., Guyatt, G. and Willan, A. *et al.* School of Nursing, McMaster University, Hamilton, Ontario, Canada.
BMJ, 324(7351): 1426-1434, 15 June 2002.

Di Censo et al. systematically review 26 RCTs investigating the effectiveness of interventions intended to lower unwanted teenage pregnancy.

- They found that primary prevention strategies did not delay initiation of first sexual intercourse, or increase use of contraception.

The authors point out that control groups in most studies received a conventional intervention, and so results do not indicate the efficacy of the strategy compared to no intervention. Additionally, lower socio-economic groups were over-represented in many of the studies; perhaps the interventions would have been more successful in other social groupings.

They conclude that there is no useful solution available to tackle the high rates of unwanted teenage pregnancy. They note that adolescent feedback on current strategies tends to focus on negative rather than positive aspects of sexual relationships, and comment that it may be helpful to involve adolescents in designing strategies to lower teenage pregnancy rates.

How do teenagers and primary healthcare providers view each other? An overview of key themes. Jacobson, L., Richardson, G., Parry-Langdon, N. and Donovan, C. Department of General Practice, University of Wales College of Medicine, Llanedyrn Health Centre, Cardiff, UK.
Br. J. Gen. Pract., 51(471): 811-816, 1 October 2001.

This combined qualitative and quantitative study uses a questionnaire, focus groups and interviews to assess teenagers and health professionals views of one another. Around 2300 teenagers were sent questionnaires and around 1100 responded. Sixteen GPs, 12 nurses and 12 receptionists also took part in the study. Some of the themes that emerged were

- Teenagers apprehension at approaching reception and being made to feel that they were bothering the doctor; and having to tell the reception about their condition.
- Some teenagers expressed concerns about being stared at or recognised in the waiting room.

- Concerns were expressed about the GP not listening or understanding about teenage problems. GPs tended to want to focus on risk taking behaviour and admitted not being knowledgeable about modern teenage issues.
- Teenagers were concerned about confidentiality.
- Teenagers had poor knowledge about available services.
- Some practices insisted on teenagers under the age of 16 being accompanied by an older adult.
- Overall, nearly 90% of teenagers said they were happy with the health care they received.

Teenage pregnancy and risk of adverse perinatal outcomes associated with first and second births: population based retrospective cohort study. Smith, G.C. and Pell, J.P. Department of Obstetrics and Gynaecology, University of Glasgow, Glasgow, UK. **BMJ, 323**(7311): 476-479, 1 September 2001.

The aim of this retrospective study was to assess the relationship between teenage pregnancy and adverse perinatal outcomes e.g. small for gestational age, still births, extreme prematurity. They compare 15-19 year olds with 20–29 year olds. Records are analyzed from the Scottish morbidity 2 (SMR 2) database.
- Compared with older mothers, there was no difference in perinatal outcomes for first births. Teenagers were less likely to have an emergency caesarean section than older mothers.
- For second births, there was a nearly three-fold increased risk for extreme prematurity and still births.
- The results were the same in smokers as well as non-smokers.

Does bullying cause emotional problems? A prospective study of young teenagers. Bond, L., Carlin, J.B. and Thomas, L. *et al.* Centre for Adolescent Health, Royal Childrens Hospital, Victoria, Australia. **BMJ, 323**(7311): 480-484, 1 September 2001.

The aim of this 2-year prospective Australian study, was to assess the relationship between victimization (bullying) e.g. being teased, excluded, threatened in year 8 students and onset of anxiety and depression in year 9. The study was part of a randomized trial of an intervention to promote wellbeing in young people. Around 2600 children took part in the study. They were surveyed twice in year 8 and again in year 9.
- One third reported victimization in year 8.
- Of those victimized in year 8, two thirds reported victimization in year 9.
- After adjustments for confounders, there was a significant association between victimization in year 8 and onset of anxiety/depression in year 9 (for girls but not for boys). This study confirms similar findings in other studies. It is contrary to studies suggesting that poor initial emotional health invites victimization.

Cross sectional study of young peoples awareness of and involvement with tobacco marketing. MacFadynen, L., Hastings, G. and MacKintosh, A.M. Centre for Tobacco Control Research University of Strathclyde, Glasgow, UK.
BMJ, **322**(7285): 513-517, 3 March 2001.

This cross sectional quantitative study looks at the involvement of 1516 year olds with tobacco marketing devices such as point of sale promotion, and coupon schemes. Over 600 young people participated in this survey carried out in Northeast England (response rate, 48%). They gain information from interviews and self-completion questionnaires.

- The number of tobacco marketing devices the young person is actively aware of was positively associated with being a current smoker.
- Almost all participants had been exposed to cigarette advertising on bill boards or at point of sale and these had the greatest influence on raising awareness of cigarettes in young people.
- Less commonly recognized forms of cigarette promotion are brand stretching (attaching tobacco brands to non-tobacco products, new pack designs, free gifts on packets, competitions, recognisable people smoking on television or movies).
- Half of the respondents had been involved in coupon schemes, special price offers for cigarettes or seen cigarette advertising in the press.
- Coupon scheme and brand stretching specifically and tobacco marketing in general are associated with a positive smoking status.
- Twice the number of smokers than non-smokers had actively engaged in tobacco marketing.

FURTHER READING

See 'Children' for

Effect of seeing tobacco use in films on trying smoking among adolescents: cross sectional study. Department of Pediatrics, Dartmouth Medical School, USA
BMJ, **323**(7326): 1394-1397, 15 Dec. 2001.

WOMEN'S HEALTH

URINARY SYMPTOMS
- A Finnish study found that cranberry juice reduced recurrences of UTIs by 20%
- A 3-day course of antimicrobials in acute uncomplicated urinary tract infection in adult women is of proven efficacy, even without bacteriological laboratory diagnosis, as compared to placebo.
- By clearly defining the management of urinary tract infection in the community we can decrease morbidity and reduce antibiotic resistance.

GYNAECOLOGICAL ISSUES
- In one study the prevalence of chronic pelvic pain in the preceding 3 months was 24% (around 17% if those with ovulation related pain are excluded)
- A study by Warner *et al.* found a discrepancy between GPs' and patients' views on menstrual problems
- An audit of east Anglian practices concerning the management of menorrhagia shows that a change in behaviour can be brought about by educational interventions
- For the management of spontaneous first trimester miscarriage women should be offered a choice between expectant management and surgical evacuation
- A prospective cohort study did not find history taking and physical examination to be of diagnostic value in the investigation of first trimester vaginal bleeding.
- Bacterial vaginosis is not a strong predictor of miscarriage; the risk increases, however, moving from the first to second trimester.

URINARY SYMPTOMS

Randomised controlled trial of nitrofurantoin versus placebo in the treatment of uncomplicated urinary tract infection in adult women. Christiaens, T.C.M., Meyere, M.D. and Verschraegen, G. *et al.* Department of General Practice and Primary Health Care, 1K3 UZG, De Pintelaan 185, B9000 Ghent, Belgium.
Br. J. Gen. Pract., 52(482): 729-734, 1 September 2002.

The increasing requirement for evidence based practice raises questions regarding the management of uncomplicated urinary tract infection in adult women, which routinely involves prescription of antibiotics without laboratory culture and sensitivity. This study across 17 practices in Belgium compared nitrofurantoin with a placebo in clinically suspected but undiagnosed acute urinary tract infection in non-pregnant adult women. The outcome was measured in terms of clinical symptoms and bacteriological culture.
- Significant clinical and microbiological improvement was seen with nitrofurantoin as compared with placebo.
- Optimal treatment duration was 3 days.

It is important to inform patients that symptoms may persist after this time even if bacteriological cure has occurred. It was concluded that bacteriological culture is only required in the general practice setting if complicated urinary tract infection is suspected.

Urinary tract infections in adult general practice patients. Hummer-Pradier, E. and Kochen, M.M. Department of General Practice, University of Gottingen, Gottingen, Germany. **Br. J. Gen. Pract., 52**(482): 752-761, 1 September 2002.

By establishing a more defined approach to investigation and management of urinary tract infection in primary care, we can reduce inappropriate prescribing and help to curb the increase of antibiotic resistance.

This study was a review of the extensive worldwide literature available regarding urinary tract infection in adults in the general practice setting. Results:

- It is important to distinguish between complicated and uncomplicated urinary tract infection.
- Prognosis in uncomplicated urinary tract infection in females is excellent.
- A good history is central to differentiating between complicated and uncomplicated urinary tract infection.
- There is no evidence to support physical examination when the history is good.
- Many countries accept that urine microscopy and culture is not necessary in most cases. Many advocate dipstick testing only, if at all.
- An important aspect of treatment is counseling the patient about their condition.
- 1st choice antibiotics remain trimethoprim or nitrofurantoin with 2nd choice including cotrimoxazole or cephalosporins.

The scope for further research in this area remains vast.

Randomised trial of cranberry–lingonberry juice and *Lactobacillus* GG drink for the prevention of urinary tract infections in women. Kontiokari, T., Sundqvist, K. and Nuutinen, M. *et al.* Department of Pediatrics, University of Oulu, Oulu, Finland. **BMJ, 322**(7302): 1571-1573, 30 June 2001.

This was a Finnish RCT involving 150 women (average age 32 years). The aim of the study was to determine whether UTI recurrences can be prevented with cranberry-lingonberry juice or with lactobacillus GG drink. Women who had *E. coli* UTIs and were not taking antimicrobial prophylaxis, were randomized to one of three groups either: (1) 50 ml of cranberry-lingonberry juice concentrate a day for 6 months; (2) 100 ml of lactobacillus GG drink 5 days a week for 1 year; (3) control group. They found:

- a 20% reduction in absolute risk in the cranberry group compared with the control group (NNT = 5).

This study adds to the current body of evidence and the authors conclude that cranberry-lingonberry juice taken daily reduces recurrence of urinary tract infection. It prevents UTI either by selecting less adhesive bacterial strains in the stool, or by directly preventing *E. coli* from adhering to uro-epithelial cells, or by both of these mechanisms.

EDITORIAL – Postpartum urinary incontinence. Brubaker, L. Professor and Fellowship Director Department of Ostetrics and Gynaecology and Urology, Female Pelvic Medicine and Reconstructive Surgery, Maywood, Illinois, USA.
BMJ, **324**(7348): 1227-1228, 25 May 2002.

One in three mothers become incontinent of urine. Many factors are thought to be associated with postpartum urinary incontinence, including large babies and long labours. No single factor has been shown to be causative. Studies have shown that advice concerning bladder care and postpartum rehabilitation have not been useful in preventing this condition. The most effective preventative measure is abdominal delivery which cannot be recommended as a routine choice. Further research is required to give us a deeper understanding of this issue.

GYNAECOLOGICAL ISSUES

Association between bacterial vaginosis or chlamydial infection and miscarriage before 16 weeks gestation: prospective community based cohort study. Oakeshott, P., Hay, P. and Hay, S. *et al.* Department of General Practice and Primary Care, St Georges Hospital Medical School, London, UK.
BMJ, **325**(7376): 1334-1338, 7 December 2002.

This study examined whether bacterial vaginosis or chlamydial infection before 10 weeks gestation was associated with miscarriage before 16 weeks. Just over 1200 women initially provided a self-administered vaginal swab, vaginal smear and first pass urine sample, and completed a postal questionnaire at 16 weeks. The prevalence of bacterial vaginosis was 14.5%, and a further 4.5% were intermediate for this infection. The prevalence of chlamydial infection was 2.4%. Ten percent of women miscarried before 16 weeks.

- Relative risk of miscarriage in women with chlamydial infection was 0.32.
- The overall relative risk of miscarriage in women with bacterial vaginosis, compared to those intermediate or negative for the infection, was 1.15. This did not alter significantly when adjusted for miscarriage risk factors or concurrent chlamydial infection, however in the second trimester (weeks 13–15) it rose to 3.45.

The authors conclude that while bacterial vaginosis is not a strong predictor of miscarriage, the risk varies with the length of gestation. It is unlikely that screening and treatment of asymptomatic bacterial vaginosis would decrease miscarriage rates, particularly in the first trimester.

The community prevalence of chronic pelvic pain in women and associated illness behaviour. Zondervan, K.T., Yudkin, P.L. and Vessey, M.P. *et al.* Department of Public Health, Institute of Health Sciences, Oxford, UK.
***Br. J. Gen. Pract.*, 51**(468): 541-547, 1 July 2001.

This study describes the results of a postal questionnaire survey (around 4000 women, response rate 74%): The Oxford Women's Health Study. The aim of the study was to evaluate the prevalence and disability associated with chronic pelvic pain in the community.

- The prevalence of chronic pelvic pain in the last 3 months was 24% (around 17% if those with ovulation related pain are excluded).
- Most also had other types of pain e.g. dysmenorrhoea or dyspareunia.
- Caucasian women were more likely to have pain than non-Caucasian women.
- A third of women had had pain for at least 5 years.
- Just over half of the women with pain described the severity as moderate or severe.
- Only a quarter had sought medical advice in the preceding year. Yet many were anxious about their pain
- More women with chronic pelvic pain took time off work than those without chronic pain.
- General wellbeing was poorer in those with chronic pelvic pain.

Referral for menstrual problems: cross sectional survey of symptoms, reasons for referral and management. Warner, P., Critchley, O.D. and Lumsden, M.A. *et al.* Public Health Sciences, Department of Community Health Sciences, University of Edinburgh Medical School, Edinburgh, UK.
***BMJ*, 323**(7303): 24-28, 7 July 2001.

This study examines the reasons for referral to secondary care for menstrual problems. Over 900 women attending three gynaecology clinics in Glasgow completed questionnaires.

- Most (76%) of the women were referred because of menorrhagia.
- However, less than 40% of women said that their bleeding was a severe problem.
- Pain and cycle related problems were of equal importance in terms of reason for actually attending the clinic.
- A referral reason of menorrhagia was more likely to be associated with hysterectomy than other reasons for referral, regardless of whether or not the women said that excessive bleeding was a severe problem.

They conclude that there is a discrepancy between GPs' and patients' views of menstrual problems. They state that this raises concerns about the correct provision of services for women with menstrual problems.

CLINICAL REVIEW SECTION – **Management of spontaneous miscarriage in the first trimester: an example of putting informed shared decision making into practice.**
Ankum, W., Wieringa-de Ward, M. and Bindels, P.J.E. Department of Obstetrics and Gynaecology, Academic Medical Centre, University of Amsterdam, The Netherlands.
***BMJ*, 322**(7298): 1343-1346, 2 June 2001.

This discussion paper examines the options for the management of first trimester spontaneous miscarriage.

Studies performed in primary care
These showed that expectant management (i.e. conservative, 'wait and see') is feasible. Between one quarter and a half of spontaneous first trimester miscarriages are managed this way in general practice in the UK and north America.

Hospital based studies
Studies comparing expectant management with surgical management show no difference in terms of complications, bleeding, pain, and time off work.

Medical vs. expectant and surgical management
Medical management involves giving a prostaglandin analogue e.g. misoprostol. Medical management is no better than expectant or surgical management. In addition, 50% of women using medical management experience gastrointestinal side effects.

They conclude that women should be given the choice between expectant and surgical evacuation. Medical management offers no advantages over the other two strategies.

Management of menorrhagia: an audit of practices in the Anglia menorrhagia education study. Fender, G.R.K., Prentice, A. and Nixon, R.M. *et al.* Department of Obstetrics and Gynaecology, School of Clinical Medicine, University of Cambridge, Cambridge, UK.
***BMJ*, 322**(7285): 523-524, 3 March 2001.

This was an audit of practices in east Anglia before and after receiving educational packages concerning the management of menorrhagia. One hundred practices (intervention and control) were involved in the study.
- There were no before and after differences in the control groups.
- In the intervention group, after receiving the educational material, women were more likely to receive tranexamic acid as first line treatment. They were less likely to receive norethisterone as first line treatment.
- Referrals for surgery in the intervention groups were reduced after the intervention.
- However, the odds of having a hysterectomy were increased in the intervention group after receiving the educational packages.

They conclude that a change in behaviour can be brought about by educational interventions.

Threatened miscarriage in general practice: diagnostic value of history taking and physical examination. Waard, M.W. and Ankum, W.M. *et al.* Academic Medical Centre-University of Amsterdam, Department of General Practice/Family Medicine, Division of Public Health, Amsterdam, The Netherlands.
Br. J. Gen. Pract., 52: 825-829, 1 October 2002.

Ultrasonography is used to ascertain the diagnosis in first trimester vaginal bleeding, but this investigation is not always available. Therefore this study aimed to investigate whether history taking and physical examination improved the efficiency of referral for ultrasonography in first trimester women with vaginal bleeding. This is a prospective population based cohort study involving 204 patients from 74 general practices in Amsterdam. These patients were seen by their GPs, who formed provisional diagnoses and predicted viability of pregnancy. They were then referred for early ultrasound testing. With the results two statistical diagnostic models based on signs and symptoms were constructed: Model 1 predicted the presence of viable pregnancies and Model 2 predicted complete miscarriages versus all remaining diagnoses.

- Model 1 increased pre-test probability from 47% to a post-test probability of 70%.
- Model 2 increased pre-test probability from 25% to a post-test probability of 41%.
- Tentative diagnosis from GPs based solely on clinical judgement, changed a pre-test probability of 47% to a post-test probability of 58%.

The authors conclude that neither statistical models nor clinical judgement are valid replacements for ultrasound testing in first trimester vaginal bleeding.

INDEX

ACE inhibitors, 1-3
  diabetes, 2-3
  heart disease, 184
  hypertension, 202
  stroke, 2-3
Alcohol, 4-9
  cancer, 4
  coronary heart disease, 6-7
  GP knowledge of patient consumption, 6-7
  ischaemic heart disease, 4
  management, 8
  mortality, 6-7
  reducing consumption, 4-5
  screening, 5-6, 7
Antibiotics, *see* antimicrobials
Antidepressants, 234-5
Antimicrobials, 10-15
  acute bronchitis, 12
  background, 10-11
  conjunctivitis, 14
  patterns in prescribing, 13
  resistance, 10, 14
  respiratory infections, 12, 322-3, 324-7, 330-1
  urinary tract infections, 10, 11
Antiplatelet therapy, 16-20
  aspirin, 16-20
  clopidogrel, 18, 20
  heart disease, 16-20
  myocardial infarction, 16-18, 20
  stroke, 16-18, 20
Aromatherapy, 93
Aspirin
  stroke, 16-18, 20, 338
Asthma, 21-36
  background, 22-3
  beta2-agonists, 21, 26, 27, 28
  budesonide, 21, 23, 29
  in children, 21, 22-3, 28-33
  corticosteroids, 23-4, 27, 30
  drugs, 22, 25-7
  dysfunctional breathing in, 25
  education, 26, 30-1
  inhaler devices, 27-8
  ipratropium bromide, 21
  leukotriene antagonists, 22
  management, 23-4
  nedocromil, 29
  non-drug management, 22
  risk factors, 23
  screening, 31-2
  self-management, 22
  undiagnosed, 22-3, 36

Back pain, 37-42
  acupuncture, 40
  exercise programmes, 39
  outcome, 39
  prediction, 39
  radiography, 41-2
Benign prostatic hypertrophy (BPH), 319
Bereavement, 43-4
Beta2-agonists
  asthma, 21, 26, 27, 28
Beta-blockers
  heart disease, 172
  hypertension, 202, 203
Blood pressure, 115, 120-1, 125
  hypertension, control, 205, 206
  in type 2 diabetes mellitus, 115, 120-1
Breast cancer, 45-50
  deprivation, 46
  hormones, 48
  mammography, 47-8
  screening, 49
  tamoxifen, 45-6
Bronchitis, acute, 12, 327
Budesonide, 21, 23, 29
Burnout, 51-53
  personal style, 51
  workload, 51-52

Calcium channel blockers, 202
Cannabis, 54-57
  mental health, 54-55
  nausea and vomiting, 56-57
  young people, 54-55
Cervical cancer, 58-61
  cervical smear, 61
  human papillomavirus, 58-9, 60
  screening, 59-61
Cervical smear
  cervical cancer, 61
Children, 62-70
  asthma, 21, 22-3, 28-33
  diarrhoea, 62-3
    racecadotril, 62-3
  ethnic minorities, 162
  head lice, 63, 65
  headache, 65
  type 2 diabetes mellitus, 118
Chlamydia, 71-3
  home sampling, 71-2
  screening, 73
Chronic disease, 74-81
  advances in management, 79-81
  patients as partners, 75, 78-79

Chronic fatigue syndrome, 82-5
  aetiology, 82
  counselling, 85
  exercise, 83-4, 85
  GP attendance, 84
  management, 82-3
Chronic obstructive pulmonary disease
  (COPD), 86-87
  physical activity, 86
  pulmonary rehabilitation, 86-87
Common cold, 322, 323-4
Complementary medicine, 88-93
  access, 88
  aromatherapy, 93
  herbal/plant remedies, 90-1
  homeopathy, 92
  integrated medicine, 89-90
Conjunctivitis, 14
Continuing professional development
  (CPD), 94-9
Contraception, 100-4
  background, 100-1
  emergency, 104
  ischaemic stroke, 103
  teenagers, 341-2
  thromboembolism, 101-2, 103
Coronary heart disease
  deprivation, 106-7
Corticosteroids, 23-4, 27, 30

Depression, 231-8
  antidepressants, 234-5
  cognitive therapy, 236
  counselling, 234-5
  detecting, 233
  hypericum, 231
  management, 235-8
  postnatal, 297-8
Deprivation, 105-10
  cancer, 108
  coronary heart disease, 106-7
  mental illness, 107
  morbidity, 108-10
  mortality, 108-10
Diabetes mellitus, 111-27
  ACE inhibitors, 2-3
  background, 112
  blood glucose control, 122-3
  care in general practice, 121-2, 124
  glycated haemoglobin, 127
  quality of life, 116-7
  type 1, 112-3
    intensive therapy, 113
    microalbuminuria, 112-3
  type 2, 113-24
    blood pressure, 115, 120-1
    CALM study, 112, 119
    in children, 118

    glycaemia, 119-20, 125
    metformin, 116, 122-3
    microalbuminuria, 113, 119
    prevention, 114-5, 117, 118
    risk factors, 118, 123-4
    screening, 117
    thiazolidinediones, 121
Diarrhoea, 62-3
Diet, 128-129
  cardiovascular disease, 219
  dementia, 128
  folic acid, 128
  polyunsaturated fatty acids, 219
  zinc, 128-129
Diltiazem, 203
Doctor-patient relationship, 130-44
  consultation length, 134-5
  frequent attenders (FA), 131, 141-3
  heart sink (HS) patients, 131
  information, 132
  patient-centred approach, 133-4, 138-9
  removal of patients from lists, 133, 140
  self-management, 132
Drug misusers, 145-7
  difficult behaviour, 146
  methadone, 145
  recreational drugs, 146
Dyspepsia, 192, 194-5, 196

Elderly patients, 148-61
  education, 153, 155-6, 159-60
  falls, 148, 150-4
  urinary incontinence, 153, 159
Ethnic minorities, 162-5
  children, 162
Evidence-based medicine, 166-70
  otitis media, 170
Exercise, 39, 238

Familial hypercholesterolaemia, 220-2
Five-Shot alcohol questionnaire, 4, 6
Fractures
  osteoporosis, 291

Glue ear, 322, 324-5
Glycaemia, 119-20, 125
Gynaecological issues, 346, 348-51

Head lice, 63, 65
Headache, 65
Heart disease, 171-89
  ACE inhibitors, 1, 184
  beta-blockers, 172
  heart failure, 171-2, 183-5
  mortality, 171, 179-83
  primary care, 183
  primary prevention, 174-8
  risk factors, 174, 175-6, 179-83

secondary prevention, 173, 174-8
sex inequalities, 187, 188
see also coronary heart disease; myocardial infarction
Heart failure, 171-2, 183-5
Helicobacter pylori, 190-6
  cost effectiveness, 191, 193
  epidemiology, 190
  noninvasive diagnosis, 190-1
  treatment, 192, 194
Herbal/plant remedies, 90-1
Heroin, 146
Homeopathy, 92
Hormone replacement therapy, 197-9
Human papillomavirus, 58-9, 60, 61
Hypercholesterolaemia, familial, 220-2
Hypericum, 231
Hypertension, 200-9
  ACE inhibitors, 202
  beta-blockers, 202, 203
  blood pressure control, 204-5, 206
  calcium channel blockers, 202
  diltiazem, 203
  drug therapies, 201-3
  elderly hypertensives, 201, 204-6
  nifedipine, 202-3
  salt, 200, 208-9
  thiazides, 201
  white coat, 205

Immunisations, 210-7
  influenza, 210-2
  MMR, 210, 212-5
    autism, 212-4
    bowel problems, 212
  pertussis, 216
  pneumococcal vaccines, 215
  varicella zoster, 216
Incontinence
  elderly patients, 153, 159
  women, 348
Influenza, 322, 325-6
Inhaler devices, asthma, 27-8
Ipratropium bromide, 21
Irritable bowel syndrome, 228
Ischaemic heart disease (IHD)
  alcohol, 4

Lactobacillus GG, 13, 347
Levonorgestrel, 102-3
Lipids, 218-24
  diet, 219
  drug therapies, 219-20
  familial hypercholesterolaemia, 220-2
  mortality, 221-2, 223-4
Lung cancer, 108

Medicalisation, 225-9
Menorrhagia, 350
Menstruation
  problems, 349
Mental illness, 230-49
  deprivation, 107
  medically unexplained physical
    symptoms, 239-40
  physical health, 249
  suicide, 232, 240-2
  see also depression
Microalbuminuria
  in type 1 diabetes, 112-3
  in type 2 diabetes, 113, 119
Miscarriage, 348, 350, 351
Musculoskeletal, 250-8
  COX inhibitors, 250-3, 255
  knee pain, 255
  lateral epicondylitis (tennis elbow), 252,
    258
Myocardial infarction, 259-64
  antiplatelet therapy, 16-20
  pre-hospital management, 259, 260

Nedocromil, 29
NHS, 265-84
  assessment of need, 266-7
  quality and clinical governance, 267-75
  rationing, 274
Nifedipine, 202-3
Nurses, 299-300

Obesity, 285-9
Osteoporosis, 290-2
  fractures, 291
Otitis media, 322, 324-5
  evidence-based medicine, 170
Out-of-hours care, 293-6
Ovarian cancer, 108

Pain
  back, 37-42
Penicillin, 10
Postnatal depression, 297-8
Pregnancy
  smoking, 335
  teenagers, 341-2, 343, 344
Premenstrual syndrome
  complementary medicine, 91
Prescribing, 301-5
  PACT data, 301-2
Primary care, 306-18
  NHS, 270-1, 274, 281-2
Prostate cancer, 320-1
Prostate disease, 319-21
  benign prostatic hypertrophy (BPH),
    319
  prostate cancer, 320-1

Racecadotril, 62-3
Renal failure
  ACE inhibitors, 3
Respiratory infections, 322-31
  antibiotics, 323, 326-7, 330-1
  common cold, 322, 323-4
  glue ear, 322, 324-5
  influenza, 322, 325-6
  otitis media, 322, 324-5
  prescribing for, 330
  sinusitis, 329-30
  sore throats, 322-3

Sinusitis, 329-30
Smoking, 332-7
  cessation, 335-7
  mortality and morbidity, 333-5
  passive, 334
  in pregnancy, 335
  teenagers, 345
Sore throats, 322-3
Stroke, 338-40
  ACE inhibitors, 2-3
  anticoagulation, 338
  antiplatelet therapy, 16-20

blood pressure, 338
contraception, 103
prevention, 339-40

Tamoxifen, 45-6
Teenagers, 341-5
  contraception, 341-2
  pregnancy, 341-2, 343, 344
  primary care services, 343
  smoking, 345
Telephone consultations, 294
Thiazides, 201
Thromboembolism
  oral contraception, 101-3
Tinnitus, 91

Women's health, 346-51
  gynaecological issues, 348-51
  incontinence, 348
  menorrhagia, 350
  menstrual problems, 349
  miscarriage, 348, 350, 351
  pelvic pain, 349
  urinary symptoms, 346-8